Back Pain

OTHER TITLES IN THE ACP KEY DISEASES SERIES

ASTHMA
Edited by Raymond G. Slavin and Robert E. Reisman

DEPRESSION
Edited by James L. Levenson

DYSPEPSIA
Edited by David A. Johnson, Philip O. Katz, and Donald O. Castell

HYPERTENSION
Edited by Matthew R. Weir

LYME DISEASE
Edited by Daniel W. Rahn and Janine Evans

OBESITY
Edited by Barry Gumbiner

For a catalogue of publications available from ACP, contact:

Customer Service Center
American College of Physicians
190 N. Independence Mall West
Philadelphia, PA 19106-1572
215-351-2600
800-523-1546, ext. 2600

Visit our Web site at www.acponline.org

Back Pain

A Guide for the Primary Care Physician

Andrew J. Haig, MD

The Spine Program
Department of Physical Medicine and Rehabilitation
University of Michigan, Ann Arbor

Miles Colwell, MD

The Spine Program
Department of Physical Medicine and Rehabilitation
University of Michigan, Ann Arbor

AMERICAN COLLEGE OF PHYSICIANS
PHILADELPHIA

Clinical Consultant: David R. Goldmann, MD
Manager, Book Publishing: Diane McCabe
Developmental Editor: Victoria Hoenigke
Production Supervisor: Allan S. Kleinberg
Senior Production Editor: Karen C. Nolan
Interior Design: Kate Nichols
Cover Design: Elizabeth Swartz

Printed in the United States of America
Printed by Versa Press
Composition by Scribe

ISBN: 1-930513-59-3

The authors and publisher have exerted every effort to ensure that drug selection and dosage set forth in this book are in accordance with current recommendations and practice at the time of publication. In view of ongoing research, occasional changes in government regulations, and the constant flow of information relating to drug therapy and drug reactions, the reader is urged to check the package insert for each drug for any change in indications and dosage and for added warnings and precautions. This care is particularly important when the recommended agent is a new or infrequently used drug.

05 06 07 08 09 / 10 9 8 7 6 5 4 3 2 1

Acknowledgments

Vicki Hoenigke, developmental editor, made hundreds of improvements that resulted in a more comprehensive, logical, and readable book.

AJH & MC

My wife, Brigit Jensen, and my children, Molly and William, are gratefully thanked for their patience as I worked on this book that stole their Saturdays.

AJH

Contributors

Michele Bird, PT
Physical Therapist
The Spine Program
Department of Physical Medicine
  and Rehabilitation
University of Michigan
Ann Arbor, Michigan

Christopher M. Brammer, MD
Chief of Rehabilitation Medicine
Huntington VA Medical Center
Huntington, West Virginia

Wing K. Chang, MD
Attending Physician
Piedmont Hospital
Atlanta, Georgia

Anthony Chiodo, MD
Clinical Assistant Professor
Department of Physical Medicine
  and Rehabilitation
The University of Michigan
Ann Arbor, Michigan

Miles Colwell, MD
Clinical Assistant Professor
The Spine Program
Department of Physical Medicine
  and Rehabilitation
The University of Michigan
Ann Arbor, Michigan

Anita S.W. Craig, DO
Clinical Instructor
Department of Physical Medicine
  and Rehabilitation
University of Michigan
Ann Arbor, Michigan

Lisa DiPonio, MD
Clinical Instructor
Department of Physical Medicine
  and Rehabilitation
University of Michigan
Ann Arbor, Michigan

Sandra Dodge, COTA
Occupational Therapy
The Spine Program
Department of Physical Medicine
  and Rehabilitation
The University of Michigan
Ann Arbor, Michigan

Michael E. Geiser, PhD
Associate Professor
Department of Physical Medicine
  and Rehabilitation
The University of Michigan
Ann Arbor, Michigan

Craig Goodmurphy, PhD
Department of Anatomical
  Sciences
St. George's University Medical
School
True Blue Campus, Grenada

Andrew J. Haig, MD
Associate Professor
The Spine Program
Department of Physical Medicine
  and Rehabilitation
The University of Michigan
Ann Arbor, Michigan

Mark A. Harrast, MD
Physical Medicine and
  Rehabilitation Specialist
University of Washington
  Medical Center
Seattle, Washington

Anne G. Hartigan, MD
Clinical Instructor
The Spine Program
Department of Physical Medicine
  and Rehabilitation
University of Michigan
Ann Arbor, Michigan

Deborah S. Heaney, MD, MPH
Clinical Instructor
Department of Emergency
  Medicine
Department of Occupational
  Health and Health Promotion
University of Michigan
Ann Arbor, Michigan

Julian Hoff, MD
Professor of Neurosurgery
Department of Neurosurgery
University of Michigan Hospital
Ann Arbor, Michigan

Joyce Huerta, MD
Physiatrist, Private Practice
Central Virginia Orthopaedics
Lynchburg, Virginia

Mara Isser, DO
Physical Medicine and
  Rehabilitation Physician
Durango Orthopedics
Durango, Colorado

Kimberly Ivy
Certified Qigong/Tai Chi
  Instructor
Seattle, Washington

Richard W. Kendall, DO
Assistant Professor
Department of Physical Medicine
  and Rehabilitation
University of Utah
Salt Lake City, Utah

Sean Kesterson, MD
Clinical Assistant Professor
Department of Internal Medicine
University of Michigan
Ann Arbor, Michigan

John M. Koch, MD
Physiatrist
Prevea Clinic
Green Bay, Wisconsin

Ann Laidlaw, MD
Clinical Lecturer
Department of Physical Medicine
  and Rehabilitation
University of Michigan
Ann Arbor, Michigan

Andrew Marsh, PT
Pediatric Spine Therapist
The Spine Program
Department of Physical Medicine
  and Rehabilitation
University of Michigan
Ann Arbor, Michigan

Quaintance L. Miller, MS, OTR
Occupational Therapist, Clinical
  Specialist
The Spine Program
Department of Physical Medicine
  and Rehabilitation
University of Michigan
Ann Arbor, Michigan

Joseph Niester, MHA
Project Manager
Trinity Information Services
Farmington Hills, Michigan

Vladimir Ognenovski, MD
Clinical Assistant Professor
Department of Internal Medicine
University of Michigan
Ann Arbor, Michigan

Paul Park, MD
Department of Neurosurgery
University of Michigan
Ann Arbor, Michigan

Ebony Parker
Medical Student
University of Michigan
Ann Arbor, Michigan

Douglas J. Quint, MD
Professor of Neuroradiology and
  Magnetic Resonance Imaging
Department of Radiology
University of Michigan
Ann Arbor, Michigan

James K. Richardson, MD
Associate Professor
Department of Physical Medicine
  and Rehabilitation
University of Michigan
Ann Arbor, Michigan

Diane Rufe, MHS, PT
Physical Therapist II
The Spine Program
Department of Physical Medicine
  and Rehabilitation
University of Michigan
Ann Arbor, Michigan

Oren Sagher, MD
Associate Professor
Department of Neurosurgery
University of Michigan
Ann Arbor, Michigan

William M. Scelza, MD
Clinical Instructor
Department of Physical Medicine
  and Rehabilitation
University of Michigan
Ann Arbor, Michigan

Susan Schmitt, MD
Physiatrist
Certified Feldenkrais Practitioner,
The Everett Clinic
Everett Washington

J. Steven Schultz, MD
Associate Clinical Professor
Service Chief, The Spine Program
Department of Physical Medicine
  and Rehabilitation
University of Michigan
Ann Arbor, Michigan

Matthew W. Smuck, MD
Clinical Assistant Professor
The Spine Program
Department of Physical Medicine
  and Rehabilitation
University of Michigan
Ann Arbor, Michigan

Andre Taylor, MD
Physiatrist
Bronx, New York

Mary E. Theisen-Goodvich, PhD
Clinical Associate
The Spine Program
Department of Physical Medicine
  and Rehabilitation
University of Michigan.
Ann Arbor, Michigan

Henry C. Tong, MD
Assistant Professor
The Spine Program
Department of Physical Medicine
  and Rehabilitation
University of Michigan
Ann Arbor, Michigan

Robert Werner, MD
Department of Physical Medicine
  and Rehabilitation,Department of
  Environmental Health Sciences,
  School of Public Health, Center
  for Ergonomics, and Industrial
  and Operations Engineering
University of Michigan
Ann Arbor, Michigan
Veterans Affairs Medical Center
Ann Arbor, Michigan

Elizabeth A. Wiggert, PT
Occupational and Physical
  Therapy Supervisor
The Spine Program
Department of Physical Medicine
  and Rehabilitation
University of Michigan
Ann Arbor, Michigan

Nancy E. Wirth, MD
Department of Physical Medicine
  and Rehabilitation
University of Michigan
Ann Arbor, Michigan

Irene A. Young, MD
Clinical Assistant Professor
Department of Rehabilitation
  Medicine
University of Washington
Kirkland, Washington

Carolyn R. Zaleon, PharmD
Clinical Pharmacy Specialist
Chronic Pain Clinic
Department of Veterans Affairs
Ann Arbor Healthcare System
Adjunct Clinical Assistant
  Professor of Pharmacy
University of Michigan College of
  Pharmacy
Ann Arbor, Michigan

Contents

INTRODUCTION

■ ■ ■

Back Pain: A New Way of Thinking

Andrew J. Haig, MD

Do You Hyperventilate over Back Pain?

Probably not. You know back pain. You've seen it every day in your office since you got out of school. You have a comfort level with it. It's not like malignant hypertension or sudden onset aphasia. Nothing to get excited about. You haven't lost sleep over a back pain case since the time you strained your back golfing.

So if you're not worried, how are Miles and I going to engage you? To teach you a new way of thinking? New ways of practicing? If this book is really going to change your practice for the better, we've got to make you just a little uneasy first.

At the American College of Physicians Annual Session a few years ago, I asked some questions of the 300 people packed in the auditorium.

"Who's been down to radiology this week to review a chest x-ray?"

Maybe half of the audience.

"Who's been down to PT this week to check on a patient's progress?" "This month?" "This year?"

Silence.

"Okay, who has spent an hour in their entire lives in the PT gym, just talking to the therapists or watching the treatment happen?"

I got a few hands. So I continued. "Let's list some drugs for hypertension."

We got to about 15 before I cut them off. I know the guy in the back row was disappointed I didn't call on him, because his hand stayed up for a while.

"Let's list some specific physical therapy exercises for low back pain."

The guy in the back row dropped his hand like a rock. After a few moments, I heard . . . "weight training." Finally, someone mentioned McKenzie exercises, then I got on with my lecture.

That evening, an editor from ACP approached me and asked if I'd write a book on back pain: a general review for internists and other primary care physicians. I was honored, of course. But I got excited when I realized that this book could be something different because of my team back at Michigan.

A few years earlier I quit my day job—a private practice in northeastern Wisconsin—when the University of Michigan offered me a unique chance to organize an interdepartmental spine program. At Michigan I found a very odd but wonderful team. All of the MDs were well-versed in manual or manipulative medicine. The therapists kept referring to "Miles" as if there was a prophet in their midst. The field of academic physiatry is pretty small, but I'd never heard of this Miles guy. Miles, it turned out, was Miles Colwell, a Architectural engineer by trade, who became an MD, specialized in physical medicine and rehabilitation, then spent 2 years at the osteopathic school at Michigan State under someone I did know quite well, Philip Greenman, DO, one of the world's great osteopathic teachers.

On the surface, we made an odd pair. I came from a private practice in industrial rehabilitation. My background included a trail of research grants, various publications, and training at Northwestern and Vermont with some of the foremost spine surgeons in the country. Miles was an academic who had never written a paper but who was well versed in the treatments that I was taught were just a bit flaky. But I saw that they worked for certain people. And he came to understand that my treatments worked for some of the patients that he struggled with. We gained each other's respect, and he became my partner in building Michigan's Spine Program.

Within a few years, we had a facility to house the 10 physiatrists who comprised the Spine Program. Specialists from other departments joined us in spirit, if not in space. Because of the eclectic and sharing academic approach to back pain, our fellowship grew into one of the most demanded training programs in the country. We obtained several million dollars in NIH and NIDRR research funding, and soon the team was turning out dozens of papers and a handful of new academic and clinical leaders. When the request came to write a book, I felt that there was no better mix of experts than our team to do the job.

So I twisted Miles' arm, and he agreed to co-edit the book. We didn't want it to fall into the trap of becoming a literature dump. So we struggled to build consensus about what should be covered and who would best teach about different concepts. Every Tuesday evening for months, while my daughter Molly was at gymnastics practice, we hashed out the concepts. To an outsider—even to our Spine Program team—it must have seemed that our opposite approaches would be in constant conflict. But these Tuesday evenings never led to conflict. The more we looked, the more we found the commonalities that make both of our approaches useful to the right patient at the right time.

It was easy to find authors. In forming the Spine Program, we had assigned small teams to develop subspecialty expertise in areas such as geriatric and athletic back pain, back pain in pregnancy, and prevention and education. The assignments succeeded wonderfully, turning "general" rehabilitation doctors into academic experts, and building programs that remain to this day. Some chapters were obvious team assignments. Our fellows and former fellows all shared the basic program philosophy of Spine, so they were great choices for other chapters. Finally, we were fortunate that a number of consultants had consistently partnered with us as we built Spine. Thus our choices for authors for chapters on rheumatology, pharmacology, radiology, surgery, internal medicine, and other specialties were simple.

We were fortunate to have a team of the best experts, who had spent real time together in the same environment and shared a common understanding of the problem of low back pain. So, with lots of help and encouragement, the book was written.

Case Study 1

A 35-year-old male from Elm Street and a 42-year-old male from a block away arrived by bus in the emergency room on the first Monday of the month, both complaining of back pain so severe that they could not attend job interviews at the local welfare office. A medical student conducted an exam that showed both men squirming around with substantial verbal pain behavior, but no neurologic deficits. Five minutes later, the staffing resident found the younger man pulseless and not breathing. Attempts at resuscitation were not successful.

I was the medical student. In this case, the 35-year-old *had* a backache. It was from an aortic aneurysm, but he didn't know that. Both he and his friend saw an opportunity to take advantage of the system. The obvious lesson here is that even "crazy" people can have bad disease. There is a more subtle and important lesson. The intern and students will remember this if it happens again. But it's unlikely they'll ever see another case like this. On the other hand, thousands of people with back pain and disability will go through their offices during their careers, but until they get additional perspective they will be satisfied with their roles as lifesavers and downplaying their important roles in preventing and treating disability.

For all their exposure to the problem, primary care physicians often have little formal education on the management of back pain. Although the numbers are increasing, most medical students are not required to take a rotation in physical medicine and rehabilitation. In some institutions, internal medicine residency requires a single lecture on back pain. So young doctors learn from their primary care faculty, who learned from perhaps Galen himself. Maybe they'll catch a few ideas from an orthopedics rotation or maybe in the emergency department or on rheumatology service.

The deficit shows. Don't tell anyone, but when it comes to back pain, the primary care physician is seen by the public as the evil gatekeeper, not the expert. When the Harvard Community Health Plan allowed enrollees free access to specialists, there wasn't a big shift (1). People with diabetes, heart disease, and so forth, continued to see their primary doctors. The only exception was back pain. As soon as the gates were open, back pain patients bolted for the specialists. The community thinks orthopedists, neurosurgeons, rheumatologists, physiatrists, chiropractors, physical therapists, and their grandmother all know more than you.

I am impressed with the ability of primary care physicians to make a diagnosis and outline medical treatments. Here at Michigan we studied our family doctors' compliance with back pain practice guidelines. Across the board they did great. Hardly a break from the rules. (They also all rotate through Spine before they finish their residencies . . . .) Although we shall discuss these guidelines, we have thought of these chapters as reviews, not new learning.

What is there to know that you don't already know? When people with acute back pain showed up in offices in Vermont and Texas, your colleagues were able to predict only 40% of those who would go on to become chronically disabled (2). Spine specialists predicted 80%. So did a one-page questionnaire. If you were to ask the policymakers, they would tell you that back pain disability is one of America's highest health care costs. Not the x-ray, not the choice of anti-inflammatory drug: the disability itself.

A Physiatry Sort of Thing?

Back pain is a physiatry sort of thing—the kind of complex intertangling of social, psychological, physical, and medical that frustrates disease-oriented physicians and excites physical medicine and rehabilitation types. For this problem, "diagnose-treat-cure" is supplanted by rehab strategies to minimize impairment, disability, and handicap. Physical medicine approaches to cure and rehabilitation approaches to quality of life are centerpieces of back pain management. Why not diagnosis-treat-cure? Here's why:

Diagnosis? There is only a 10-20% chance that an anatomically valid diagnosis can be made. And in the long term, the anatomic diagnosis may not even be a crucial factor in success or failure, because rehabilitation-improving-function regardless of pain is currently the standard.

Treatment? Choosing a treatment leads to similar frustrations. Practice parameters for back pain treatment remind the experienced clinician of the old joke about the guy looking for his lost quarter under the street lamp. He lost it over in a dark corner but is looking under the lamp because the light is better. In fact, very few back pain treatments have been scientifically validated. The easy-to-study ones, such as pills and simplistic therapies, have been shown to have only moderate effect. Yet the complex anatomy of the spine suggests that detailed, individualized treatment (read here as "experience dependent") may be the best bet. Surgery, one of the most crucial and costly treatments, is lacking substantial validation. But we do not seriously doubt that operation is the right choice for a minority of patients. Such a quagmire breeds both alternative and quack treatments. How can the generalist tell the difference?

Cure? It's a verb here. As in "I cured the patient." Too bad our actions seldom cause a cure. The natural history is so benign for most patients that, like the common cold, their problem will go away with time (and like the cold, come back again!). Before we fall back on the "Take two aspirin and call me in the morning" approach, however, we recall that some back problems can kill. When pain becomes chronic, too, it ruins lives despite our best attempts to cure.

So back pain is a physiatry sort of thing. Exactly what is that? It's a whole-patient approach. A look not just at the disease but at the varied ways it may limit people (impairment), the things they can't do in life as a consequence (disability), and the impact on their role in society (handicap). As a primary care physician you can be good treating back pain—just as you're good at some other specialty areas. However, you must be able to juggle many balls at once. And that's against William Osler's insistence on finding a single unifying diagnosis.

I tell my students, "Surgeons use knives, internists use pills, psychiatrists use their mouths, and physiatrists use . . . people." We work with a team: allied health professionals; PT, OT, and psychology experts; vocational rehabilitation counselors; social workers;, exercise physiologists; and others. People who are smarter than us in specific areas, but who aren't trained to look at the whole picture. Your role in managing back pain is as a member of a team. Some physicians we talk with struggle to know the difference between OT and PT. They have no idea how to access a vocational rehabilitation counselor. Even if they know who these people are in their community, they don't know how to judge their effectiveness and certainly aren't in the business of sitting down with a group of them to coordinate the care of a suicidal, deconditioned, work-disabled woman who's had three lumbar fusions. To treat effectively, the physician needs to work with these experts or at least understand how the process is happening around them.

Admittedly, back pain is not all rehab. There's a part of back pain that fits quite nicely into the "diagnose-treat-cure" mindset. Tumors, infection, and fractures happen. Surgical cures sometimes are miraculous. You should learn more about MRIs, EMGs, and a myriad of blood tests. We've asked some of the best people in the country to write chapters on these. Have a read.

But then let's get right back to the other 97% of your patients. Take a look at next week's clinic schedule. A patient who has been out of work for 2 years and is on a heavy dose of Prozac. The pregnant woman whose backache is worsening with 3 months to delivery. The 75-year-old whose legs are so bad you gave him a wheelchair. (Is it his arteries or his back?) Worst of all, there's your wife's brother's biking partner. You saw him as a favor. You fought the HMO for another month of PT. He's still on the schedule. He'll be at a family wedding next week. He'll ask you if yoga can help. And you honestly just don't know.

You Need to Reclaim Your Reputation!

In truth, I can't think of a better doctor to triage back pain than a generalist. You know these patients. You can put their complaints in the context of all the other problems they've had. You're the best doctor to screen for the serious conditions. You're the most powerful, unbiased source of information patients can have. And, of course, you're there for them in the end. After we specialists have conducted our tests and given our diagnoses, you're the one who manages the case year after year.

You need to reclaim your role as an expert for people with back pain. How? You need to think like an expert.

You need to be sure you know the basics: anatomy, physiology, pathophysiology, diagnoses, interventions. Take a look through the chapters in Section I for a review.

Then you need to develop a new framework for managing back pain. We've organized the rest of the book according to that framework. Sections II to IV are not organized according to diagnosis; there is no chapter on spinal stenosis, for instance. Instead, they are organized according to time frame (i.e., acute, subacute, and chronic presentation). You will learn soon enough that time, not diagnosis, drives most decision making. Medical, surgical, and rehabilitation interventions for back pain are organized according to the time frame in which they are most appropriate. Therefore those are intermingled in the three sections.

Section V deals with special circumstances, again relating to function, not disease. The chapters on back pain in older people, in the pregnant patient, and in those with other major disabilities may be the first reviews of these topics ever written. There are chapters on athletes and children. In this section, we also deal with challenges you may face in your community: prevention, public health, and the legal aspects of care. Primary care physicians often have important administrative roles (e.g., as clinic director, dean, HMO or insurance administrator, policymaker), so the final chapter discusses these important jobs.

Case Study 2

A 34-year-old construction worker has been out of work for 6 months with radiating pain. Magnetic resonance imaging (MRI) and electromyography (EMG) are negative. He has an excellent work history and enjoys his work. He is the sole provider for his 5-year-old daughter after a divorce. On exam you find that his right sacroiliac joint does not move. You note that this can be a cause for pain, but there are no obvious risk factors for disability. On further inquiry, you find that 3 months ago his ex-wife got out of jail after a conviction for child abuse, and he has no safe haven for his daughter while he is working. In debt and on workers' compensation, he can not afford to send her to afterschool care. You call the insurance case manager who goes "out of contract" to provide one month's afterschool care for the daughter. You send your patient to an out-of-the-way therapist who is good at manual medicine and direct him to return to work after the second week of therapy. He returns to work without incident.

This real case illustrates how back care is multidimensional. Diagnostic tests may lead to specific treatment, but here the problem with the sacroiliac joint did not show up on diagnostics. The problem is readily treatable but not by the average therapist. We know that the extent of pain does not correlate with disability. When known risk factors for disability are not found, further inquiry is needed. Finally, the solution required "out of the box" thinking by the physician, who knew how to work with the legal/insurance system.

Finally, the chapters in this text are generally short and all aim to be to the point. Put *Back Pain* on your night table and knock off a chapter or two each evening. And please feel free to let the editors know what you think!

■   ■   ■

REFERENCES

1. **Ferris TG, Chang Y, Blumenthal D, Pearson SD.** Leaving gatekeeping behind—effects of opening access to specialists for adults in a health maintenance organization. N Engl J Med. 2001;345(18):1312-7.

2. **Hazard RG, Haugh LD, Reid S, Preble JB, MacDonald L.** Early prediction of chronic disability after occupational low back injury. Spine. 1996;21(8):945-51.

SECTION I

BACK PAIN BASICS

1

◼ ◼ ◼

Back Pain Algorithms

Andrew J. Haig, MD

Miles Colwell, MD

This chapter presents six algorithms that introduce the reader to the basic decisions involved in the diagnosis and treatment of patients with back pain. As such, the chapter serves as a handy reference to the remainder of the book.

It must be emphasized that *Back Pain* is not intended for a practice guideline. Numerous evidence-based guidelines exist, of course, including one written by our group at the University of Michigan (1). The most commonly quoted guideline for back pain is that devised by the Agency for Health Care Policy and Research (2), but it has been criticized to the point where its remaining value may be to justify future research.

Too often, practice guidelines draw conclusions from *what* researchers have studied, rather than *how* experts in back pain diagnose and treat. Most areas of back pain management have not been subjected to randomized controlled studies; consequently, important factors are often minimized, whereas other areas, minor but well covered, carry too much importance. In fact, research has shown that robotic compliance with low back pain practice guidelines can actually increase the cost of treatment with no substantial benefit to the patient (2).

Practitioners who treat back pain are of three kinds. Novices are those who are learning the categories of back pain and the rules and procedures involved in its treatment. Competent practitioners are those who know all of these. Experts have sufficient knowledge and intuition to recognize the exceptions to the rules and procedures that are commonly used. We begin with the premise that our readers have basic competency in treating back pain. Our goal is to help them attain the level of expert.

Categories of Back Pain

Time is the primary element in the categorization of back pain: *acute* pain is defined as present for less than 6 weeks, *subacute* pain as lasting for 6 to 12 weeks, and *chronic* pain as present for more than 12 weeks. These categories may be considered standard (Figure 1-1). Certainly, some patients who present with new-onset back pain have many attributes of a chronically disabled person, and occasionally a patient presents with long-standing pain that is amenable to simple interventions. But these exceptions are few and far between.

Acute Back Pain

Patients with acute back pain, almost regardless of its cause, have an outstanding chance of getting better. In cases other than disk herniation or specific muscular injury, it is hard to make a concrete diagnosis and is not, in fact, cost-effective to do so. The physician's main role in evaluating most cases of acute back pain is not the traditional "diagnose, treat, cure"; rather, it is "screen for danger, look for factors that may cause disability, and reassure."

The major clinical decision for most episodes of acute back pain is whether the pain is radiating. Radiating pain implies but does not always mean disk herniation or radiculopathy. A large percentage of disk herniations respond to nonsurgical intervention but, collectively, patients with radiating acute low back pain have a somewhat poorer prognosis and slower recovery than those with nonradiating pain. Many effective treatments are available, however. Figure 1-2 shows the basic algorithm for acute back pain.

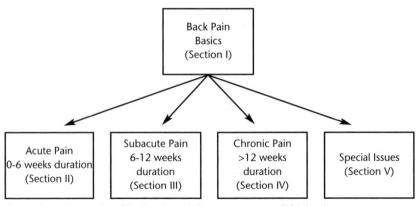

Figure 1-1   Categories of back pain and the arrangement of this book.

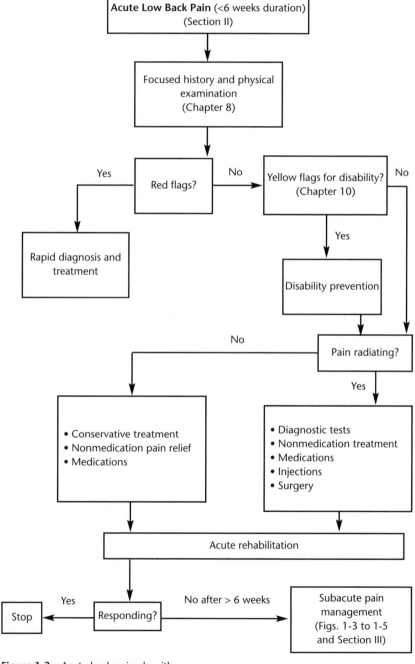

Figure 1-2   Acute back pain algorithm.

Subacute Back Pain

At the subacute level, the odds of spontaneous improvement are less than for acute pain, and the odds that the patient has a specific treatable lesion are greater. This patient, however, has not yet acquired the comorbidities of chronic back pain disability. It is at this level where the "diagnose, treat, cure" physician should be most comfortable. Guided by patient symptoms and physical examination findings, the physician can often successfully use diagnostic tests.

Especially if there is work or lifestyle disability associated with the pain, patients should not leave this time frame (6 to 12 weeks of pain) without either a diagnosis or substantial comfort that no dangerous or specifically treatable pathology exists. Physical examination techniques beyond those taught in medical school come into play here. Because subacute neurogenic pain suggests radiculopathy, usually from disk herniation, the aforementioned diagnostic tests, including magnetic resonance imaging (MRI) and electromyography (EMG), will confirm or refute that diagnosis. Positive tests lead toward specific physical therapy, injections, and perhaps surgery.

In this phase, the physician must reckon with the fact that there is not just pain, but disability. Simple rehabilitation measures are important to maintain function. Work restrictions may be required because of the risk (however remote) of progression of neurologic deficit. Figure 1-3 gives the algorithm for subacute neurogenic back pain.

Much has been made of radiating versus nonradiating pain in the subacute phase. Most subacute back pain is nonradiating. Diagnostic tests are typically negative for nonradiating pain, but, depending on symptoms, it may be important to rule out disease and reassure the patient that nothing serious has been missed. Here is where the physician focused on the "diagnose, treat, cure" role can easily become frustrated. It is the back pain specialist who has the dedicated clinic time, physical examination skills, particular knowledge, and multidisciplinary contacts and procedures that are necessary for this group of patients.

To help the reader get a handle on subacute nonradiating pain, we further divide it into myofascial versus structural or biomechanical. The concepts are somewhat intertwined, but the flow of patients through the process of care is distinctly different. Patients with pain that is reproducible on specific maneuvers that suggest pathology in a specific anatomical structure have mechanical pain (Figure 1-4). Patients whose pain is vague or generalized with fairly normal biomechanical examination are somewhat more likely to have myofascial pain (i.e., pain caused by systemic disease or psychiatric overlay) (Figure 1-5).

Subacute structural or myofascial pain is the kind of pain that "makes sense" to a clinician who is familiar with the anatomy of the spine. On examination, ligaments hurt when stretched, joints hurt when compressed, and muscles ache when activated. After a thorough physical examination,

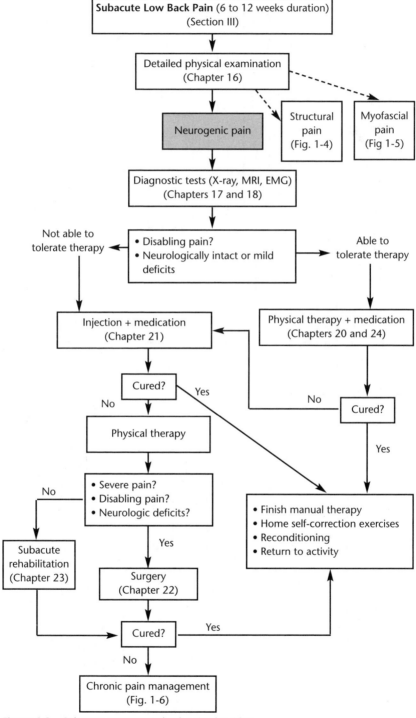

Figure 1-3   Subacute neurogenic back pain algorithm.

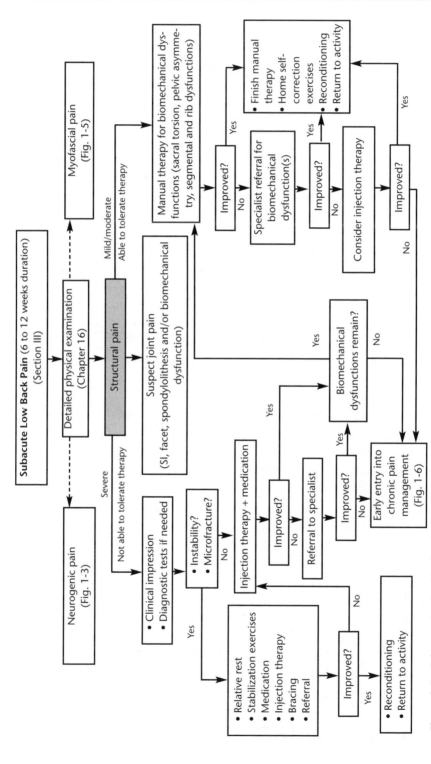

Figure 1-4 Subacute structural back pain algorithm.

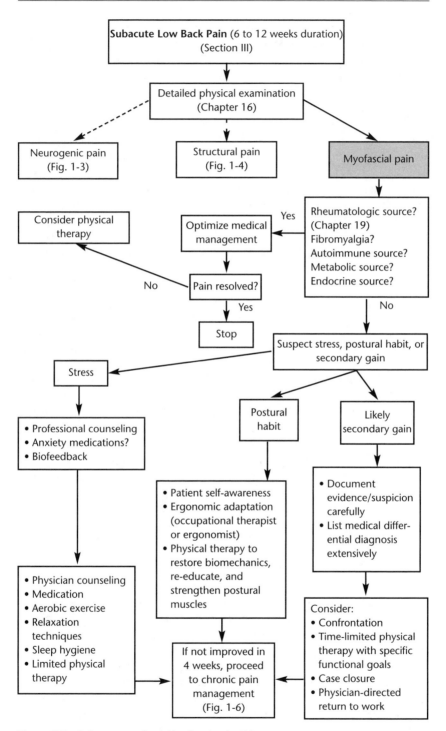

Figure 1-5   Subacute myofascial back pain algorithm.

the clinician should have a good idea of what is causing the pain. The decision will then need to be made whether this cause is more biomechanical due to focal structural asymmetries, muscle imbalance, and misalignments or is diffusely myofascial. If diffusely myofascial, rheumatologic, autoimmune, metabolic, and endocrine causes should be explored; stress or overuse as the cause of pain must also be considered.

Severe musculoskeletal pain from joint or biomechanical dysfunctions may need a more aggressive approach, including various injection procedures. Less severe pain can initially be treated with a specialized group of exercises known collectively as manual therapy. If response is insufficient, the primary care physician must ask himself or herself some hard questions: "Was this the right set of therapy techniques to use? Was the therapy technically well done? Do biomechanical asymmetries remain? Am I misreading the diagnosis? Is there a hidden factor causing disability?" Depending on his or her experience, this may be where the physician refers the patient to a specialist.

Subacute myofascial pain is troubling to the physician. This category encompasses diffuse tenderness or aching. Although there may be pain reproduction on examination, the main aspect of the pain does not seem to relate to a specific joint or ligament. Muscle strains always heal within weeks after an injury and should be significantly improved or resolved at this stage.

The first consideration is the possibility of generalized physical disease. Next to be considered are psychosocial factors such as stress, depression, and anxiety. These can cause muscle tension and increase patient vigilance toward otherwise trivial discomfort. Severe psychiatric disease can present with bizarre or inconsistent pain behaviors. Then, one must recognize the great social rewards for back pain disability. Often, patients who are malingering (premeditated fictitious pain behavior) or exaggerating the pain that they really feel will present with more diffuse complaints. Finally, many patients with myofascial-type pain of a nonsystemic disease etiology may still have hidden biomechanical asymmetries perpetuating a component of their pain and disability.

Chronic Back Pain

Chronic back pain is one of society's most costly disorders. Back disability lasting 12 weeks or more that is improperly treated can ruin a person's life forever. Aggressive treatment can reverse the natural history, but the "diagnose-treat-cure" paradigm does not get the job done at this stage. Separation of the *three p's* (pain, pathology, performance) becomes important. Chronic back pain management is often a rehabilitation process more than a medical one.

The first step in managing chronic back pain is confirming that all potentially treatable etiologies have been evaluated, therapy has been provided as appropriate, and a "cure" does not exist. It is emotionally difficult for a patient to accept the fact that there is no cure for the pain if at the same time the doctor is continuing to pursue various diagnostic tests or proposing other pain interventions. Pain cannot be equated across patients, and disability is not just a medical issue, it also relates to psychosocial factors. The next stages require the physician and the patient to embark on a process of rehabilitation.

Research has shown unequivocally that treatment of chronic pain and disability requires a coordinated multidisciplinary approach from an expert team. An algorithm in Chapter 25 (Figure 25-2) outlines the decision-making responsibilities of such a team. During this phase, the primary care physician's role becomes supportive, encouraging the patient's efforts to increase his or her level of function and allaying fears about the significance of pain. Providing focused follow-up examinations to confirm that there is no progressive medical diagnosis or medical harm occurring is helpful; repetitive conversations about the patient's pain are not helpful.

Patients whose pain is less disabling or severe are often managed in the primary care setting. If progress is slow or insufficient or if third-party verification to bring case closure is needed, referral to a specialist may be indicated. Perhaps the toughest decisions are those that involve discontinuing treatment. Figure 1-6 outlines the primary care physician's decision making for chronic back pain.

Special Circumstances

Many areas of back pain management are best dealt with separately. Certain life circumstances, such as pregnancy or major disability, may make treatment different than the norm (Table 1-1), and unique physician roles deserve special attention (Table 1-2).

Table 1-1   Special Populations

Population	Unique Issues
Children	Developmental stages, increased risk of tumor, teaching future adults
Athletes	Value of performance more than comfort, body mechanics of specific sports, reconditioning
Pregnant women	Progressive nature of pain, some tests and medications contraindicated
People with major disabilities	Challenging biomechanics, complex medical history, progression of deformities
Older persons	Different life roles, exercise tolerance, complex medical history

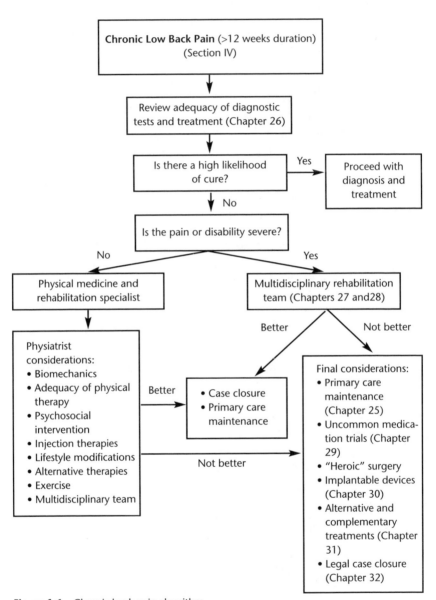

Figure 1-6   Chronic back pain algorithm.

Table 1-2   Unique Physician Roles

Physician Role	Challenges
Determination of disability	Legal vs. medical certainty, ethical considerations, different statutes and contracts
Prevention and public health	Prevention of disability not only pain, ergonomic considerations, community education
Medical administration	Spine program development, health system disease management, insurer policy development, government stewardship.

▨   ▨   ▨

REFERENCES

1. **Chiodo A, Haig AJ, Standiford C, Alvarez D, Graziano G, Harrison V.** Acute Low Back Pain. University of Michigan Health System Guidelines for Clinical Care. Ann Arbor: University of Michigan Health System; 1997. Updated April 2003, available at http://cme.med.umich.edu/pdf/guideline/backpain03.pdf.

2. Acute Low Back Pain Problems in Adults: Assessment and Treatment. Clinical Practice Guideline No. 14. Bethesda, MD: U.S. Agency for Health Care Policy and Research; 1994. Available at http://www.guideline.gov.

2

■ ■ ■

Epidemiology of Back Pain

Anne G. Hartigan, MD

Back pain is a pervasive health problem in the United States, occurring in 85% of all persons at some point during their lifetimes. In fact, back pain is the second most common reason for visits to the doctor (the common cold is first). Primary care physicians, therefore, are in an especially important position for helping these patients. The causes of back pain are numerous, ranging from a recent injury that is easily identified to tumors that have metastasized to the spine. For these reasons, it is especially important to understand the epidemiology of back pain. To develop the most efficient and cost-effective management approach, one should be aware of the likelihood of back pain among various populations and of its risk factors and causes:

- The annual prevalence of back pain is 15% to 20%.
- Approximately 1% of the population is chronically disabled from back pain; another 1% is temporarily disabled.
- Back pain is the most frequent cause of activity limitation in persons under age 45.
- Back pain is the fifth most common cause of hospitalization.
- The lifetime prevalence of herniated disks is 1% to 3%.
- Back surgery is the third most common surgical procedure.
- The rate of disk operations is greatest in the United States, followed by the Netherlands, Great Britain, Sweden, and Finland (24).

Low Back Pain Studies

The study of low back pain is challenging because back pain is defined in many different ways, and the definitions used by one group of specialists frequently do not match those used by another. Many studies conducted by orthopedic or neurosurgical groups use sciatica, disk herniation, or results of clinical tests such as the straight leg raise test to compare patient groups. Yet when examined more closely, it is clear that even the straight leg test does not have a single definition. Other differences are over time frame (e.g., definitions of acute and chronic back pain). Broad terms such as *musculoskeletal low back pain* can encompass a wide variety of diagnoses.

Adding to the complexity of comparing low back pain studies is the way back pain is tracked. Many studies use personal reports of back pain or measure time off from work, whereas others use the number of work-related injuries or workers' compensation claims. Even fewer studies base their low back pain analyses on physical examination findings.

In some studies, exposure (i.e., contact with a risk factor) is evaluated. There are many ways to characterize exposure. For example: "Has the patient ever been exposed to a risk factor? One time? Many times? Can the exposure be eliminated or minimized?" Job exposure may be characterized, for instance, by the amount of time spent at work in a specific posture or lifting specific objects.

Evaluation of exposure can be both subjective and objective. It can also be challenging to compare accurately even two well-planned studies because of different methodologies used to track low back pain, time frames, variations in exposure, and the effects of recall bias.

The Role of the Medical-Legal System

Studies show that 90% of low back pain episodes resolve within 6 to 12 weeks. However, data also show that 70% to 90% of patients have recurrence, and one third of patients have persistent or intermittent low back pain after their initial episode. An obvious question arises: If 90% of low back pain improves, why do we see so many repeat patients with back pain in offices and clinics across the country? What drives patients outside the expected medical algorithm and gets them caught in a cycle of poor recovery?

Because back pain is a complex issue, one in which it is difficult to isolate causality, the simple back injury does not fall neatly into the workers' compensation system. Take, for example, a woman working on an automobile assembly line who begins to experience back pain. If she feels her condition was caused or exacerbated by an occurrence at work, she can choose to file a workers' compensation claim. However, as soon she makes this choice, she becomes involved in the legal process and the intricacies and rules of the insurance system. To obtain adequate compensation benefits, she may have to be concerned not only with her real pain but with assuring her physician that the pain has incapacitated her such that she can no longer work. Such a situation is just one of the legal and financial complexities that physicians must consider. Chapter 32 provides more detail on the workers' compensation system and its role in back pain.

Costs

Low back pain is a significant problem not only in terms of patient suffering but in terms of economic impact. Annually, 2% of workers in the United States have compensable back injuries. In 1986, there were an estimated 175 million lost workdays and 20 million dollars in lost productivity, with more than 500,000 injuries. Today, the total estimated annual cost of back disorders ranges from $38 billion to $50 billion. Included in these estimates are direct medical expenses and indirect costs such as lost workdays and disability-related costs. Total indirect disability-related payments are estimated at two to four times the direct costs (1).

Using injury cost data to evaluate the magnitude of the problem may be misleading due to the litigious environment and workers' compensation system in the United States. However, several studies have demonstrated that a small percentage of back pain workers' compensation cases account for a very large percentage of the total costs (2-4). For example, in the Boeing retrospective study, 19% of cases accounted for 41% of the total injury costs (3). In California, 24% of cases made up 87% of total costs (4).

Risk Factors

Back pain and back disability are two very different entities. Because back pain is often not reported unless there is some associated disability, however, it is difficult to separate risk factors for causing pain from the risk factors that cause disability. Also, factors that may cause a single episode of back pain may be the same as those that predispose to increased susceptibility to repeated back pain episodes. For every study that supports a particular risk factor, there is probably another study that proves the opposite. Figure 2-1 illustrates some of the individual risk factors contributing to the back pain cycle. Table 2-1 lists many of the important risk factors for back pain.

Individual Risk Factors

Genetics
Personal and environmental risk factors play a larger role than hereditary factors in predicting low back pain. In a Finnish cohort study, environmental factors explained greater than 80% of the etiology of sciatica and low

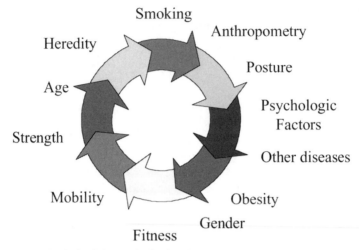

Figure 2-1   Individual risk factors for back pain.

Table 2-1   Individual Risk Factors for Back Pain

Associated with Low Back Pain	Unclear Relationship	Not Associated with Low Back Pain
Age	Obesity	Heredity
Smoking	Muscle strength	Gender
Psychological factors	Fitness	Height
• Stress		Weight
• Anxiety		Body build
• Depression		Posture (lordosis)
Pregnancy		Leg length
Severe scoliosis		Mobility
Certain sports		Flexibility
• Cross-country skiing		Certain sports
• Jogging		• Downhill skiing
		• Ice hockey
		• Snowmobiling

back pain (5); however, a familial predisposition for lumbar disk herniation has been reported.

Age

Low back pain occurs with the highest frequency between ages 35 and 55. Andersson found that back pain and symptom duration that are not associated with sickness absence increase with age (6); however, a study of Swedish women demonstrated no significant age effect (7).

For patients with lumbar disk herniation, the mean age for operation is 40 (8). The incidence of lumbar herniation above L4-5 increases with age.

In contrast, the incidence of L5-S1 disk herniation is low in children, peaks at age 35, then decreases with age.

Smoking
Many studies have found a positive correlation between smoking and low back pain and herniated nucleus pulposus. There is also evidence for a dose-response relationship. Kelsey et al. showed a 20% increased risk for herniated disk for each 10 cigarettes smoked per day for the past year (9). A combination of studies suggests a 1.4 to 2.6 increased relative risk for low back pain among smokers (10,11).

Psychological Factors
Studies have shown that psychological distress is a good predictor of the development of low back pain among persons with no previous back pain. The main three factors are stress, anxiety, and depression. The association of psychological factors and low back pain is much clearer in patients with chronic pain than with acute pain. Chapters 10 and 23 discuss the effect of psychological factors on returning to work.

Pregnancy
There is increased risk of low back pain in pregnancy (see Chapter 37). Ostgaard and co-workers reported a 9-month prevalence rate of 49% and a point prevalence rate of 22% to 28% from the 12th week until birth (12). Multiparity, young age at first pregnancy, and low back pain before pregnancy are risk factors for increased back pain during pregnancy.

Sports and Exercise
Cross-country skiing and jogging have been associated with low back pain (13). Baseball, golf, and bowling have been associated with prolapsed lumbar disks (14,15). Individuals with low back pain had less physical activity at home and more physical activity at work than those without low back pain (16).

Obesity
The relationship between obesity and low back pain is unclear. Although an association has been noted in the industrial population (17), it is believed that obesity may contribute more to the severity of the pain than to the actual onset of pain, due to the effects of spinal loading. With a larger abdomen, the person's center of gravity is pushed outward, making a larger lever arm, and increasing the counteractive dorsal force required by the back muscles.

Muscle Strength
Muscle strength and its association with back pain is another debatable issue. Is the trunk weakness observed in back pain patients primary or

secondary to the pain and injury? Study conclusions range from a theory of poor abdominal and extensor strength in back pain patients to showing no muscle strength difference compared with controls. Chaffin and co-workers studied the industrial population and demonstrated a threefold increase in back pain in individuals who did not have strength greater than or equal to the job requirements (18). In a subsequent study, subjects matched to job strength had fewer complaints (19). The Boeing study demonstrated that isometric strength was not a predictor of subsequent back injury (20).

Fitness

The effect of physical fitness on low back pain episodes has been studied in firefighters, nurses, teachers, airline mechanics, and others. A frequently referenced prospective study by Cady and co-workers followed 1652 Los Angeles firefighters between 1971 and 1974. Flexibility, isometric lifting, and performance on bicycle ergometer were among the variables compared. The study concluded that the fittest firefighters had the lowest injury rates and that conditioning has a preventive effect on back injuries (21,22). However, a study of nurses found that although physical training helped improve conditioning, it did not reduce the overall rate of injury (23). Nevertheless, the nurses in the training group did recover faster from low back pain episodes than nonparticipants. In contrast to the Cady study, the Boeing prospective study and others found that aerobic capacity was not predictive of future injury. Other studies demonstrated that insufficient exercise is associated with prolapsed lumbar disks (14,15).

Gender

Gender appears to be of little importance in low back symptoms. However, operations for disk herniation are performed 1.5 to 3 times more frequently in men than women, even though sciatica symptoms are evenly distributed. These numbers may be influenced by the large number of males who perform manual labor. Because of financial constraints requiring a quick return to work, these men may prefer surgery rather than conservative measures. In Sweden, women showed a higher absence rate than men at the same heavy jobs, but this finding may be influenced by a strength-job mismatch (24).

Previous Back Pain

Once a person has had a back pain episode, he or she is predisposed to have further episodes. This is especially true for patients with disk herniation, perhaps because of the biomechanical changes (e.g., disk space collapse) that occur afterwards, nerve damage to the stabilizing paraspinal muscles, and sensitization of the central nervous system to pain at previously injured locations. The only intervention that has been shown to decrease recurrences is reassurance and encouragement to resume usual activity (25).

Anthropometry

No strong correlation exists between back pain and height, weight, or body proportions according to the prospective Boeing study and several other studies (26). The Boeing study measured variables including standing height, sitting height, arm span, and body mass index. Measurement of tibia length, femur width, and malleoli also demonstrated no correlation with back pain (27). A few studies suggest that taller men and women are at greater risk for herniated disks and sciatica.

Posture

Postural deformities such as scoliosis, kyphosis, hypolordosis, and hyper-lordosis do not predispose adults to low back pain. Back pain may be as-sociated with severe scoliotic curves greater than 80 degrees, and some authors suggest that persons with increased curvature have increased back pain (28). Hansson et al. demonstrated radiographically in 600 subjects (comprising patients with no back pain, first episode of back pain, and chronic back pain) that there was no difference in the distribution of the lordosis angles between the three groups (29).

Leg Length

Whether leg length discrepancy predisposes to low back pain is disputed. Most studies have found that leg length is not a risk factor. Part of the diffi-culty in assessing the relation of back pain to leg length is the variety of measurement techniques used in determining the latter and differences in how much discrepancy is considered clinically significant.

Decreased Mobility

Most low back pain patients have reduced spinal mobility. However, it is unlikely that decreased mobility is the *cause* of the low back pain but rather a component that helps perpetuate the cycle. In a study in northwest England, Troup et al. demonstrated that mobility was a poor predictor of low back pain (30). The Boeing study also showed no association between flexibility and low back pain (31). There is a suggestion that decreased mo-bility leads to increased recurrence and increased risk for future low back pain (32).

Case Study 2-1

A 35-year-old woman who is a smoker visits her doctor for chronic bron-chitis on a regular basis but today adds the concern that she will de-velop back problems. "My twin sister called last night and told me she has a bad backache. Both my parents had back surgery due to arthritis. I'm worried that I'll be next."

After informing her that genetics plays a smaller role than environ-mental factors in the development of low back pain, the physician asks the patient some questions about her sister. He learns that she had her first child at the age of 18, is now in her fifth pregnancy, and had a history of low back pain before this pregnancy.

The physician tells the patient: "There are several reasons that your sister may have increased risk for back pain More importantly, however, I am right now concerned about you. You know about smoking and cancer. You know about your bronchitis. Did you also know that smokers have up to a 2.6 times greater risk for developing low back pain than nonsmokers? And that by smoking just 10 cigarettes a day for a year, you have a 20% increased risk of developing a herniated disk?"

The patient listens carefully, asks several further questions about the causes of back pain, and promises to cut back on her smoking.

Occupational Risk Factors

In addition to personal risk factors, a number of occupational risk factors contribute to the likelihood of low back pain. The National Institute for Occupational Safety and Health (NIOSH), in a summary of more than 40 articles, examined the relationship between workplace factors and low-back musculoskeletal disorders (33). The five main areas of focus were heavy physical lifting, awkward postures, lifting or forceful movements, whole body vibration, psychological factors, and static work postures (the association between the last factor and low back pain is unclear). Table 2-2 lists important occupational factors.

Heavy Physical Work

Heavy physical work for the purposes of this discussion may be defined as work that has high energy demands or requires some measure of physical strength. Heavy work has a positive correlation with low back pain, with a prevalence rate of 0.75 to 4.5. Injuries occur more frequently in blue-collar

Table 2-2   Occupational Risk Factors for Back Pain

Associated with Low Back Pain	Unclear Relationship
Heavy physical work	Static postures
Frequent bending and twisting	
Lifting, pushing, and pulling	
Vibration	
Work psychological factors	
• Job dissatisfaction	
• Poor relationships with co-workers and supervisors	
• Monotony	

workers than in white-collar workers. Herrin studied musculoskeletal injury rates among 6900 workers and found that medical problems were two times greater if predicted lumbosacral disk compression forces were above 6800 N (1500 lb) (34). In contrast, the prospective Boeing study found no difference in injury rates between light and heavy work (35).

Differences in studies regarding work exposure may relate to difficult-to-solve methodology issues. For example, persons who already have back pain may look for work that is less strenuous, and workers who develop back pain at their job may also switch or quit jobs more frequently than those who do not have back pain.

In Denmark and England, nurses have the highest injury rates of any occupation. Magora observed a higher prevalence of back injury in nurses than farmers, bus drivers, or light industrial workers (36). A study comparing occupational and nonoccupational back pain in nurses and teachers, however, did not show an overall difference between the two groups (37). Despite these discrepancies, most studies have concluded that nursing is a high-risk occupation for low back injuries.

Frequent Bending and Twisting

Keyserling and co-workers studied postures of automotive plant workers and observed that the risk for low back pain increased with exposure to multiple non-neutral postures and increasing duration of exposure. The most severe postures included mild and severe trunk flexion, trunk twist, or lateral bend (38).

Lifting, Pushing, and Pulling

Chaffin and Park observed that workers in heavy-lifting jobs had eight times more back injuries than sedentary workers (39). Snook observed that workers with excessive manual handling tasks are three times more susceptible to compensable low back injury (40).

Because of data indicating that one third of the workforce lifted in excess of what was felt acceptable, NIOSH guidelines were initiated in 1981. The NIOSH lifting equation uses object weight, location of handle on the item, travel distance, lifting frequency, and duration to calculate the safety of a lifting task.

Case Study 2-2

A 37-year-old construction worker has built houses for more than 20 years. After helping set a heavier-than-usual garage door, he develops sudden back pain with shooting pain and numbness down his right buttock, back of his leg, and into the top of his foot. After 2 weeks of pain and an inability to climb on the roof of the house he is working on, he visits his doctor.

When he comes into the office, he is angry because he has had to take time off from work. He tells the physician: "I can't believe this. I've never hurt my back before. I'm too young to have a back problem!"

After taking the patient's history and a thorough physical examination, the physician makes the diagnosis of a disk herniation. "Back pain is most common between the ages of 35 and 55," he tells the patient. "The particular type of problem you have occurs most frequently at about your age. The good news is that 90% of low back pain episodes resolve within 6 to 12 weeks."

The physician points out that construction work contains several of the most common occupational risk factors for back pain, including heavy work, heavy lifting, and frequent bending and twisting. Realizing that the patient has no intention of changing jobs, however, the physician reviews steps that may help speed his recovery and lessen the frequency of further attacks, including staying fit and stopping smoking. The patient is reminded that he should confine his work tasks to those appropriate to his strength.

Vibration

Based on the NIOSH review of 19 studies, a positive association exists between low back pain and whole body vibration. There is a large range of risk estimates, however, due to many studies with poor exposure data and few controls. Truck drivers have a fourfold risk for disk herniation. There is a twofold risk of disk herniation with a car commute of more than 20 miles (41).

Static Work Postures

There is disagreement about the relationship between static postures and the onset of low back pain. Studies show increased risk for low back pain with both predominant sitting and predominant standing. There is also increased risk with frequent posture changes. When NIOSH reviewed the topic, however, they found insufficient evidence that a relationship exists between static postures and back pain.

Repetitive Work

The sickness absence rate is higher for workers engaged in repetitive work, and a higher absence rate is seen in manual workers than in office workers.

Psychological Work Factors

Job dissatisfaction, poor relationships with co-workers and supervisors, and monotony on the job have been associated with low back pain. In the prospective Boeing study, the authors concluded that psychological work factors were more important than physical work factors as risk factors for LBP (26,42).

Conclusion

Making sense of the epidemiological studies on back pain can be overwhelming. New studies often dispute earlier work, and it is difficult to keep up with recent findings. Nevertheless, research has identified certain risk factors, including specific occupational risk factors, a history of smoking, and psychological factors (e.g., depression). Understanding of the epidemiology of back pain can not only be used to guide diagnosis and treatment decisions but also can be shared with patients to help lessen their risk of developing or exacerbating back pain.

Many patients are unaware of how common back pain is in the general population and feel that they are part of an unfortunate minority. Simply reminding them that 90% of patients with back pain do get better in 6 to 12 weeks may bring them a feeling of relief. For those patients with more stubborn back pain who are still seeking the answers to "Why me?" and "What caused this?" the clinician can explain the individual and occupational risk factors that may have predisposed them to injury. The clinician can emphasize that although some of these factors may not have been in their control at the time of the injury, perhaps lifestyle changes can be made to reduce the number of risk factors and avoid further injury.

■   ■   ■

Key Points

- Low back pain is the second most common reason for a visit to the doctor.
- Low back pain occurs with the highest frequency between ages 35 and 55 for men and women.
- Previous history of back pain, smoking, pregnancy, and psychological factors (stress, anxiety, depression) are associated with low back pain.
- Gender, heredity, body build, height, weight, posture, flexibility, and leg length are not clearly associated with low back pain.
- The relationship of obesity, muscle strength, and fitness to low back pain is less clear. However, some studies report that physically fit subjects recover more quickly from back pain episodes.
- Occupational risk factors include heavy work, lifting, pushing, pulling, non-neutral postures, and vibration.
- Psychological work factors, such as job dissatisfaction, poor relationships with co-workers and supervisors, and job monotony, also increase the risk for low back pain episodes.

■   ■   ■

REFERENCES

1. **Frymoyer JW, Durett CL.** The economics of spinal disorders. In: Frymoyer JW, Ducker TB, et al., eds. The Adult Spine: Principles and Practice, 2nd ed. Philadelphia: Lippincott-Raven; 1997:143-50.

2. **Johnson AD.** The Problem Claim: An Approach to Early Identification. Olympia, WA: Department of Labor and Industries, State of Washington [Mimeograph]; 1978.

3. **Spengler DM, Bigos SJ, Martin NA, Zeh J, Fisher L, Nachemson A, et al.** Back injuries in industry: a retrospective study. I. Overview and cost analysis. Spine. 1986;11:241-5.

4. **Leavitt SS, Beyer RD, Johnson TL.** Monitoring the recovery process. Indust Med Surg. 1972;41:25-30.

5. **Videman T, Heikkila JK, et al.** The role of environmental factors in the development of back pain and sciatica: an epidemiological study with adult twin pairs. In: Proceedings. International Society for the Study of the Lumbar Spine. Kyoto; 1989 May 15-19; Abstract 19.

6. **Andersson GB.** Epidemiologic aspects on low back pain in industry. Spine. 1981;6:53-60.

7. **Svensson HO, Andersson GB, Johansson S, Wilhelmsson C, Vedin A.** A retrospective study of low back pain in 38- to 64-year-old women: frequency and occurrence and impact on medical services. Spine. 1988;13:548-52.

8. **Spangfort EV.** The lumbar disc herniation. Acta Orthop Scand (Suppl). 1972;142:1.

9. **Kelsey JL, Githens PB, O'Conner T, Weil U, Calogero JA, Holford TR, et al.** Acute prolapsed lumbar intervertebral disc: an epidemiologic study with special reference to driving automobiles and cigarette smoking. Spine. 1984;9:608-13.

10. **Battié MC, Bigos SJ, Fisher LD, Hansson TH, Nachemson AL, Spengler DM, et al.** A prospective study of the role of cardiovascular risk factors and fitness in industrial back complaints. Spine. 1989;14:141-7.

11. **Biering-Sorensen F, Thomsen CE, Hilden J.** Risk indicators for low back trouble. Scand J Rehabil Med. 1989;21:151-7.

12. **Ostgaard HC, Andersson GBJ, Karlsson K.** Prevalence of back pain in pregnancy. Spine. 1991;16:549-52.

13. **Frymoyer JW, Pope MH, Clements JH, Wilder DG, MacPherson B, Ashikaga T.** Risk factors in low back pain: an epidemiological survey. J Bone Joint Surg. 1983;65A:213.

14. **Kelsey JL.** An epidemiological study of acute herniated lumbar intervertebral discs. Rheumatol Rehabil. 1975;14:144-59.

15. **Kelsey JL.** An epidemiological study of the relationship between occupations and acute herniated lumbar intervertebral discs. Int J Epidemiol. 1975;4:197-205.

16. **Svensson H-O, Andersson GBJ.** Low back pain in 40-47 year old men: work history and work environment factors. Spine. 1983;8:272.

17. **Tsai SP, Gilstrap EL, Cowles SR. Waddell LC Jr, Ross CE.** Personal and job characteristics of musculoskeletal injuries in an industrial population. J Occup Med. 1992;34:606-12.

18. **Chaffin DB, Herrin GD, Keyserling WM.** Pre-employment strength testing: an updated position. J Occup Med. 1978;20:403-8.

19. **Keyserling WM, Herrin GD, Chaffin DB.** Isometric strength testing as a means of controlling medical incidents on strenuous jobs. J Occup Med. 1980;22:332-6.

20. **Battié MC, Bigos SJ, Fisher LD, Hansson TH, Jones ME, Wortley MD.** Isometric lifting strength as a predictor of industrial back pain. Spine. 1989;14:851-6.

21. **Cady LD, Bischoff DP, O'Connell ER, Thomas PC, Allan JH.** Strength and fitness and subsequent back injuries in fire fighters. J Occup Med. 1979;21:269-72.

22. **Cady LD Jr., Thomas PC, Karwasky RJ.** Program for increasing health and physical fitness of firefighters. J Occup Med. 1985;27:110-4.

23. **Dehlin O, Berg S, Andersson GB, Grimby G.** Effect of physical training and ergonomic counseling on the psychological perception of work and on the subjective assessment of low-back insufficiency. Scand J Rehabil Med. 1981;13:1-9.

24. **Andersson GB.** The epidemiology of spinal disorders. In: Frymoyer JW, Ducker TB, et al., eds. The Adult Spine: Principles and Practice, 2nd ed. Philadelphia: Lippincott-Raven; 1997:93-141.

25. **Indahl A, Velund L, Reikeraas O.** Good prognosis for low back pain when left untampered: a randomized clinical trial. Spine. 1995;20:473-7.

26. **Battié MC, Bigos SJ, Fisher LD, Spengler DM, Hansson TH. Nachemson Al, et al.** Anthropometric and clinical measures as predictors of back pain complaints in industry: a prospective study. J Spinal Disord. 1990;3:195-204.

27. **Westrin CG.** Low back sick-listing: a nosological and medical insurance investigation. Scand J Soc Med (Suppl). 1973;7:1-116.

28. **Kostuik JP, Bentivoglio J.** The incidence of low back pain in adult scoliosis. Spine. 1981;6:268-73.

29. **Hansson T, Bigos S, Beecher P, Wortley M.** The lumbar lordosis in acute and chronic low back pain. Spine. 1985;10:154-5.

30. **Troup JD, Foreman TK, Baxter CE, Brown D.** The perception of back pain and the role of psychophysical tests of lifting capacity. Spine. 1987;12:645-57.

31. **Battié MC, Bigos SJ, Fisher LD, Spengler DM, Hansson TH, Nachemson AL, et al.** The role of spinal flexibility in back pain complaints within industry. Spine. 1990;15:768-73.

32. **Biering-Sorensen F.** A prospective study of low back pain in a general population. I. Occurrence, recurrence and aetiology. Scand J Rehabil Med. 1983;15:71-9.

33. **Bernard BP, ed.** Musculoskeletal Disorders and Workplace Factors: A Critical Review of Epidemiologic Evidence for Work-Related Musculoskeletal Disorders of the Neck, Upper Extremity, and Low Back, 2nd ed. Cincinnati: National Institute for Occupational Safety and Health; 1997:1-96.

34. **Herrin GD, Jaraiedi M, Anderson CK.** Prediction of overexertion injuries using biomechanical and psychophysical models. Am Ind Hyg Assoc J. 1986;47:322-30.

35. **Bigos SJ, Spengler DM, Martin NA, et al.** Back injuries in industry: a retrospective study. II. Injury factors. Spine. 1986;11:246-51.

36. **Magora A.** Investigation of the relation between low back pain and occupation. 2. Work history. Ind Med Surg. 1970;39:504-10.

37. **Cust G, Pearson JC, Mair A.** The prevalence of low back pain in nurses. Int Nurs Rev. 1972;19:169-79.

38. **Keyserling WM, Punnett L, Fine IJ.** Trunk posture and back pain: identification and control of occupational risk factors. Appl Ind Hyg. 1988;3:87-92.

39. **Chaffin DB, Park KS.** A longitudinal study of low-back pain as associated with occupational weight lifting factors. Am Ind Hyg Assoc J. 1973;34:513-25.

40. **Snook SH.** Low back pain in industry. In: White AA, Gordon SL; eds. Proceedings. Symposium on Idiopathic Low Back Pain. St. Louis: Mosby; 1982:23-8.

41. **Kelsey JL, Hardy RJ.** Driving of motor vehicles as a risk factor for acute herniated lumbar intervertebral disc. Am J Epidemiol. 1975;102:63-73.

42. **Bigos SJ, Battie MC, Spengler DM, Fisher LD, Fordyce WE, Hansson TH, et al.** A prospective study of work perceptions and psychosocial factors affecting the report of back injury. Spine. 1991;16:1-6.

■   ■   ■

KEY REFERENCES

Andersson GB. The epidemiology of spinal disorders. In: Frymoyer JW, Ducker TB, et al., eds. The Adult Spine: Principles and Practice, 2nd ed. Philadelphia: Lippincott-Raven; 1997:93-141.
More detail than most general practitioners will need but a solid summary of studies supporting/refuting risk factors contributing to back pain. Good place to start for key references.

Battié MC, Bigos SJ, Fisher LD, et al. The role of spinal flexibility in back pain complaints within industry. Spine. 1990;15:768-73.
One of several articles from one of the largest prospective studies on low back pain; researchers followed Boeing aircraft employees. Thought-provoking on the utility of lumbar range-of-motion evaluations in the office. Look for other articles in the same series as well as the earlier retrospective studies by Bigos.

Bernard BP, ed. Musculoskeletal Disorders and Workplace Factors: A Critical Review of Epidemiologic Evidence for Work-Related Musculoskeletal Disorders of the Neck, Upper Extremity, and Low Back, 2nd ed. Cincinnati: National Institute for Occupational Safety and Health; 1997:1-96.
Well-organized evaluation of occupational risk factors. Excellent tables enhance this overview of more than 40 back pain studies. Included are study design, population, outcomes, exposures, prevalence of musculoskeletal disorders, and comments.

3

■ ■ ■

Anatomy of the Spine

Craig Goodmurphy, PhD

The vertebral column is truly the core of our anatomy. It supports our body, protects our nervous system, and controls our movement. The deep back is an area that is rich with complexities and nuances, yet many people graduate medical school with a relatively rudimentary knowledge of the back. Although medical technology continues to advance at a staggering pace, with new tools becoming available regularly, there are still a plethora of conditions that affect the back and spine to which these new and emerging tools are blind. Consistently, one of the most inexpensive and best tools for the diagnosis and treatment of back pain is still a well-trained clinician with a thorough understanding of the anatomy and function of the back. This chapter will highlight the core information necessary for understanding the structural basis of the anatomic units of the spine and the functional components that govern its strengths and weaknesses.

Anatomic Subunits of the Spine

The anatomic subunits of the back are the vertebrae, intervertebral disks, ligaments, tendons, fascia, and muscles. The static nonpliable and slightly plastic components are the vertebrae and ligaments. The dynamic components are those with more elastic qualities such as the tendons, muscles, and intervertebral disks.

The Bones of the Vertebral Column

The vertebral column is composed of 33 individual bones, which can be divided into five unique regions. From superior to inferior these are composed of the 7 cervical, 12 thoracic, 5 lumbar, 5 fused sacral, and 3-4 fused coccygeal segments. There is a continuum of change that occurs as you descend the vertebral column. The shared features are structural support and shock absorption by the anterior bodies and intervertebral disks, while the posterior portions (neural arch) are involved more with neural protection and movement (Figure 3-1). The posterior arch consists of the two pedicles, two superior and two inferior zygapophysial joints, two laminae, two transverse processes, and a single spinous process. The regional uniqueness of the vertebrae helps set the functional parameters that control the movement of the vertebral column as summarized in Table 3-1. Note that C1 and C2 are often referred to as atypical vertebrae. T1 has a unifacet for the articulation of the first rib, whereas the others have demifacets. The attachment of the ribs to the thoracic vertebrae limit their motion compared to the cervical and lumbar segments.

The Vertebral Column as a Whole

The smallest functional unit of the vertebral column consists of two superimposed vertebrae with an interposed disk. This unit contains the two primary types of joints and the five primary ligaments of the movable 24 presacral vertebrae (Figure 3-2). As a whole, the 33 vertebrae of the spine are combined with joints, ligaments, and muscles to form a flexible and mechanically stable vertebral column. The posterior elements combine to form a canal for housing the spinal cord, vessels, and the three meningeal coverings. The neural canal is quite wide and pear-shaped at the level of C1, becomes triangular at C3, and transitions to a smaller, more rounded shape as it approaches the thoracic region. Until the mid-thoracic region, the canal is narrow and round then again starts to take a more triangular form as one descends to the lumbar and sacral regions (Figure 3-3).

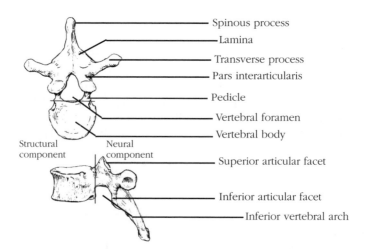

Figure 3-1   Typical vertebra.

Table 3-1   Regional Vertebrae and Their Specializations

Region and Major Landmarks	Primary Regional Features
Cervical (7 vertebrae) **C1 Atlas**—atlantooccipital joint	**C1—Atlas:** Articulates with occipital condyles. Provides 50% of flexion/extension of neck. No body and no spinous process.
C2 Axis—atlantoaxial joint of	**C2—Axis:** Odontoid process is modified body C1 and C2. Provides 50% lateral rotation of neck
C3 Level of hyoid	by allowing C1 to rotate around the odontoid like a pivot pin. No disc between C1 and
C4 Level of thyroid cartilage	**Typical:** Bifid spinous process. Foramen in transverse processes for vertebral vessels.
C5	Anterior projecting transverse processes. Small body. Large triangular vertebral foramen.
C6 Vertebrae prominens 25%; vertebral artery enters transverse foramen	Articular facets are roughly 45 degrees off the horizontal and are transversely oriented. **Predominant motions**
C7 Vertebrae prominens; 60%; vertebral vein enters transverse foramen	+++Rotation ++Flexion/extension +Side flexion
Thoracic (12 vertebrae)	**Typical:** Thoracic vertebrae have the least modification from basic vertebrae Spinous
T1 Vertebra prominens 15% **T2** **T3** **T4** Bifurcation of the trachea **T5** Root of heart and great vessels **T6** **T7** **T8** Foramen for IVC in diaphragm **T9** **T10** Esophageal hiatus **T11** **T12** Aortic hiatus	processes project inferiorly and posteriorly. Articular processes are located on both the body and the transverse processes for thoracic ribs to articulate. Thick overlapping laminae are thicker than the bodies of the vertebrae. Transverse processes project posteriorly and laterally and are long and sturdy. Articular facets are roughly 60 degrees off the horizontal and are in the frontal plane. **Predominant motions:** +++Rotation ++Side flexion +Flexion/extension
Lumbar (5 vertebrae)	**Typical:** Lumbar vertebrae are the deepest and widest of all vertebrae because they carry
L1 End of sympathetic outflow (L1/L2)	the weight of the body above them. They are thicker anteriorly than posteriorly, which adds to the lumbar curvature.
L2 End of adult spinal cord (conus medullaris)	Laminae are thinner than bodies. Transverse processes are short and thin and are positioned anterior to the articular facets.
L3 End of infant spinal cord	Articular facets are almost vertical and are oriented in the sagittal plane. The superior is
L4 Transtubercular plane/aortic bifurcation	slightly concave and the interior slightly convex.
L5 IVC formation	**Predominant motions** +++Flexion/extension +Side flexion

Table 3-1   Regional Vertebrae and Their Specializations *(cont'd)*

Sacral (5 fused vertebrae)	**Typical:** Fusion of 5 verebrae with no interposing discs.
S1	Costal elements fuse and broaden the sacrum. Four anterior and posterior sacral foramina
S2 Attachment for the dural sac	accommodate the ventral and dorsal rami of the sacral mixed nerves.
S3	Auricular surface articulates with the two os coxae (hip bones) to form the sacroiliac or SI
S4	joint. Superiorly the bodies of the vertebrae form an
S5	anteriorly projecting ridge called the *promontory* (distributes weight into the pelvis and then the lower limb).
Coccyx (usually 4 fused vertebrae)	**Typical:** Three or four fused vertebrae. Shows no development of pedicles, laminae, or spinous process. Coccygeal horns articulate with the horns of the sacrum. Vestigial tail. **Predominant motions** Minute mounts of extension, especially noticeable during defecation.

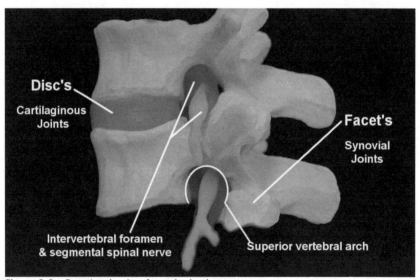

Figure 3-2   Functional units of vertebral column.

Access to and from the vertebral canal is largely through the intervertebral foramena. Exceptions are spinal nerves C1, S5, and the coccygeal nerve. The intervertebral foramena are formed by the apposition of the superior vertebrae's inferior vertebral arch and the inferior vertebra's superior vertebral arch or by the fusion of bones, such as the sacrum, where there is

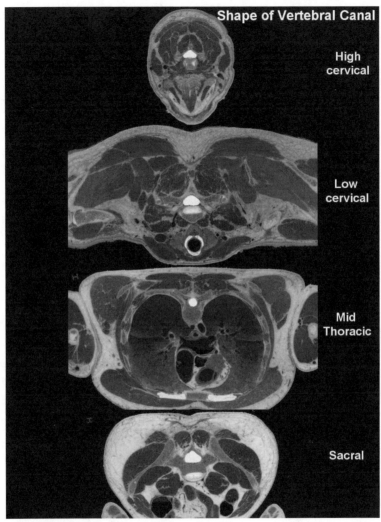

Figure 3-3 Regional shapes of the vertebral canal.

a separation from the dorsal sacral foramena and the ventral sacral foramena. The intervertebral foramena allow 28 of the 31 paired spinal nerves to pass out of the vertebral canal. In addition, they provide passage for radicular arteries traveling to the spinal cord and for anastomosis of the internal and external vertebral venous plexi. Cervical intervertebral foramena are angled anterolateraly and are smaller in relation to the size of the passing segmental nerve when compared to those in the lumbar region. The peripheral spinal nerves are susceptible to compression at the intervertebral foramena, often resulting in pain referring to the distribution of the involved nerve.

Curvatures of the Vertebral Column

The first ossification centers of the human vertebral column are seen at about the 12th week of development. This cartilaginous model has an anterior curvature (posterior convexity) along its entire length and known as the primary curvature. The primary curvature is a phylogenetic development from our ancestral quadrupeds that maintain this curvature into adult maturity. As bipeds, human adults develop a posterior curvature (anterior convexity) in both the cervical and lumbar regions and maintain a primary anterior curvature in the thoracic and sacrococcygeal regions. Clinically, a primary anterior curvature is known as a *kyphosis*, and a secondary posterior curvature is known as a *lordosis* (Figure 3-4). The development of the cervical secondary curvature is complete by birth but requires the infant to develop sufficient motor control of the cervical musculature to raise and control its head so that it may visually sample the environment. The lumbar curvature is developmentally incomplete at birth and requires approximately a year for continued growth of the lumbar vertebrae and the intervertebral disks. The anterior portions of the lumbar vertebrae and disks grow faster than the posterior elements, creating the secondary curvature. Until the secondary lumbar curvature develops, an infant has difficulty walking because the torso cannot be brought under the lower limbs for efficient weight transfer and bipedal locomotion.

In *Muscles Alive*, when discussing the efficiency of human antigravity mechanisms and the upright posture, Basmajian states that "The expenditure of muscular energy for what seems to be a most awkward position is actually extremely economical" (1). This economy of design is apparent in the spine and how it transfers the weight of the head, torso, and upper limbs into the lower limb. The line of gravity in the postural standard ideally passes through the external auditory meatus, the odontoid process of the axis and cervical bodies, through the bodies of the lumbar vertebrae (especially L5) and is distributed equally through the two halves of the pelvic ring via the sacral promontory and into the femoral head, neck, and shafts (2). The neutral pelvic alignment with anterior superior iliac spine and pubic tubercle in the same vertical plane along with the 30-degree angle between L5/S1 articulation allows the weight of the body to fall largely onto the skeletal and ligamentous framework and requires relatively little ATP expenditure (Figure 3-5).

Joints of the Vertebral Column

The adult vertebral column is composed of fibrocartilaginous joints and synovial joints (see Figure 3-2). Fibrocartilaginous symphyses exist between the bodies of most vertebrae as intervertebral disks. The synovial joints include the craniovertebral joints, costovertebral joints, zygapophyseal (facet) joints, and sacroiliac (SI) joints. Each joint provides a small amount of

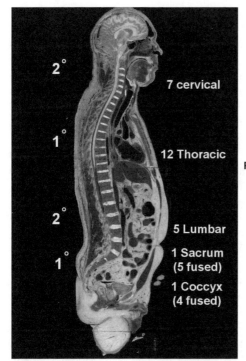

2°

7 cervical

1°

12 Thoracic

2°

5 Lumbar

1°

1 Sacrum
(5 fused)

1 Coccyx
(4 fused)

Figure 3-4   Curvatures of the spine.

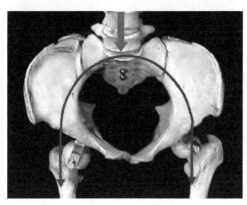

Figure 3-5   Weight distribution
from the vertebral column through
the pelvic ring.

movement, which is summated across the 24 movable presacral vertebrae.
These small summative movements result in a vertebral column with a relatively wide range of movements. As a unit, the vertebral column is capable of flexion, extension, lateral flexion, and rotation. The amount and
degree of movement possible in each region of the vertebral column is dictated by the thickness and compressibility of the intervertebral disks, the
shape and orientation of the facets, ligaments, tendons, and other imping-
ing tissues such as ribs or excessive adipose.

The zygapophyseal, or facet joints as they are clinically known, are true encapsulated joints that exist between the superior and inferior articular processes of all 24 presacral vertebrae, the occipital condyles, and the superior aspect of the sacrum. These planar joints have loose capsules that tighten as you descend the column. Lumbar facets often have reinforcing connective tissue rims and a fibroadipose menisci. The projection angles between the articular surfaces of the joints vary from region to region and therefore play an important role in the types of movement possible in each region as well as the regional susceptibility to traumatic injury.

Facets in the cervical region are roughly 45 degrees from the horizontal and are oriented in the transverse plane. This not only makes them very mobile in the primary motions but also makes them susceptible to forward displacement, hyperextension, and dislocation injuries. Articular facets of the thoracic region are roughly 60 degrees from the horizontal and are oriented in the frontal plane. They are relatively sturdy and stable and are most often involved in avulsion fractures. The thoracic region is well suited for side flexion and rotation but is limited in its flexion and extension capabilities. However, the fact that there are 12 thoracic segments still provides the thoracic region with reasonable amounts of flexion and extension movement when summated across the entire region. The lumbar articular facets are almost a vertical 90 degrees and are oriented in the sagittal plane. The superior is slightly concave and faces medially, whereas the inferior is slightly convex and faces laterally. Because the facets are oriented in the sagittal plane, this area is not well suited for side flexion or rotation but is adapted more for flexion and extension. Because the weight bore on the lumbar vertebrae is greater than other areas, this level is susceptible to crush injuries and blowout compression fractures (3).

Intervertebral Disks

The vertebral bodies contribute 75% of the overall length of the vertebral column (adult average of 72 to 75 cm), and intervertebral disks contribute the other 25% (4). The intervertebral disks are considered secondary fibrocartilaginous joints. They are positioned between the bodies of the adjacent vertebrae in all of the 24 presacral vertebrae excepting C1 and C2. They vary in size, thickness, and shape in the different vertebral regions and also within regions. In the cervical and lumbar regions, they are thicker ventrally than dorsally. However, all disks serve the same function. Intervertebral disks are designed for weight bearing, shock absorption, and small amounts of movement due to their compressibility and elasticity. Other than a thin, loose articular capsule, there are two primary parts to the disk. The annulus fibrosus makes up the outer circumference. This layer is composed of fibrous tissue and fibrocartilage arranged in lamellar and cruciform patterns to add strength and durability. The annulus fibrosus tends to be thicker as one ascends the column and is also thicker in the anterior portions of the disk. The crosshatched fibers of the annulus fibrosus give tortional stability to the disk under rotational sheering forces that are produced during either pure rotational movements or side flexion.

At the center of the disk is the nucleus pulposus. The pulp is a soft compressible mucopolysaccharide substance with a fine fibrous matrix and highly elastic properties. As a functional consideration, it is important to note that the nucleus pulposus is more posteriorly located in the cervical and lumbar regions, which is biomechanically wise, as the secondary curvature places more wight bearing strain on the posterior aspects of the disk. Within the cartilaginous gel of the nucleus pulposus there is a high water content (80%) and an independent blood supply through the second decade of life. During daily activities, the viscosity of the nucleus pulposus increases due to transient dehydration of the disk, which is replenished during the non-weight-bearing sleep phases. After the blood supply to the disk disappears, there is a continual degradation of the disk associated with a nontransient increase in the viscosity of the nucleus pulposus and a decrease in its elastic properties. By the seventh decade of life, this degenerative process leaves people up to an inch shorter than they were in the second decade. As the water level and protein structure of the disk change, the disk necessarily loses its capacity to function in shock absorption. Ensuing microtrauma or acute injury damage begins to accumulate in the disk tissues, leading to instability and potentially, but not necessarily, pain. This degenerative cascade was first described in the 1970s by Kirkaldy-Willis. The cascade describes a cycle of initial degeneration and acute pain followed by a relatively long period of instability and intermittent pain. In the final stages of the degenerative cycle, the disks restabilize due to a thickening of the disk and eventual fall in the amount of inflammation associated with the proteins present (5). Evidence to support this theory comes from longitudinal studies that show that persons in their 30s and 40s are more likely to suffer from disk-associated pain symptoms that those in their 60s. It is also very important to know that degenerative disk disease does not necessarily result in pain, as there are many MRI-based studies that show up to 30% of young individuals with evidence of degenerative disk disease do not experience any back pain or associated symptoms (6). When disk material is lost, there is an increased susceptibility to spinal nerve compression due to the reduced separation of the vertebral arches forming the intervertebral foramen. This leads to the classic symptoms of radiating neuralgic pain along the myotome and dermatomal distribution patterns of the nerve being compressed.

Ligaments of the Vertebral Column

Excluding the specialized ligaments associated with C1, C2, and their attachments to the base of the skull, there are five primary ligaments that connect the vertebrae to one another. Two of the five connect the bodies and three of the five connect the vertebral arches. The bodies are attached by the anterior and posterior longitudinal ligaments. The anterior longitudinal ligament is a strong band of tissue that runs from the anterior basi occiput attaching to the anterior arch of C1 as well as the bodies and disks of all vertebrae to the level of the superior sacrum. The posterior longitudinal ligament runs in the anterior vertebral canal along the posterior aspects of the vertebral bodies and disks. Superiorly, it is continuous with the tectorial membrane, which helps anchor and stabilize the vertebral column to the skull. Both ligaments serve to protect from sheering forces that would result in vertebrae gliding anteroposteriorly upon one another. They attach firmly to the intervertebral disks with the posterior longitudinal forming lateral projections across the posterior aspects of the disks to reinforce the annulus fibrosus. When a herniated nucleus pulposus protrudes into the vertebral canal, the thickness of the cruciform reinforcement from the posterior longitudinal ligament helps to direct the protrusion to the posterior lateral portions of the canal. Using a clockface analogy with 12 o'clock being the anterior portion of the disk, herniations tend to occur most frequently at 5 and 7 o'clock positions (Figure 3-6).

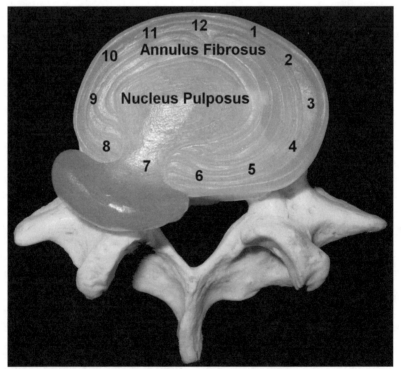

Figure 3-6   Clockface view of a lumbar intervertebral disk showing the classic herniation at 7 o'clock (or 5 o'clock) position. This posterior lateral position is typically the thinnest and weakest part of the annulus fibrosus, as the medial portion is reinforced by the posterior longitudinal ligament.

The ligamentum flavvum and interspinous and supraspinous ligaments serve to connect the vertebral arches of opposed vertebrae. Some authors include these as accessory ligaments of the facet joints, and others consider them proper and named syndesmotic joints of the vertebral column (3,4). Either way, they serve to direct and limit the movements between adjacent vertebrae. The supraspinous ligament is a tough cord-like structure attaching from the tips of the spinous processes extending from the sacrum to the base of the skull. In the lumbar and cervical regions, there are fascial thickenings and specializations of this structure known as the thoracolumbar fascia and the ligamentum nuchae, respectively. Some texts consider the ligamentum nuchae a separate structure extending from the base of the skull to C7 vertebrae, but functionally, the ligamentum nuchae and the thoracolumbar fascia act as a low-energy (ATP) method of maintaining secondary curvatures. Because secondary curvatures are an adaptation to the evolutionarily new bipedal walking stance, these fascial thickenings serve to reduce the ATP requirements of standing by supporting the curvatures with little need for muscular effort. Postural degeneration and the increased strain on muscles as well as disks that occurs as we move away from the static supports of the vertebral column and ligaments is theorized to be a root cause of low back injury and pain. Both the thoracolumbar and ligamentum nuchae serve as attachment sites for the large superficial back muscles such as latissimus dorsi and trapezius. The interspinous ligaments are positioned from root to tip as a membranous structure between the spinous processes of adjacent vertebrae. They are thicker and more developed as one descends the vertebral column. The most unique of the vertebral ligaments is the ligamenta flava. These bilateral, yellow ligaments attach to the lamina of adjacent vertebra at the posterior aspect of the spinal canal from the axis to the first sacral segment. Like the interspinous ligaments, they too thicken as you descend the vertebral column. They are yellow because of their high elastin fiber content. Besides limiting motions of flexion like the other ligaments posterior to the vertebral canal, their elastic qualities allow them to deform and reform during flexion and extension movements in which the distance between lamina of adjacent vertebra must necessarily increase. The elastic properties enable the movements of the vertebral column to be smooth and less abrupt in nature.

Muscles of the Back

The muscles of the back can be divided into four groups. There are the prevertebral muscles, superficial or migratory back muscles, intermediate back muscles, and deep, or true, back muscles. The prevertebral, superficial, and intermediate groups of muscles are all innervated by ventral rami of the segmental nerves or spinal accessory nerve. The prevertebral muscles are flexors of the neck and head and include muscles such as the longus colli, longus capitis, rectus capitis anterior and lateralis. The superficial back muscles are the trapezius, latissimus dorsi, rhomboid major and minor, and levator scapulae. They are considered migratory in that they have at some point shifted from the shoulder region, where they exist in quadrapeds, to the dorsal regions of the back, where they help in the movement and maintenance of an upright posture and the shoulder girdle. There are only two members in the intermediate muscle group: the superior and inferior serratus posterior muscles. These muscles are accessory respiratory muscles but may also play a role as contractile bands that help to hold the true back muscles close to the vertebral bodies during flexion and extension. These intermediate muscles are in good position to prevent the underlying true back muscles from bow stringing, which would result in a loss of muscular mechanical advantage.

The deep back muscles are innervated by dorsal rami only and can be broken into two primary groups: the erector spinae and the transversospinalis group. These muscles attach to the axial skeleton or os coxae and insert back onto the axial skeleton via ribs, other vertebrae, or the posterior skull. They are encased by posterior and anterior layers of the thoracolumbar fascia as it attaches to the spinous and transverse processes, respectively. They sit along the vertebrocostal gutter formed between the transverse and spinous processes of the vertebral column and ascend in this gutter or they extend out to the ribs (Figure 3-7). The lumbar region is composed of larger muscles and motor units, whereas the more cephalad portions area arranged in smaller slips and motor units. The increase in the number of muscles and the decrease in their size results in providing us with an increase in the complexity of control in the neck. This allows us to take advantage of the increased range of motion available in the cervical regions. As always, with increased mobility there is decreased stability and an accompanying increase in the complexity of control. This can be evidenced by the increase in cervical vertebral specializations such as the anterior and posterior tubercles on the transverse processes and the bifid spinous processes, not to mention the orientation of cervical facets. Most of the deep muscles of the back regardless of their size and position are bilateral extensors and unilateral side flexors and/or rotators. Their major role is in maintenance of the upright posture and the movements of

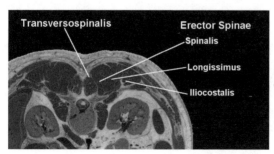

Figure 3-7 Deep back muscles in cross section.

the vertebral column and head. They contain many slow oxidative fibers and are well vascularized from numerous segmental arteries.

The erector spinae is a complex muscle that sits more superficial and lateral than the transversospinalis group (Figure 3-8). The impressive muscle mass of the erector spinae has a common attachment to the iliac crest, the posterior sacrum, posterior sacroiliac ligaments, as well as to the sacral and inferior lumbar spinous processes and intervening ligaments. The iliocostalis is the most lateral of the three primary portions of the erector spinae, and it ascends laterally from the common attachment to attach to the angles of the ribs. The longissimus is the middle portion of the erector spinae, and it ascends laterally to transverse processes. The spinalis is the most medial portion of the erector spinae and the smallest. It ascends from the common muscle belly up to the spinous processes in the thoracic and cervical regions as well as sending slips up to the base of the skull.

The transversospinalis muscle group sits deep and medial to the erector spinae. The muscles of this group are so named because they predominantly attach on the transverse process medially to the spinous process of vertebrae above. The semispinalis arises from half of the vertebral column and traverses four to six vertebrae. It is responsible for extension bilaterally, and unilaterally it causes rotation to the opposite side. The multifiidus (from the term multiple segments) extends across the lamina from S4 to C2 levels. It spans one to three vertebral levels and is responsible for extension bilaterally and side flexion to the same side and rotation to the opposite side unilaterally. The rotatores muscles are short, crossing only one or two vertebral levels. They are poorly developed or not present in the lumbar regions, as the facet joint orientations do not lend themselves well to

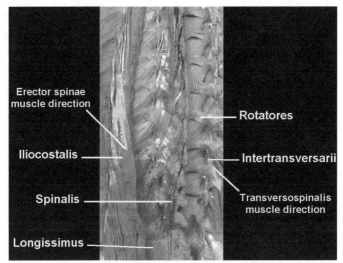

Figure 3-8 Deep back muscles dissection. (Republished with permission from McMinn's Color Atlas of Human Anatomy, 5th ed. St. Louis: Mosby; 2002.)

rotational movements. They are best developed in the thoracic regions attaching from the transverse process up to the base of the spinous process of closely adjacent vertebrae. Besides rotating to the opposite side, they stabilize the vertebral column. The interspinales and intertransversarii are small muscles that attach from spinous to spinous process and transverse to transverse process of adjacent vertebrae. They function to extend the vertebral column bilaterally and side flex it unilaterally. Table 3-2 further breaks down the regional specialization and subsections of the erector spinae and transversospinalis groups.

Nerves of the Spine and Spinal Cord Coverings

The spinal cord is covered by three meningeal layers. The outer covering, often called the thecal sac, is composed of a dense and fibrous connective tissue sheet called dura mater, which translates to "tough mother." The dura is continuous with the dura of the cranial vault but differs in that there is only one layer of dura around the spinal cord, and the dura of the spinal cord is not as intimately connected to the bones of the vertebral column as it is with the bones of the cranial vault. Therefore, there is a space external to the dura but within the vertebral canal that is called the epidural space. The epidural space is filled with fat, connective tissue, and the internal vertebral venous plexus. This plexus is clinically important because it has no

Table 3-2   Subdivisions of Deep Back Muscles

Erector Spinae Subdivisions

General description: Lies superficial and lateral to the transversospinalis group in the paravertebral gutter between the transverse and spinous processes. Muscles travel superiorly and laterally and, when combined with the other side, the muscles form a V-shape.

i. Iliocostalis	Iliocostalis lumborum	Iliocostalis thoracic	Iliocostalis cervicis
i. Longissimus	Longissimus thoracis	Longissimus cervicis	Longissimus capitis
i. Spinalis	Spinalis thoracis	Spinalis cervisis	Spinalis capitis

Transversospinalis Subdivisions

General description: Lies deep and medial to the erector spinae in the paravertebral gutter between the transverse and spinous processes. Muscles travel superiorly and medially and, when combined with the other side, the muscles form an inverted V-shape.

i. Semispinalis	Semispinalis thoracis	Semispinalis cervicis

Semispinalis Capitis

i. Multifidus	Multifidus	Multifidus	Multifidus
i. Rotatores	Rotatores lumborum	Rotatores thoracis	Rotatores cervicis
i. Interspinales	Interspinales	Interspinales	Interspinales
i. Intertransversarii	Intertransversarii	Intertransversarii	Intertransversarii

valves and can act as a conduit for metastasis of cancerous cells. The dura itself attaches to the foramen magnum where the two layers of cranial dura rejoin together as one layer and extends to the level of the S2 vertebrae where it attaches and ends. Directly under the dura is the second meningeal layer. This thin, cellophane-like layer has spider web-like projections emanating from its deep surface and is therefore called the arachnoid mater, or "spidery mother." The spider-like space under the arachnoid mater is called the subarachnoid space and is the area where the cerebrospinal fluid (CSF) is contained to bathe and protect the spinal cord and brain. The third meningeal layer is attached intimately to the spinal cord and brain. This meningeal layer is very thin and delicate and is called the pia mater, or "soft mother" (Figure 3-9). The pia has two specialization that help maintain the spinal cord in the proper positioning so that it can be efficiently bathed in the CSF. The first specialization is a set of bilateral projections of pia that anchors to the dura in a horizontal plane. They are tooth-like and are therefore called denticulate ligaments. There is one denticulate ligament on each side of the spinal cord, but each ligament has 21 of these tooth-like specializations. These denticulate ligaments serve as landmarks, as dorsal to the ligaments is the sensory half of the spinal cord and ventral to the ligaments is the motor half of the spinal cord. The second pial specialization is the filum terminale. This is a vertically traveling extension of pia that continues after the spinal cord proper ends. The filum terminale passes down and through the dural (thecal) sac to attach to the coccyx as the coccygeal ligament.

The 31 segmental spinal nerves that project from the spinal cord are mixed nerves that are formed from the combination and mixing of the

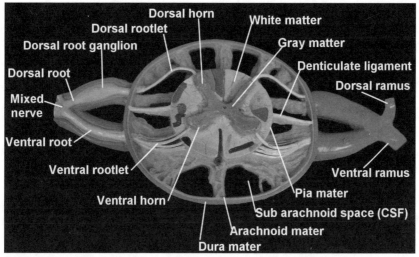

Figure 3-9   Schematic model of a typical segmental spinal nerve and the three meningeal coverings.

dorsally located afferent (sensory) information and the ventrally located efferent information. This uniting of information occurs after the dorsal root ganglion at the region of the intervertebral foramena. The mixed nerve divides into mixed dorsal rami and mixed ventral rami (see Figure 3-9). The dorsal rami and their branches innervate the true back muscles and the skin above them. The dorsal rami also provide branches to the zygapophyseal joints. The ventral rami supply structures that are not supplied by either cranial nerves or dorsal rami. Of special note, the recurrent meningeal branch (of Lushka) supplies the intervertebral disk and is usually from the ventral ramus. This nerve may also carry somatic afferent information from the anterior thecal sac. Thirty-one pairs of spinal nerves exit the vertebral canal and are numbered according to which vertebral region they originate from. There are 8 cervical, 12 thoracic, 5 lumbar, 5 sacral, and 1 coccygeal nerves. Eight cervical nerves are counted because the first cervical nerve exits above the C1 vertebrae and the eighth cervical nerve, and all nerves afterward exit below the vertebrae for which they are numbered. Each nerve except C1 (which is motor only) and the coccygeal nerve (which is sensory only) has motor and sensory components. All will carry both somatic and visceral fibers, though some will not receive their visceral components until after the nerve has exited the intervertebral foramen. The ventral rami braid together to form plexi such as the cervical, brachial, and lumbosacral plexi and innervate regions not supplied by dorsal rami or cranial nerves. The smallest segmental nerve is the coccygeal nerve, which is predominantly somatic sensory from the skin overlying the coccyx. The largest segmental nerve is the S1 nerve that contributes ventral ramus fibers to the sciatic and gluteal nerves and dorsal ramus fibers to the true back muscles over the sacrum and the skin of the gluteal region.

The spinal cord proper contains segmental representation for all 31 levels but only extends from the foramen magnum to the L1/2 vertebral level in adults. The infant spinal cord projects lower to the L3 level, and the fetal cord extends to the end of the forming vertebral canal. The difference is due to the growth rates of the skeletal system and nervous system. Fetally, the nervous system is one of the first and fastest systems to form, but the skeletal system is very slow to develop. After birth the reverse is true. Because the nervous system is almost complete by birth, its growth rates are very slow compared to that of the skeletal system. As a child grows, their distal cord is in effect pulled upward by the growth. Thus, the cervical spinal cord is almost in line with the segmental nerve projecting from it. As you descend the cord, the projection angles of the nerves fall from almost 90 degrees to almost 0 degrees (Figure 3-10). It is because of the postpartum growth of the skeletal system that the distal end of the spinal cord tapers and ends at the conus medullaris located at the L1/L2 vertebral level. After the spinal cord proper terminates, the remainder of the segmental nerves head to their appropriate intervertebral foramina arranged inside the dural sac as the cauda equina, or "horse's tail." At the center of the cauda equina is the filum terminale.

■   ■   ■

REFERENCES

1. **Basmajian JV, De Luca DJ.** Muscles Alive, 5th ed. Baltimore: Williams & Wilkins; 1985:255, 414.
2. **Kendal FP, McCreary EK, Provance PG.** Muscles Testing and Function. Baltimore: Williams & Wilkins; 1993:73-9.
3. **Williams PK, Warlock R, Tyson M, Banister LH.** Gray's Anatomy, 38th ed. London: Churchill-Livingstone; 1995:490-550.
4. **Wordburne RT, Burkel WE.** Essentials of Human Anatomy. New York: Oxford University Press; 1988:334-5.

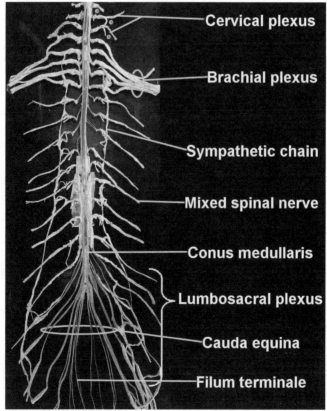

Figure 3-10   Peripheral spinal nerves as they exit the spinal cord. The cauda equina has been teased apart for demonstration purposes.

5. **Kirkaldy-Willis WH, et al.** Pathology and pathogenesis of lumbar spondylosis and stenosis. Spine. 1978;3(4):319-28.

6. **Vanharanta H, et al.** Pain provocation and disc deterioration by age. A CT/discography study in low-back pain population. Spine. 1989;14:420-3.

7. **Moore KL.** Clinically Oriented Anatomy, 3rd ed. Baltimore: Williams & Wilkins; 1992:351-69.

■   ■   ■

KEY REFERENCES

Basic Text

Moore KL and Agur AM, eds. Essential Clinical Anatomy, 2nd ed. Philadelphia: Lippincott Williams & Wilkins; 2002.
Sound information and good clinical cases.

Detailed Text

Woodburne RT, Burkel WE, eds. Essentials of Human Anatomy, 9th ed. New York: Oxford University Press; 1994.
Not as complete or verbose as Gray's but gives good anatomical detail. Does not put the same focus on clinical information as Moore and Agur above but is useful if you want to learn more anatomy.

Atlas

Clemente CD. Anatomy: A Regional Atlas of the Human Body, 4th ed. Philadelphia: Lippincott Williams & Wilkins; 1997.
I love this book because of the excellent Sobotta images, but more importantly the text that accompanies the images helps you to focus on the important relationships and structures that make the images useful. Many atlases are confusing and difficult to follow because of the overabundance of labels, cross-referencing numbers, and so forth. Clemente gives a nice balance of information and ease of use.

Web Sites

ANATOMY
Integrated Medical Curriculm by Gold Standard, available at www.imc.gsm.com, is a pay site but has all kinds of information including anatomic, histologic, pharmacologic, and so forth. Excellent value.

CLINICAL
A good source for easy-to-read and fairly up-to-date information about the spine is www.spine-health.com. It is a site that both clinicians and lay persons can learn from.

4

■　■　■

Pain Pathophysiology

Andrew J. Haig, MD

ain is a difficult and complex concept. In answer to the question "What is pain?" specialists love to quote a definition by the International Association for the Study of Pain: "Pain is an unpleasant sensory and emotional experience associated with actual or potential tissue damage or described in terms of such damage." However, clinicians are inclined to scratch their head at this academic theory and ask the more important questions: Is my patient in pain? Why? How much? What can I do about it?

Clearly, pain is what the patient says it is-assuming honest reporting, of course. There are many ways to measure pain, but they all depend on communication from the patient (1). Pain is not contained in any single anatomical structure. Rather, it is up to us to find pathways that lead to a particular patient's pain complaints. In recent years, there has been a deepening of our understanding of pain pathophysiology, which has led to new treatments and a better understanding of diagnoses and treatments. By understanding these mechanisms, the clinician can rationally understand many of the issues presented later in this book-ranging from new medications to the relatively benign natural history to the complexities of false positive and false negative imaging tests. In this chapter, we will discuss the pathophysiology of pain as it relates to the spine, local biochemical changes, pain pathways, and neurochemical changes related to chronic pain. Finally, we will review the somewhat complex terminology used in pain management.

The Spinal Degenerative Cascade

This chapter outlines the anatomy of the "perfect" spine, but not the anatomy of the *normal* spine. As we have come to learn, the spine changes with age. It is normal for an older person to have substantial degeneration without any evidence of dysfunction or pain. It is well-known that one third to two thirds of asymptomatic persons have degenerative changes and that this number increases with age. A smaller percentage (perhaps 5%) have extruded or severely herniated disks; again, with no pain. Facet joint arthritis and spinal canal stenosis are also common in people without symptoms.

William Kirkaldy-Willis first described this process as a rational progression of maturation of the spine (2). Figure 4-1 illustrates the sometimes, but not always, painful degenerative cascade. His "degenerative cascade" is a good framework for understanding pathophysiology (Figure 4-1). The degenerative cascade begins early-in the teen years. Autopsies on young victims of the Korean War showed tears in the annulus fibrosus fibers that surround the gel-like nucleus pulposus. The lower disks degenerate earlier than the higher disks, probably related to the increased force on the lower disks. Some contend that tears in the annulus occasionally irritate the sparse nerves fibers that are present in the outer annulus. Thus, they theorize, some annular tears are painful, whereas others are clearly not.

There has been a flurry of activity trying to show that annular tears are the cause of back pain. A plain x-ray finding of disk collapse is not related to pain. An exception is collapse of a disk above L5-S1 before that lowest level has shown collapse. For example, if the L2-3 disk is collapsed, while the disks below remain normal, there is an increased chance that that person has pain. The so-called painful white bodies seen in the posterior annulus on magnetic resonance imaging (MRI) have not been shown to be specific for pain. Diskograms show annular tears, but the anatomy shown on a diskogram does not relate to diskogenic pain. Subjective pain reproduction on provocative diskography has been used for some time as proof, but most recently, research shows that the patient's response to diskogram is predicted primarily by psychological status, not spinal factors.

Over time, more cracks occur in the annulus as dehydration and collagen changes take their toll. These cracks may cause diffuse bulging (not associated with pain, but seen often on MRI scans) or focal protrusions or herniations. Herniations upwards through the vertebral end plate (Schmorl's nodes) may relate to transient pain. By the time they show up on x-ray as calcified indentation in the vertebra, they are painless. Anterior herniations are not thought to be painful. Clearly, many people with posterior disk herniation have no pain. But there are a number of persons with severe debilitating pain and neurologic deficit that we call sciatica. We know that the pain of sciatica is not caused by direct pressure "pinched nerve" in most cases but rather by inflammation of the nerve root sheath. (We will discuss this in more detail later.) Proof that a disk herniation is causing sciatica is demonstrated via electromyography or perhaps selective nerve root blocks. Nevertheless, at this time we do not know why some disk herniations are painful, whereas others are not.

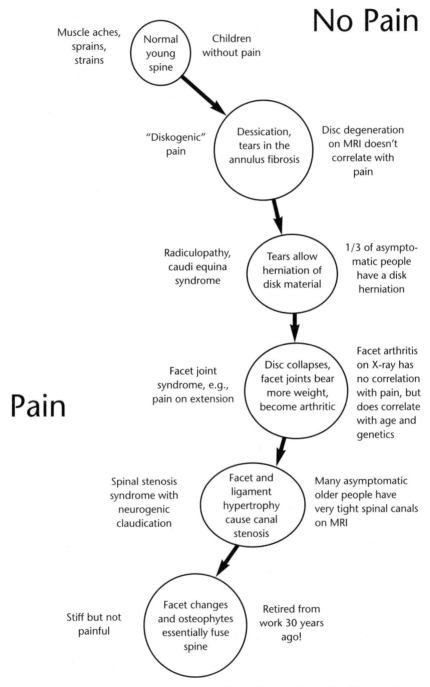

Figure 4-1   The degenerative cascade of Kirkaldy-Willis. At each level in this normal process there may or may not be pain.

With or without herniation, all disks slowly degenerate and collapse. This collapse brings facet joints closer to each other. The facet joints change from guiding movement to bearing weight. This weight bearing, in turn, causes degenerative changes in the joints. Again, facet joint arthritis on an x-ray is not an epidemiologic marker for pain. Still, many believe that facet joints can be the cause of substantial pain. Injection with local anesthetic under fluoroscopy is one standard used to determine if a certain facet joint is causing pain.

Facet arthritis causes the joints to get larger. The ligaments surrounding the facet get thicker. All of this means there is less room in the spinal canal for the nerve roots. This is called spinal stenosis. Although there is a statistical relationship between spinal canal size and pain, there is substantial variation. In a prospective study we are working on, some people with radiologically severe stenosis have no symptoms whatsoever. Symptoms associated with spinal stenosis may result from any of several factors: The geometry of the canal (a "trefoil" shaped canal is more at risk than a rounded one, a flexed spine opens up the canal compared to MRI imaging when lying down), the quality of the arterial supply of the nerve roots, venous congestion of the nerve roots, spinal segmental hypermobility causing transient worsening of symptoms, or the presence of fat or other contents in the canal. The leg cramping and weakness characteristic of spinal stenosis is often described as neurogenic claudication to differentiate from peripheral vascular disease, but in fact these symptoms may be vascular claudication of the nerve roots.

Case Study 4-1

A 65-year-old male volunteered for a research project. His MRI showed severe degenerative changes and moderate-to-severe spinal stenosis. The research surgeon, blinded to clinical information, believed that the findings were severe enough for an operation. In fact, the research subject was himself a physician. He worked full-time and walked 4 miles a few times each week for exercise with no back pain or disability. A physical examination was unremarkable, and electromyography (EMG) was negative. He performed well on a 15-minute laboratory test of ambulation and a week-long pedometer test of functional ambulation.

Of course, outside of a research situation, the surgeon would have inquired about symptoms and performed a physical examination. But the case illustrates how crucial the clinical presentation is. In fact, imaging tests in isolation are *not* considered gold standards for most spine syndromes.

People who are fortunate to live long enough experience the final stage of the degenerative cascade. Disk collapse and facet hypertrophy, along with the immobility typical of older persons, leads to great stiffness or fusion of the spine. The fused or stiff spine is typically not painful, although it may be somewhat disabling and may put pressure on other structures.

There are other variations to the degenerative cascade. Denervation of the back muscles occurs naturally and frequently. This may lead to increased instability, thus speeding up the degenerative process. Related to this process, neuromuscular diseases frequently result in scoliosis. Postoperative patients who have had more soft tissue damage are more likely to have chronic pain. Fusion results in hypermobility of adjacent spinal segments, increasing the speed of the degenerative cascade in these areas.

A number of other factors further speed up spinal degeneration. Cigarette smoking and repetitive twisting, bending, or lifting are some of the factors that are controllable. Twin studies show genetics is an important predictor of degeneration. Focal trauma to a joint may cause segmental changes. Perhaps most common, yet least studied, is the effect of local biomechanics, such as tightness in rotating one segment or another, on both degeneration and pain.

Local Biochemical Changes

The term *pinched nerve* is commonly used by patients to describe back pain. It is used by the public to describe two different types of pain:

1. *Pain that is sharp and reproducible, yet localized.* We think this is usually not related to an anatomic nerve at all but is instead related to ligament or joint irritation. Nerves certainly transmit this sharp sensation, but patients are relieved to learn that sharp reproducible pain is usually not related to paralysis.

2. *Sciatica, or pain that radiates down the leg.* Surprisingly, sciatica is seldom related to mechanical pinching of the nerve. Often, it is actually referred pain from another structure. The sacroiliac joints, the facet joints, ligaments, tendons, and muscles in the lumbar region are well established as causes for pain that radiates down the leg-even below the knee. Sometimes, sciatica is not truly from the back. Mechanical back pain is so common that lower limb nerve problems ranging from peroneal nerve palsy to polyneuropathy to compartment syndromes have a good chance of occurring coincident to mechanical low back pain.

Even when there is clear consensus from MRI and EMG that a disk herniation is the cause of the pain, it is uncommon for the nerve to be "pinched." A pinched nerve root causes paresthesias and weakness. An inflamed nerve root sleeve, on the other hand, causes pain. Recent research has shown that most disk herniations cause pain through inflammation. The nucleus pulposus has no vascular supply, so its tissues are viewed by the immune system as foreign bodies. With painful disk herniation there is an immense outpouring of phospholipase A2, tumor necrosis factor alpha, and numerous other immune products in an attempt to attack the foreign body. These cause inflammation of the nerve root sleeve, and the inflammation causes a pain sensation to travel through the vasa nervorum in the nerve root sheath to the spinal cord.

Epidural or oral steroids are used to attack this inflammatory cascade. A number of products are being developed to have a more specific effect on the inflammation of a disk. This inflammation successfully dissolves the herniated material. The larger the herniation, the more inflammation and the faster it disappears. Both the clinical literature and laboratory studies suggest that patients will undergo diskectomy regardless of treatment- whether caused by a knife or caused by the inflammatory cascade. In the long term, there is no difference in outcome.

Perhaps the most exciting new evidence that pain from a disk herniation is *not* from pressure is a study that shows that an inhibitor of tumor necrosis factor alpha, given intravenously essentially cured the pain of disk herniation in a group of 10 subjects.

The Pain Pathway

Tissue damage or irritation in the low back causes depolarization of a number of nerve fibers, most importantly the myelenated A-delta fibers, which cause a sharp focused pain sensation, and the unmyelinated C fibers, which cause a dull, diffuse pain sensation. These travel to the dorsal horn of the spinal cord.

The role of the spinal cord in the pain pathway is complex. Countless axons interact with nerve transmission, activated or inhibited by a number of chemicals including substance P, beta endorphins, enkephalins, amino acids, and other neuropeptides. Proof that a disk herniation is causing sciatica is demonstrated via electromyography or perhaps selective nerve root blocks. In the cord, the gate theory of Melzack and Wall, a long-held but still unproven theory, may play itself out. According to Melzack and Wall, if a distracting stimulus heads up fast myelenated fibers from the limb, the pain fibers are "beat to the pass," and the pain is not as bad. A phenomenon called *wind up* involves facilitation of transmission and increased sensitivity to pain. This occurs primarily in the spinal cord, although the pathways are complex and not perfectly well understood. Wind up means repeated pain hurts more than a single episode; that pain hurts more when the patient is anxious or attentive to the stimulus.

At the brainstem, the spinothalamic tract attaches to the lateral thalamic nuclei (thus the uncommon procedure of thalamotomy for intractable pain). The rubrospinal tract goes to the medial thalamic nuclei. Pain is modulated by countless inputs to the thalamus from other brain areas. The thalamus sends fibers to a number of sites, most importantly the sensory cortex where pain is "felt." In the secondary sensory cortex and related area, pain is evaluated and judged. Somewhere in here is where that spacey definition of pain resides.

But it does not end here. Pain behavior is what the clinician sees. In this sense, then, pain behavior is as much a reflection of the clinician's subjective input and judgment as it is the display of pain on the part of the patient himself. The clinician's past experiences, alertness status, and social context are all integrated into this judgment.

Adaptation to Chronic Pain

Once pain is chronic, research has shown that it becomes a learned behavior. At the nerve root level there is a "memory" for pain, so that stimulating a normal root causes tingling, but stimulating a previously operated root causes radiating pain. Factors in the spinal cord and brainstem, discussed above, are amplified in favor of increased pain perception.

There is increased vigilance or attention to detect painful stimuli. Tenderness occurs in a wider area. Pain is sensed over a larger surface area than the stimulus would normally evoke. Autonomic responses may increase, resulting in reflex sympathetic dystrophy (complex regional pain syndrome, for those in the know). Eventually, adaptation of the system occurs at many levels, so that, even when the original stimulus is removed or lessened, the perception of pain persists. The reader may recall stories of the old days when they would unsuccessfully treat chronic foot pain with nerve blocks, leg amputation, thigh amputation, and even spinal cord lesioning-to no avail. Such lessons should not be lost on those of us who hope the fifth-lumbar fusion will do the trick. Pain probably causes neurochemical changes that result in anxiety and sleep disturbances, leading to depression.

This cascade seems depressing to the clinician as well as the patient. But an understanding of the process can reassure us that we and the patient can work to reverse it. Unlearning pain involves substituting other experiences. Getting up and about, exercising and stimulating painful parts, can have an effect on pain. (Of course, back pain often involves ongoing "acute" local irritation so that this is not easy.) Effective treatment of depression, anxiety, and sleep disturbances can also have a real effect. Education and pain counselling aren't just niceties-they attack the pathophysiology of the disease itself. Biofeedback, relaxation, and other means of refocusing may help. Numerous medications attack different aspects of the pain cycle, too.

Pain Definitions

The language of pain has become more sophisticated as we understand more about its pathophysiology. The International Association for the Study of Pain has come up with a classification and some definitions (3). A brief review of some of the words will help the physician communicate with others who use precise terminology.

Allodynia: Pain related to a stimulus that usually does not cause pain (e.g., allodynia occurs when a light touch causes substantial pain to a burn patient).

Causalgia: Same as CRPS II (below).

Complex regional pain syndrome I (CRPS I): Pain, allodynia, or hyperalgesia greater than expected for the tissue injury.

Complex regional pain syndrome II (CRPS II): Pain, allodynia, or hyperalgesia greater than expected and not limited to the distribution of a traumatized nerve.

Dysesthesia: An abnormal sensation, whether spontaneous or evoked, which is unpleasant.

Hyperalgesia: Exaggerated response to a stimulus that is usually painful.

Hyperpathia: Exaggerated pain (especially in duration) in response to a stimulus.

Nociception: The sensation that a stimulus is painful.

Pain: "An unpleasant sensory and emotional experience associated with actual or potential tissue damages or described in terms of such damage" (IASP).

Paresthesia: An abnormal sensation, whether spontaneous or evoked, which is not unpleasant.

Radiating pain: Pain in a nerve distribution, caused by stimulation of that nerve.

Referred pain: Pain in an area where the stimulation is not occurring, but not radiating pain (not in the distribution of a *nerve* that is irritated).

Reflex sympathetic dystrophy: Pain, vasomotor insufficiency, and dystrophy. Numerous other synonyms exist. The entity is poorly defined, and other terms (CRPS) are preferred.

Sympathetically mediated pain: Pain associated with sympathetic phenomenon such as redness or sweating.

Sympathetically nonmediated pain: Pain not associated with sympathetic phenomenon.

■   ■   ▩

Key Points

- Anatomical derangement of the spine follows an orderly degenerative cascade.
- Pain does not correlate well with anatomical disruption.
- Numerous factors in the nerve, spinal cord, and brain modulate pain.
- The language of pain is becoming more complex.

▦   ▦   ▦

REFERENCES

1. **Turk DC, Melzack R.** Handbook of Pain Assessment. New York: The Guilford Press; 1992.
2. **Kirkaldy-Willis WH, Wedge JH, Yong-Hing K, Reily J.** Pathology and pathogeneiss of lumbar spondylosis and stenosis. Spine. 1978;3:319-28.
3. **International Association for the Study of Pain Subcommittee on Taxonomy.** Classification of chronic pain: descriptions of chronic pain syndromes and definitions of pain terms. Pain Suppl. 1986;3:S1-S225.

▦   ▦   ▦

KEY REFERENCES

Bonica JJ. The Management of Pain, 2nd ed. Philadelphia: Lea and Febiger; 1990.
A huge text on pain, including chapters on pathophysiology and treatment.

Woolf CJ, Mannion RJ. Neuropathic pain: aetiology, symptoms, mechanisms, and management. Lancet. 1999;353:1959-64.
Volume 353 of Lancet (full text on Medline) has a strong series of articles that review many aspects of pain and pain management.

5

■ ■ ■

Diagnoses: A Glossary Approach

Joyce Huerta, MD

The diagnostic terminology for back pain is substantial and confusing. Readers will find it useful to review this list and to refer to it throughout the book.

Acquired stenosis: *See* Spinal stenosis.

Anterior herniated disk: Very uncommon condition in which the intervertebral disk herniates anteriorly; it is not thought to be a painful condition and is not associated with radiculopathy or myelopathy, as there are not anterior neural structures.

Arachnoiditis: A condition in which the arachnoid membrane becomes inflamed and may eventually become fibrotic. Usually, it is a rare, self-limited process that may be a complication of epidural steroid injections, myelography, or surgery. It may result in disabling pain if it becomes chronic in nature.

Arthritis: Inflammation of a joint or a state characterized by inflamed joints in the body, often leading to swelling, pain, stiffness, and the possible loss of function. *See* Osteoarthritis, Nonspondylitic spondylolisthesis, Spondylosis, Spondylitis, Spondyloarthritis, Spondyloarthropathies, Spondylolysis, Spondylolisthesis, Spondyloptosis, Spondylolisthesis aquista.

Axial pain: Low back pain that does not radiate into the limb.

Bursitis: Inflammation of the bursa. Trochanteric bursitis is often a cause of "false radiating" pain after recovery from disk herniation.

Burst fracture: *See* Fracture.

Cauda equina syndrome: A syndrome of low back pain, progressive bilateral lower extremity motor weakness (even paraplegia), radicular pain, saddle anesthesia, urinary retention, and bowel incontinence. The syndrome is caused by external compression of the cauda equina due to such conditions as a large central herniated disk, tumor, epidural hematoma or abscess, trauma, and so forth. This condition requires emergent surgical decompression to stop the progression of neurologic loss.

Central canal stenosis: *See* Spinal stenosis.

Central herniation: A midline herniation of the nucleus pulposus through the posterior longitudinal ligament. This may affect the roots on either side or both sides and may affect multiple roots including those that exit the spinal canal a few segments below. It can result in cauda equina syndrome.

Claudication: *See* Vasogenic claudication.

Congenital stenosis: *See* Spinal stenosis.

Contained herniation: The nucleus pulposus ruptures through the inner annular fibers but does not rupture through the outer annular fibers.

Compression fracture: *See* Fracture.

Degenerative disk disease: A condition of the intervertebral disk in which small tears in the annulus fibrosus form and the water content of the nucleus pulposus decreases. It is caused by the normal wear and tear of the disk and may be due to aging or trauma, thus the term *disease* may be misleading. Degenerative disk disease may lead to diffuse disk bulging, bone spurs, decreases in disk height, and narrowing of the intervertebral space.

Disk bulge: Diffuse expansion of the annular fibers beyond the contour of the vertebral body, usually related to loss of disk height from degenerative disk disease. Disk bulge is a normal finding not associated with low back pain, but occasionally a disk herniation will be misread as a bulge on imaging studies.

Diskitis: An infectious disorder of the axial skeleton affecting the intervertebral disk that may be due to hematogeneous spread through the bloodstream as a complication of vertebral osteomyeltis or due to direct penetration from surgery or other spinal procedures. Sterile diskitis is a nonpurulent inflammation of the disk, sometimes occurring postoperatively.

Diskogenic pain: Pain arising in the intervertebral disk caused by trauma or excessive degeneration of the disk. The pain is thought to increase with increased intradiskal pressure with such activities as sitting, flexion, standing, lifting, and valsalva. Proof that a certain disk is causing pain is problematic. Some believe that pain reproduction on diskogram is useful but others do not.

Enthesitis: Inflammation of the area of attachment of a tendon to a bone. Enthesitis, which can occur alone (e.g., tennis elbow), is also associated with some seronegative spondyloarthropathies.

Facet joint disease: Arthritis of the facet joints; the intervertebral synovial joints that receive innervation from the median branch of the dorsal rami.

Facet syndrome: Consists of pain originating at the facet joint due to facet degeneration and/or hypertrophy that may compress a nerve root or may refer pain to the gluteal region or lower extremities.

Failed back surgery syndrome: Chronic and persisting back pain or increased neurological deficit after back surgery, most commonly after disk surgery. Previously called *failed back syndrome*, it is associated with surgical misadventure and complications, intraoperative damage to the paraspinal muscles, and psychosocial barriers to recovery.

Far lateral disk: A herniation that traps the nerve root lateral to the central canal and is located in the intervertebral foramen.

Fibromyalgia: A soft tissue pain syndrome characterized by chronic generalized aches, pains, or stiffness in discrete tender point areas. The symptoms involve more than three anatomic sites for greater than 3 months and are not associated structural abnormalities of the muscle, bone, cartilage, or other systemic conditions to account for the multiple complaints. Other additional symptoms may include disturbed sleep, generalized fatigue or tiredness, subjective swelling, numbness, pain in the neck and shoulders, chronic headaches, and irritable bowel symptoms.

Foraminal stenosis: *See* Spinal stenosis.

Fracture: Traumatic bone disruption. Fractures are considered unstable if two of the three stabilizing "columns" of the vertebrae are disrupted (anterior, middle, and posterior aspects of the vertebrae). Mechanisms may include flexion-distraction, extension, and fracture dislocation.

> *Compression fracture:* Compression of the vertebral body without substantial displacement into the spinal canal and without destabilization of the posterior elements. Compression fractures typically occur in relationship to osteoporosis but can occur in normal vertebrae with substantial trauma. They are typically biomechanically and neurologically stable.

> *Burst fracture:* A fracture that disrupts the posterior longitudinal ligament. These can compromise the spinal canal and cause neurologic deficit.

Herniated disks (also known as **herniated nucleus pulposus,** or HNP): Focal protrusion of the nucleus pulposus through the annular fibers of the disk. Posterior disk herniations may cause the sciatic syndrome commonly recognized as *disk herniation*. Anterior disk herniations are asymptomatic. Superior or inferior disk herniations, *Schmorl's nodes*, may cause acute nonradiating pain at onset.

> *See also* Anterior herniated disk, Central herniation, Contained herniation, Disk bulge, Disk sequestration (noncontained herniated disk), Far lateral disk, Posterolateral herniation, Schmorl's node.

Infections: *See* Diskitis, Osteomyelitis.

Kyphosis: Curve of the spine with the concavity facing anteriorly. (The normal curvature of the spine includes a cervical and lumbar lordosis and a thoracic kyphosis.)

Leg length inequality: Leg length inequality may be functional or anatomic. *Anatomic* leg length inequality is due to a long or short tibia or femur. *Functional* leg length inequality is a difference in apparent leg length due to an adaptive curve of the lumbar spine, a pelvic asymmetry, or a sacroiliac joint dysfunction.

Lordosis: Curve of the spine with the concavity facing posteriorly. (The normal curvature of the spine includes a cervical and lumbar lordosis and a thoracic kyphosis.)

Manipulable lesion: (osteopathic lesion, somatic dysfunction): This refers to an alteration in the mobility, alignment, and function of the musculoskeletal system. Malalignment and restriction to movement are the easiest lesions of this category to understand, though it also includes hypermobility and muscle imbalance. A formal definition per the Glossary of Osteopathic Terminology is as follows: Somatic dysfunction: Impaired or altered function of related components of the somatic (body framework) system: skeletal, arthrodial, and myofascial structures and related vascular, lymphatic, and neural elements. The positional and motion aspects of somatic dysfunction may be described using three parameters: (1) the position of the element as determined by palpation; (2) the direction in which motion is freer; (3) the direction in which motion is restricted.

Mechanical back pain: An overuse injury of a normal anatomic structure, or an injury causing the alteration of the normal anatomic structure and function. These injuries may then cause work to be shunted to other nearby structures, which in turn become overloaded and painful. Mechanical injuries include such conditions as muscle strain, muscle imbalance, impaired mobility and alignment of the spine and related structures, herniated nucleus pulposus, osteoarthritis, spinal stenosis, spondylolysis, spondylolisthesis, scoliosis, and so forth The term *mechanical back pain* is used generally for back pain not caused by a systemic disorder and not related to nerve injury.

Muscle spasm: A poorly defined entity apparently not related to spasticity and debated to be voluntary or reflexive splinting of the back muscles.

Musculoligamentous back pain: Back pain that may result from injury to the muscles and ligaments. Sprains of muscles may occur in any of the spinal musculature including the multifidus, quadatus lumborum, piriformis, and others. Ligament sprains can occur at any of the spinal ligaments including the supraspinous ligaments and the interspinous ligaments.

Myofascial pain: Pain emanating from muscular or fascial structures.

Myofascial trigger point: A taught palpable band in a muscle that is painful with palpation and refers pain to a distant reference zone, in a characteristic distribution to other nearby body areas. The presence of trigger points may be associated with autonomic symptoms such as sweating, salivation, localized vasoconstriction, pilomotor activity, proprioceptive disturbances, dizziness, tinnitus, and so forth.

Neurogenic pain: Pain intensified by sensory stimulation of a damaged nerve in the distribution of the neural structure. The pain typically is described as a burning, tingling, or skin-crawling sensation. The term *neurogenic back pain* is typically used in contrast to *mechanical back pain.*

Nonspondylitic spondylolisthesis: A degenerative spondylolisthesis that is caused by degenerative facet joints rather than a fracture of the neural arch (pars intraarticularis). A spondylolisthesis without spondylolysis.

Osteoarthritis: The most common form of arthritis; it is a degenerative process including spondylosis and spurring of the vertebral bodies. The hallmark of cartilage degeneration.

Osteomyelitis: An infectious disorder of the bones of the axial skeleton, most commonly due to hematogenous spread. The patient may have a history of an invasive procedure or a recent primary infection. Pain may be present weeks to months before a diagnosis is established. The pain may be intermittent or constant and may be present at rest. The most common affected area of the spine is the lumbar spine followed by the thoracic spine, sacrum, and cervical spine. *Staphylococcus aureus* is the most frequent infecting organism. Other organisms may include *Staphylococcus epidermidis, Streptococcus pneumoniae, Escherichia coli, Pseudomonas, Klebsiella, Pasteurella,* or *Salmonella* spp., *Proteus mirabilis, and Bacteroides fragilis.* Less frequent causes of infection include anaerobic bacteria, mycobacteria, fungi, spirochetes, and parasites.

Osteoporosis: A metabolic bone disease causing loss of bone mass predominantly occurring in the axial skeleton, femoral neck, and pelvis. The loss in bone mass may then result in vertebral fracture, pain, and deformity.

Posterolateral disk herniation: This is the most common type of herniation and is a condition where the nucleus pulposus herniates around the posterior longitudinal ligament. A posterolateral herniation typically affects the exiting nerve root; for example, an L4-L5 posterolateral herniation would affect the L4 more than the L5 root.

Pregnancy: Back pain occurs in approximately 50% of pregnant women. The pain may be located to the low back, sacroiliac joints, and may radiate to the buttocks or thigh. Possible causes of low back pain in pregnancy may be a hyperlordotic posture, muscular fatigue, ligamentous hyperlaxity, bulging intervertebral disks, direct fetal pressure on the lumbosacral plexus, vascular obstruction, or other metabolic causes.

Psychogenic pain: Pain originating in the cerebral cortex. May imply hysteria, malingering, or somatization disorder. Purely psychogenic pain is hard to prove and thought to be rare. The term is often used incorrectly to describe pain with associated psychological factors that exaggerate but do not cause pain (depression, anxiety, etc.).

Radicular pain: Pain radiating from the back to the lower extremity and/or foot in the distribution of the effected spinal nerve root. It is typically described as a lancinating, shooting, burning, or sharp type of pain.

Radiculopathy: The dysfunction of a nerve root associated with radiating pain, numbness or tingling, in a dermatomal distribution, with or without weakness in the myotome supplied by that nerve root. Aside from spinal disorders, radiculopathy can be a presentation of polyneuropathy, especially from diabetes or inflammatory disorder.

Referred pain: Pain originating in one body part but perceived in another. Numerous structures in the spine can cause referred pain down the leg, even below the knee. These include facet joints, sacroiliac joints, muscle, or ligament. Referred pain is frequently confused clinically with radiating pain from irritation of a nerve root.

S-curve: A type of scoliosis containing both a *major curve* and a *minor curve;* a minor curve is a small curve that has developed to compensate for the larger major curve. The minor curve is in the opposite direction of the major curve and occurs to keep the shoulders and pelvis level.

Sacroiliac dysfunction: A biomechanical dysfunction of the sacroiliac (SI) joint altering the normal SI joint movement. The SI joint is a synovial joint between the sacrum and ileum. The SI joint may be hypo- or hypermobile. SI joint dysfunction may or may not cause pain.

Sacroiliac joint syndrome: Pain arising from the SI joint and may include referred pain to the anterior thigh, pain in the SI joint, and may involve pain in the muscles that cross the SI joint and pelvis. Cracking or popping of the joint may occur.

Sacroilitis: Inflammation of the sacroiliac joint. This finding is typically seen in seronegative spondyloarthropathies. For example, it is the hallmark finding of ankylosing spondylitis.

Schmorl's node: Herniation of the disk up through the bony end-plate into the vertebra above. The onset of a Schmorl's node as seen on MRI may be painful, but by the time the node is calcified and detected on plain x-ray, these are incidental findings.

Sciatica: An inaccurate term commonly used to refer to pain radiating from the back to the lower extremity. *See* Radicular pain.

Scoliosis: An abnormal lateral curvature of the spine with or without a rotational component to the curve. Structures on the concave side of the

curve are tight, and structures on the convex side of the curve are weak.
See also S-curve.

Spina bifida occulta: A defect in the neural arch with no protrusion of neural elements. Spina bifida occulta most commonly occurs at L5 and S1. It is not associated with low back pain.

Spinal stenosis: Narrowing of the spinal canal. This can be defined radiologically (e.g., (12 mm anterior-posterior spinal canal diameter) or clinically (a syndrome of neurogenic claudication). These two trend together, but many people with "small canals" have no symptoms, and many people with larger canals have symptoms.

Central canal stenosis: Narrowing of the central spinal canal due to pseudohypertrophy of the ligamentum flavum, facet joint hypertrophy, disk degeneration, or spondylosis.

Foraminal stenosis: Decrease in the size of the intervertebral foramen (where the nerve exits the spinal canal) due to hypertrophy of the superior facet.

Congenital (developmental) stenosis: Narrowing of the spinal canal due to underdevelopment of the vertebrae or short pedicles, but is not related to trauma.

Acquired stenosis: Stenosis in the central portion of the spinal canal, the peripheral portion of the canal, the lateral recesses, and/or nerve root canals caused by degenerative changes.

Spinal malalignment: *See* kyphosis, lordosis, scoliosis.

Spondylitis: Inflammation of the facet joints. This typically occurs in association with sacroilitis in seronegative spondyloarthropathies such as ankylosing spondyitis.

Spondyloarthritis: An arthritic condition of the spine.

Spondyloarthropathies: A group of related arthritic conditions of the spine that are characterized by peripheral inflammatory arthritis, diffuse spinal involvement, inflammation of the sacroiliac joints, are seronegative (negative rheumatoid factor), and may include extra-articular features such as uveitis or conjunctivitis. Examples include ankylosing spondylitis, psoriatic arthropathy, enteric arthropathies, and Reiter's syndrome.

Spondylolisthesis: A spinal segment that has slipped on another, commonly related to a defect in the pars (spondylolysis). The vertebrae may be an anterolisthesis (moved forward relative to the vertebrae above or below it) or a retrolisthesis (moved posteriorly compared to the segment above or below it). Graded I to V depending on the percentage of slipping over the vertebra below. Grade I (< 25% slippage) is not associated with pain in adults.

Spondylolisthesis aquista: Spondylolisthesis that occurs above or below a fused level due to shunting of biomechanical forces related to the fusion.

Spondylolysis: A defect in the pars intraarticularis, which may range anywhere from an elongated but intact pars to a complete fracture of the pars. Spondylolysis is associated with pain in children and teens but not in mature adults.

Spondyloptosis: A severe spondylolisthesis (grade V), where one vertebrae has completely slipped off another.

Spondylosis: Osteoarthritis of the facet joints. It is a normal finding associated with age and in most cases not related to increased risk of back pain. It results in osteophytes formation, decreased disk height, a narrowed foramen, and hypertrophied facet joints.

Stenosis: *See* Spinal stenosis.

Subluxation: Displacement of a joint that disrupts the opposition of cartilage surfaces. In chiropractic terminology, subluxation is used differently, to suggest minor misalignment or dysfunctional movement of a joint.

Traumatic injury: *See* Fracture.

Tumors: There are two major types of tumors: extradural (50-60% of all tumors) and intradural. Intradural tumors are further divided into intramedullary (30-35% of all tumors) and extramedullary (10-20% of all tumors). Tumors that commonly metastasize to the spine are thyroid, prostate, breast, and lung tumors.

Vasogenic claudication: Cramping of the legs due to vascular insufficiency in the legs. Differentiated from neurogenic claudication of spinal stenosis.

Visceral disease and viscerogenic pain: Pain arising from the abdominal or pelvic viscera, lesions of the lesser sac, or retroperitoneal organs; for example, the pancreas, duodenum, ascending/descending colon, rectum, kidney, ureter, uterus, cervix, and prostate. The pain arises from the abnormalities in the organs that share segmental innervation with structures in the lumbosacral spine. An abdominal aortic aneurysm may cause thoracic or low back pain and should be considered in older populations.

Whiplash: A sprain or strain of the cervical spine caused by a hyperextension-hyperflexion injury. It most commonly results from motor vehicle accidents. The sternocleidomastoid, longus colli, anterior longitudinal ligament, or cervical disks may be injured. Not used to describe a similar lumbar spine injury.

▦   ▦   ▦

BIBLIOGRAPHY

Bartley R, Coffey P. Management of Low Back Pain in Primary Care. Oxford: Butterworth Heinemann; 2001.

Borenstein D, Weisel S, Boden S. Low Back Pain: Medical Diagnosis and Comprehensive Management, 2nd ed. Philadelphia: WB Saunders; 1995.

Centeno C. The Spine Dictionary: A Comprehensive Guide to Spine Terminology. Philadelphia: Hanley & Belfus, Inc.; 1999.

Floman Y. Disorders of the Lumbar Spine. Rockville, MD: Aspen Publishers, Inc.; 1990.

Jayson M. The Lumbar Spine and Back Pain, 4th ed. Edinburgh: Churchill Livingstone; 1992.

Macnab I, Transfeldt E. Macnab's Backache, 3rd ed. Baltimore: Williams & Wilkins; 1997.

Rothman R, Simeone F. The Spine, Vol. II. Philadelphia: WB Saunders; 1975.

Seimon L. Low Back Pain Clinical Diagnosis and Management, 2nd ed. New York: Demos Medical Publishing; 1995.

6

■   ■   ■

Diagnostic Tests for Back Pain:
A Glossary Approach

Mara Isser, DO

n general, unless there are compelling reasons, diagnostic tests should only be considered with symptoms lasting greater than 1 month. This is because most patients improve within this period. Also, because there are often pathological imaging findings in asymptomatic patients, some uncertainty exists regarding the value of abnormal findings in low back pain (LBP) patients.

To optimize the results of diagnostic tests, the ordering physician must include a description of the presenting symptoms, clinical impression, and diagnosis to be ruled out. Increasingly, cost is a factor as well. Table 6-1 lists approximate costs of various diagnostic tests discussed in this chapter. This chapter provides an overview of diagnostic tests discussed elsewhere in the book. Along with definitions and brief introductions, examples of appropriate referral requests are provided.

Types of Diagnostic Tests

Physiologic tests provide evidence for physiologic dysfunction such as infection, malignancy, neurological deficits, inflammation, or other systemic illness and include blood tests, urinanalysis, and electrodiagnostic exams. *Anatomic tests* show anatomic abnormalities such as spinal stenosis, herniated lumbar disk, tumor, abdominal mass, and infection. Abnormal findings on these studies must be supported by history and clinical exam because many of these findings can also be seen in asymptomatic patients. (These studies are limited because there are no reference standards to determine whether an anatomic abnormality seen on imaging study is the actual cause of symptoms.)

Table 6-1   Estimated Hospital Charges for Back Pain Diagnostic Tests

CBC	$133
Urinalysis	$20-$25
ESR	$27-$33
Electrodiagnosis	$500-$1000
Whole body bone scan	$950
Lumbar spine x-ray	$133
SPECT scan	$1100
MRI lumbar spine noncontrast	$1415
MRI lumbar spine with contrast	$1579
MRI lumbar spine with and without contrast	$2221
CT lumbar diskography	$845
CT lumbar spine noncontrast	$845
CT lumbar spine with contrast	$958
CT lumbar spine with and without contrast	$1171
Injection studies under fluoroscopy	$1400

Physiologic Tests

Bone scan: *See* Nuclear scinitigraphy.

CBC: Complete blood count. This test is used to detect an anemia or leukocytosis from a suspected occult neoplasm or occult infection that could cause back pain such as a genitourinary infection or spinal abscess.

Electrodiagnostic tests: Often referred to as electromyography (EMG), electrodiagnostic testing, neurodiagnostic testing, and so forth. In contrast to imaging studies, electrodiagnosis is though to have rare false positive results. It has similar sensitivity to magnetic resonance imaging (MRI) or computed tomography (CT) and also detects peripheral nerve lesions (e.g., sciatic nerve tumor) and nonanatomic lesions (e.g., polyneuropathy) that are not found on spine MRI. The test, more properly a consultation, may include a number of different components including needle electromyography, nerve conduction studies, somatosensory evoked potentials, and motor evoked potentials. They are used to assess myelopathy, radiculopathy, generalized peripheral neuropathy, mononeuropathy, and myopathy. EMG can be useful in assessing radiculopathy in patients with symptoms greater than 4 weeks if the diagnosis is not obvious by physical exam.

When ordered, electrodiagnostic tests can but do not necessarily include all the following individual exams. It is not necessary to request each of the following exams, as this is decided by the electromyographer during the study.

Needle electromyography: Requires insertion of a needle into muscle to look for spontaneous activity and motor unit recruitment to assess acute and chronic nerve root dysfunction, myelopathy, and myopathy.

H-reflex: Measures sensory conductions through nerve roots; however, it is dependent on the integrity of the spinal reflex arc and therefore mostly assesses radiculopathy and neuropathy. It is generally used to assesses S1 radiculopathies because it is recording the tibial nerve response.

F-wave response: Used to assess proximal nerve segments by measuring proximal motor conduction through nerve roots, it is a muscle action potential resulting from supramaximal stimulus of a motor nerve that occurs after the muscle action potential. It can be, but is not necessarily prolonged in radiculopathy, motor neuron disease, Guillain-Barré syndrome, diabetic neuropathy, and some hereditary neuropathies.

Surface EMG: Assesses acute and chronic recruitment patterns during static or dynamic tests instead of needle insertion but is not indicated for assessment of low back pain.

Sensory evoked potential: Electrophysiologic examination of sensory function by tracing the afferent impulses produced by peripheral nerve stimulation through the plexus and root into the spinal cord, brainstem, and cerebrum. Sensory evoked potentials essentially are brain waves that occur in response to small shocks on a nerve. By averaging the response hundreds of times, the larger brain waves disappear and only the sensory response occurs on the screen. They are used to assess sensory neurons in peripheral and spinal cord pathways, especially in spinal stenosis and spinal cord myelopathy.

Nerve conduction studies: Induce and detect depolarization along the nerve axon by stimulating either a sensory, motor, or mixed nerve and recording the conduction velocity, amplitude, and latency of the response. These tests are used to evaluate nerve injury due to acute or chronic nerve root dysfunction and acute and chronic peripheral entrapment neuropathies that may mimic radiculopathies. Nerve conduction studies are usually normal in radiculopathy, therefore an abnormal test usually indicates another process other than nerve root dysfunction.

Example Requisition

A 33-year-old male with lower left back pain and parasthesias radiating into dorsal aspect of left foot for 6 weeks and new onset left foot drop. Rule out L5 radiculopathy.

The time frame of 6 weeks ensures that the EMG will be positive if there is nerve damage. The EMG is as sensitive as MRI and is less expensive as a first diagnostic test for radiculopathy. It picks up lesions away from the spine such as sciatica or peroneal nerve lesions.

Electromyography: *See* Electrodiagnostic tests.

Erythrocyte sedimentation rate (ESR): Blood test used as a marker of inflammation in many disease processes including infection, hematologic or neoplastic process, and collagen, renal, or endocrine diseases. Usually ordered in combination with plain films to rule out tumor or infection in patients with acute low back pain and prior history of cancer, recent infection, fever above 100°F, IV drug abuse, prolonged steroid use, low back pain worse with rest, and recent weight loss.

Nuclear scintigraphy (bone scan): A type of radionuclide imaging using IV injection of radioactive compounds (usually technetium-99m) that can adhere to metabolically active bone with areas of increased uptake recognized by gamma detectors. Increased uptake of radionuclide indicates increased bone blood flow and increased bone osteoblastic activity due to new bone formation, which can be indicative of, but not specific for, fracture, degenerative spine disease, metastasis, synovitis, infection, or neoplasm. A three-phase bone scan including blood flow, blood pool scans, and static scans 2 to 4 hours after injection can be used to evaluate localized bone or joint pain. Radiation exposure is similar to that from radiographs of lumbar spine. It is the study of choice in evaluation of skeletal and spinal metastasis. Although MRI can better detect some tumors such as myeloma, and MRI can define the anatomy better, scintigraphy allows a better global assessment of whether a bony tumor exists. Scintigraphy is contraindicated during pregnancy.

Example Requisition
A 67-year-old male with history of prostate cancer and previous wrist fracture, with more than 1 month duration of low back pain. Rule out spinal metastasis.

Serum protein electrophoresis: Blood test used to detect monoclonal patterns of serum proteins when multiple myeloma is suspected cause of back pain. The serum protein electrophoresis can detect myeloma when the plain x-rays and bone scans are negative.

Thermography: A noninvasive exam that involves measuring small temperature differences between both sides of the body and evaluating the patterns on infrared thermographic images of back and lower extremities. This test is not recommended to assess acute low back pain, as it does not precisely predict the presence of nerve root impingement and has been found to be abnormal in asymptomatic patients.

Urinalysis: Used to evaluate urine to detect if urinary tract infection or renal disease is a cause of back pain.

Case Study 6-1

A 57-year-old female has a 3-month history of low back pain radiating into the right lateral and medial lower leg (not improving with physical therapy) and abnormal electrodiagnostic testing performed at 6 weeks (showing normal nerve conduction studies of the right leg, increased spontaneous activity in the right L5 innervated muscles, and normal

F-wave response). She now complains of acute foot drop. An MRI without contrast was done at this time showing L4-L5 disk bulging with right L5 nerve root compression.

Anatomic Tests

Computed tomography: *See* MRI, CT, and CT myelography.

CT diskography: *See* Injection studies.

CT myelography: *See* MRI, CT, and CT myelography.

Facet joint blocks: *See* Injection studies.

Fluoroscopy: Used to determine the position during invasive radiologic procedures (i.e., myelography, diskography, and SI joint, facet joint, and nerve root injections). Flouroscopy can be used for evaluation of motion and to determine spinal stability. The main disadvantage is excessive radiation exposure. This test is ordered only in combination with other diagnostic exams, therefore there is no reason to order a separate requisition.

Injection Studies

These tests, usually done under fluoroscopy, are designed to detect actual pain generators by eliciting and/or relieving the patient's pain. These studies and therapeutic injections should only be obtained after consulting with a spine specialist. These tests have been regarded as more capable of finding the patient's actual pain generator, as imaging abnormalities can be seen in both symptomatic and asymptomatic individuals (see Chapter 24, Part III, for details).

CT diskography: Combination of CT and diskography that can show disk disease and herniation (see below).

Facet joint blocks: The facet joint suspected as a source of pain is injected with a corticosteroid and a local anesthetic as a diagnostic and/or therapeutic method to relieve pain caused from facet joint pathology.

Example Requisition

A 75-year-old male with L4-L5 facet degenerative joint disease and right-sided low back pain with extension and lateral sidebending. Perform diagnostic therapeutic L4-L5 facet joint injection and record pain changes.

The facet joint block may afford temporary pain relief while confirming the pain generator. Repeated positive facet blocks may lead to selective dorsal rhizotomy.

Provocative diskography: Involves the injection of a water-soluble imaging material directly into the nucleus pulposis of the disk in order to evaluate the disk damage and see if the disk is the actual pain generator. The examiner records the amount of dye accepted, the resistance during injection, the configuration created by the dye, and reproduction of patient's pain. A symptomatic degenerative disk will show dye distributed in an abnormal pattern reaching the outer margins of the annulus and occasionally the epidural space. Several studies show that abnormalities are found in asymptomatic individuals, but pain can only be elicited in symptomatic patients, therefore some examiners only consider it positive if similar pain results from the injection. Although some studies suggest that this is the best diagnostic test for symptomatic disk degeneration, the AHCPR clinical practice guidelines do not recommend diskography because interpretation is equivocal and complications can be avoided using less invasive techniques.

Example Requisition

A 65-year-old male with axial low back pain not relieved with L5-S1 facet joint injection and equivocal degenerative facet joint disease on MRI at L5-S1. Failed conservative treatment. Diskography to rule out diskogenic back pain.

Diskography is not indicated to merely prove the location of pain. Because of its invasive nature, it should be used only in preparation for a major intervention such as fusion.

Nerve root blocks: A diagnostic and/or therapeutic test that is used as an adjunct to imaging studies showing nerve root impingement by provoking and possibly palliating a patient's pain while injecting anesthetic and/or corticosteroid. This can be helpful to distinguish multilevel disease or indistinct nerve root impingement seen on imaging studies.

Example Requisition

A 50-year-old male with pain over right sacroiliac joint with palpation reproduced with FABERE test. Perform right sacroiliac (SI) joint injection for diagnostic and therapeutic purposes. Record pain relief.

It is unclear whether sacroiliac joint blocks can cause permanent pain relief, but they can help get therapy started and can isolate the pain generator, avoiding other diagnostic and treatment interventions.

Sacroiliac (SI) joint blocks: An injection with anesthetic and corticosteroid into the sacroiliac joint that is diagnostic and/or therapeutic, as joint changes can be a substantial source of pain. Some studies suggest that this is the gold standard for diagnosis of SI joint-generated pain.

Example Requisition

A 50-year-old male with pain over right sacroiliac joint with palpation reproduced with FABERE test. Perform right SI joint injection.

Spondylolysis blocks: An injection of the facet joint adjacent to the area of pseudoarthrosis in the pars defect caused by spondylolysis and spondylolisthesis (causing possible foraminal stenosis and irritation of the exiting nerve root). It is thought that injection of the adjacent facet joint with anesthetic (after contrast material has extended into the pars defect) can relieve pain. However, its diagnostic value is questionable, because the anesthetic also affects surrounding structures such as facet joints and nerve roots.

Example Requisition
A 30-year-old male with known chronic L5 spondylolysis and foraminal stenosis per MRI with L5 radicular pain. Perform spondylolysis block at L5 with anesthetic and steroid for diagnostic and therapeutic purposes.

Spondylolysis and spondylolisthesis occur so commonly that they cannot be presumed to be the cause of the pain. When there is a question, an injection can clarify the pain generator.

Case Study 6-2

An 18-year-old male former gymnast presents with dull aching low back and buttock pain after a motor vehicle accident. Anterior to posterior (AP) and lateral x-rays were normal. A bone scan showed equivocal findings of a spondylolytic lesion. A SPECT (single photon emission computed tomography) scan was recommended; it showed increased radioisotope uptake in the region of the right pars interacularis.

MRI, CT, and CT Myelography

In the presence of red flags suggesting cauda equina syndrome or progressive motor weakness, immediate use of any of these tests is indicated, however, MRI is the gold standard in imaging lumbar spine and the study of choice to evaluate radicular pain. MRI is noninvasive and does not expose the patient to ionizing radiation.

Magnetic resonance imaging (MRI) without contrast: This is a noninvasive method to image lumbar spine using pulse sequence parameters in combination with multiplanar imaging capabilities. By producing computer-generated axial and sagittal cross-sectional images of the body, this study can show details of the intervertebral disk, spinal nerves, dural sac, and surrounding structures. MRI is the study of choice for neoplasm and infection. MRI is insensitive for demonstrating cortical bone or osteophytes. Contraindications to MRI include presence of internal metallic objects, pacemaker, surgical clip, metal objects/fragments in eyes, and claustrophobia. Figures 6-1 and 6-2 show an MRI film.

Example Requisition

A 65-year-old male with chronic low back pain and parasthesias radiating into lateral foot and absent Achilles' reflex. Rule out left S1 root lesion.

The MRI is the standard for evaluating the presence of disk herniation, spinal stenosis, and tumor but is not perfect in any of these.

MRI with contrast: MRI enhanced with gadolinium-DPTA. It does not provide further diagnosis of symptomatic disk herniation. However, contrast is indicated in the face of previous back surgery to distinguish scar tissue from disk herniation. Contrast is also appropriate if a noncontrast MRI is negative in suspected infection or extramedullary or intramedullary intradural neoplasm.

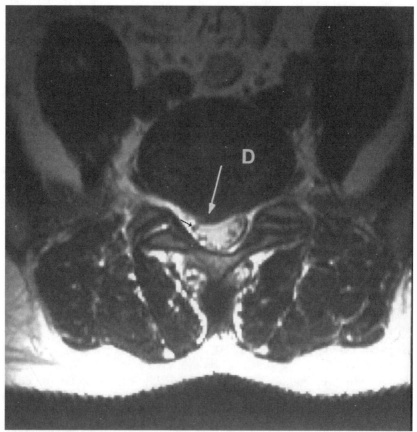

Figure 6-1   MRI axial view: herniated disk. Axial T_2-weighted lumbosacral spine magnetic resonance scan demonstrates a large herniated disk (white arrow) extending to the right side of the spinal canal at the L5/S1 level compressing the right S1 nerve root (black arrow); D = L5/S1 intervertebral disk. (Courtesy of Douglas Quint, MD, Ann Arbor, Michigan.)

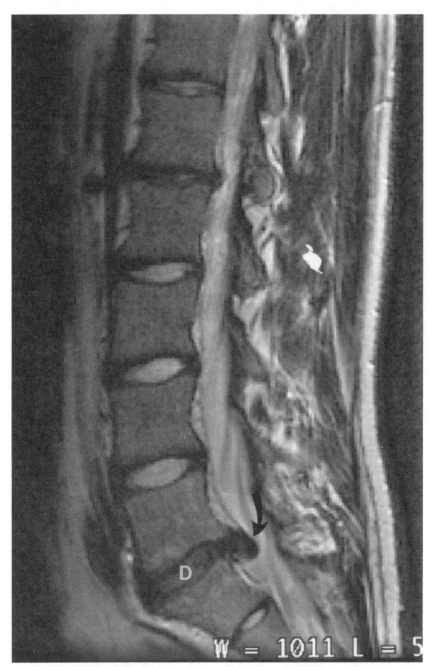

Figure 6-2 MRI sagittal view: herniated disk (black arrow). D = degenerated intervertebral disk. (Courtesy of Douglas Quint, MD, Ann Arbor, Michigan.)

Example Requisition

A 65-year-old male with history of L4-L5 posterior fusion and low back pain radiating into lateral foot described as numbness and burning and absent Achilles' reflex. Evaluate for S1 root lesion secondary to scar tissue versus recurrent disk material.

On plain MRI, it is sometimes difficult to differentiate between scar and disk, but because scar is vascular, the contrast MRI can help.

Computed tomography: Also known as CT, this test creates computer-generated axial cross-sectional images of the body by using multiple x-ray beams projected at different levels and angles. Demonstrates bone and soft tissue of lumbar spine and is superior to MRI for detecting bony abnormalities such as central and lateral facet joint arthrosis, calcifications, osteophytes, fractures, bone destruction secondary to tumor or infection.

Example Requisition

A 70-year-old male with low back pain and nonspecific facet joint changes per MRI. Characterize osseous abnormalities of lumbar facet joints.

CT better demonstrates the anatomy of bony structures. Here, the clinician must consider whether CT findings will change treatment plans.

Myelography and CT myelography: Myelography creates images of the contents and borders of the dural sac using plain x-rays taken after a non-ionic water-soluble contrast media is injected into the spinal canal through a lumbar puncture needle (Figure 6-3). Myelography permits direct identification of spinal stenosis and indirect identification of abnormalities such as herniated disks, compression of nerve roots, and other soft tissue lesions. It is used for lumbar spinal functional assessment such as effects of axial loading, flexion, extension, and lateral bending, especially in lateral stenosis.

Myelography is limited, as images can only be obtained in the frontal and lateral views (i.e., no axial imaging) and does not *directly* visualize most pathologic processes. It is also an invasive test, as placement of a spinal needle can cause bleeding, infection, and trauma to nerve roots; performing a lumbar puncture below the level of a spinal cord compression can exacerbate patient symptoms; injection of contrast material can cause arachnoiditis; patients may be allergic to the iodinated contrast material; patients can have post-myelogram/LP headaches; and there is the risk of radiation exposure.

Myelography is almost always followed (within several hours) by CT scanning, which is performed in the axial plane and allows better delineation of soft tissue and osseous abnormalities including direct visualization of many pathologic processes (Figure 6-4). The combination of CT with myelography creates axial cross-sectional images of the spine that enhance the difference between the dural sac and surrounding structures. Although it surpasses the ability of MRI to assess spinal stenosis because it allows

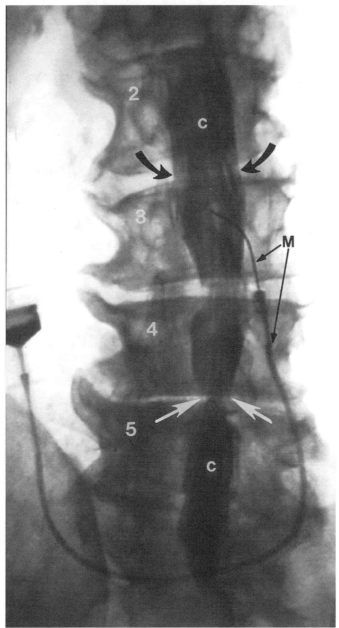

Figure 6-3   Spinal stenosis: myelography. Frontal lumbar myelogram demonstrates extradural narrowing at the L4/5 level (*white arrows*) resulting in spinal stenosis. The L2/3 level (*curved black arrows*) demonstrates no spinal stenosis. M = myelographic needle and tubing; 2 = L2 level; 3 = L3 level; 4 = L4 level; 5 = L5 level; c = contrast material in the thecal sac. (Courtesy of Douglas Quint, MD, Ann Arbor, Michigan)

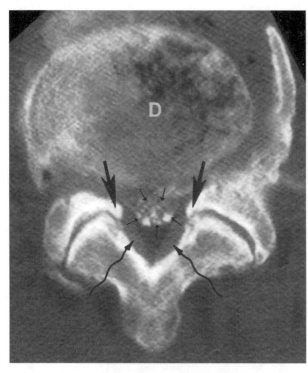

Figure 6-4 Spinal stenosis: post-myelogram CT. Axial CT scan obtained after injection of subarachnoid contrast for a myelogram demonstrates central spinal stenosis resulting in a small contrast-filled thecal sac (*small straight arrows*); D = degenerated intervertebral disk; *large straight arrows* = hypertrophic facet joint spurs; *wavy arrows* = thickened ligamentum flavum. (Courtesy of -Douglas Quint, MD, Ann Arbor, Michigan)

multiplanar views, it is rarely the first study ordered to evaluate low back pain. Because both myelography and CT myelography are invasive, they are only used as an alternative to MRI and CT when there are contraindications to MRI or CT and sometimes for perioperative planning. Figures 6-3 and 6-4 illustrate a myelo-CT study.

Example Requisition
A 70-year-old male with history of L4-L5 posterior spinal fusion with right ankle dorsiflexion weakness and parasthesias of bilateral lateral legs. Rule out spinal stenosis.

In this case, CT myelopathy can identify impingement of the nerve roots more precisely than MRI. If there is suspicion of hypermobility, then the myelogram portion could be performed in flexion and extension—something that other tests cannot do.

Nerve root blocks: *See* Injection studies.

Provocative diskography: *See* Injection studies.

Radiography: An imaging modality that uses an x-ray beam directed through the back to a sensitized plate where part of the beam is absorbed by the body, producing a shadow on the plate.

AP and lateral views evaluate lumbar alignment, vertebral body and disk space size, bone density and architecture, and gross evaluation of soft tissue structures. Although tissue differentiation is limited, x-ray is relatively inexpensive, and this is the best initial screening to rule out fractures and visualize hardware after surgery. Plain x-rays are not recommended for routine evaluation of low back pain within the first month of symptoms unless there is a red flag warning sign as described below:

Radiographs are recommended for ruling out fractures in patients with low back pain and recent significant trauma (at any age), recent mild trauma (age above 50 years), history of prolonged steroid use, osteoporosis, or in any patient above 70 years of age. In young persons, spondylolisthesis is almost always detected on lateral film. Given the increased radiation to the gonads, oblique films should not be ordered for suspected spondylolisthesis unless the lateral film is negative.

Plain x-rays in combination with CBC and ESR can assist in detecting infection or tumor when the following red flags are present: fever, IV drug abuse, unexplained weight loss, prolonged steroid use, or low back pain worse with rest. Figure 6-5 shows a plain x-ray (lateral view).

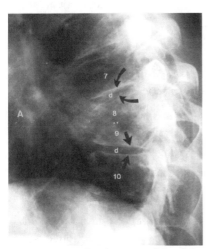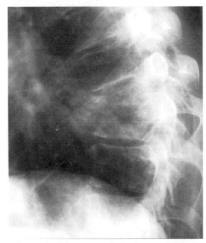

Figure 6-5   Diskitis/osteomyelitis: plain x-ray. Lateral plain x-ray of the lower thoracic spine demonstrates absence of the inferior T8 and superior T9 end plates consistent with diskitis of the T8/9 intervertebral disk with spread to the contiguous TS and T9 vertebra (osteomyelitis). Note the normal superior T8 end plate and inferior T7 end plate (*curved arrows*) and the normal inferior T9 end plate and superior T1O end plate (*straight arrows*). Also note the normal disk space between the T7 and T8 vertebral bodies (d) and also between the T9 and TI 0 vertebral bodies (d) and the absence of such a space at the T8-T9 level (*). A limitation of plain radiographs is that one cannot detect spread of infection to the spinal canal. (Courtesy of Douglas Quint, MD, Ann Arbor, Michigan.)

In presence of red flag warning signs with normal x-rays, use of other imaging studies are indicated such as bone scan, MRI, or CT.

Oblique films, although not routine, are the best views for facet pathology and can sometimes show facet joint degenerative disease, spondylolysis, or tumor. Oblique views double a patient's x-ray exposure, therefore unless the physician is ruling out spondylolisthesis that has not been detected with a lateral film, with symptoms lasting more than 3 months, there is no need to obtain these films.

Sacroiliac views are special views that can detect sacroiliitis before it is reliably seen on AP and lateral views.

Functional x-ray views during spinal flexion and extension are thought to measure spine motion and lumbar instability; however, insufficient data exists to establish efficacy.

Example Requisition

A 76-year-old female with history of osteoporosis, history of long-term steroid use for asthma, and new onset lumbar back pain after recent fall landing on low back. Rule out fracture. Plain x-rays will pick up any significant compression fracture.

Reverse straight leg raise test: While prone, with the knee bent at 90 degrees, the patient's foot is lifted up, causing stretching of the anterior thigh. This test detects about 50% of disk herniations found on higher lumbar roots (L1, L2, L3, and L4).

SPECT: Single Photon Emission Computed Tomography (SPECT) uses scintigraphy and CT to evaluate overlapping structures in healing spondylotic defects. It is helpful in diagnosing acute traumatic spondylosis, pars stress fracture, acute or old fractures.

Example Requisition

A 19-year-old female gymnast with acute onset of dull aching low back pain and pain with palpation of L4 spinous process. Negative radiographs. Bone scan with SPECT to rule out spondylolisthesis.

Often, plain bone scans are negative for spondlolisthesis. The SPECT image should be ordered. Activity on the scan documents a lesion but does not predict pain or instability.

Sacroiliac joint blocks: *See* Injection studies.

Spondylolysis blocks: *See* Injection studies.

Ultrasound: Also known as sonography, ultrasound is the delineation of anatomical structures by measuring the reflection of ultrasonic waves directed into the underlying tissue. It can be used to evaluate soft tissue masses and characterize them as cystic or solid. It cannot evaluate internal bony structures because ultrasound waves are deflected by bone. There are currently no practical uses for ultrasound in low back pain.

Specific Physical Exam Tests and Signs

FABERE test: The Flexion, ABduction, External Rotation, Extension (FABERE) test, also known as Patrick test, can detect pathology in the hip and/or sacroiliac joint. The patient lies supine on the table, and the knee of the involved leg is placed on the opposite knee. Then the examiner passively flexes, externally rotates, and abducts the hip. Pain produced in the groin is usually indicative of intrinsic hip pathology or surrounding hip musculature. Pain reproduced in the lateral low back with the hip further placed in this position of external rotation, flexion, and abduction is more indicative of sacroiliac joint pathology. Figure 6-6 shows the FABERE test.

Palpation: The application of variable manual pressure through the surface of the body for the purposes of determining the shape, size, consistency, position, mobility, and health of the tissues beneath. Specifically, the examiner can check for tender or trigger points, local tenderness with percussion, or muscle spasm.

Somatic dysfunction: Impaired or altered function of related components of the somatic (body framework) system; skeletal including arthroidal and myofascial structures; and related vascular, lymphatic, and neural elements. The three diagnostic criteria quantifying somatic dysfunction are asymmetry, range of motion abnormality, and tissue texture abnormality. These three criteria are also known as ART.

Asymmetry: Usually measured by observation and palpation, it is absence of symmetry of position or motion; for example, unequal shoulder heights, iliac crest heights, or thoracic cage contour.

Range of motion (ROM) abnormality: Alteration of range of motion of a joint determined by observation, palpation, and active and passive movement through a joint's range. ROM should be assessed for lumbar flexion, extension, lateral sidebending, and rotation. Normal values for lumbar motion include flexion, 40 degrees; extension, 15 degrees; lateral bending, 30 degrees; lateral rotation, 40 degrees to each side. It can be described as either restricted (decreased range or hypomobility) or having increased mobility.

Tissue texture abnormality: Also known as TTA. Any palpable change in tissues from skin to periarticular structures that represents any combination of the following signs: vasodilation, edema, flaccidity, contraction, contracture, fibrosis; and the following symptoms: itching, pain, tenderness, and parasthesias. Types of TTAs include: bogginess, thickening, stringiness, ropiness, firmness, increased/decreased temperature, or increased/decreased moisture.

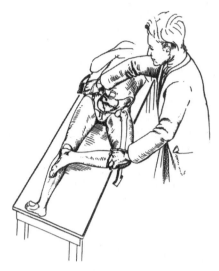

Figure 6-6   FABERE test.

Straight leg raise: This test, also known as Lasègue's test, is designed to reproduce back and leg pain to determine its cause. With the patient lying supine, the examiner lifts the patient's extended leg off the table. It is positive for radicular pain when symptoms are reproduced down the same leg at an angle between 35 and 70 degrees. However, it can also indicate hamstring tightness when pain is described as a "stretch" and only felt in posterior thigh. Figure 6-7 illustrates a straight leg raise test.

   Crossed straight leg raise: Same as above, except examiner lifts asymptomatic leg. The test indicates radicular pain if there is reproduction of pain down the symptomatic leg with straight leg raising of contralateral leg.

Tender point: A localized area of muscle that with palpation reveals only local discomfort without referral of pain. Needling of a tender point never causes a twitch response (transient reaction of a taut band of muscle fibers), whereas it can cause this response with a trigger point.

Trigger point: A localized area (about 1 cm) of muscle usually located in the belly of a taut muscle that with flat palpation of the relaxed muscle and sustained pressure (10 seconds) or needle injection causes referred pain. There may or may not be a palpable nodule or taut band at this site.

Visual analog scales: A scale allowing the patient to quantify their pain by marking a line that on one end signifies no pain and the other end signifies severe pain.

Waddell's sign: Physical signs that indicate a nonorganic source of low back pain.

1. Nonanatomic weakness or sensory loss.
2. Overreaction: exaggerated pain response to a nonpainful stimulus.

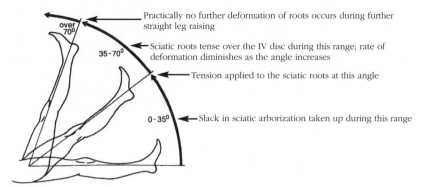

Practically no further deformation of roots occurs during further straight leg raising

over 70°

35-70° Sciatic roots tense over the IV disc during this range; rate of deformation diminishes as the angle increases

Tension applied to the sciatic roots at this angle

0-35° Slack in sciatic arborization taken up during this range

Figure 6-7   Straight leg raise test for nerve root tension.

3. Stimulation: low back pain with axial loading or simulated rotation of the spine.
4. Nonanatomic or superficial tenderness such as with skin rolling.
5. Distraction: inconsistent physical findings with distracting motions.

If three of the above signs are positive, then a nonorganic basis for the patient's low back pain is more likely (see Table 8-5 in Chapter 8).

◼   ◼   ◼

BIBLIOGRAPHY

Bigos S, Bowyer O, Braen G, et al. Acute Low Back Problems in Adults. Clinical Practice Guideline No. 14. AHCPR Publication No. 95-0642. Rockville, MD: Agency for Health Care Policy and Research, Public Health Service, U.S. Department of Health and Human Services; December 1994.

Boos N, Hodler J. What help and what confusion can imaging provide. Bailliere's Clin Rheumatol. 1998;12(1):115-39.

Braddom RL. Physical Medicine and Rehabilitation, 2nd ed. Philadelphia: WB Saunders; 2000.

Herkowitz HN, Garfin SR, Balderston et al. The Spine, 4th ed. Philadelphia: W.B. Saunders; 1999.

Hoppenfeld S. Physical Examination of the Spine & Extremities. Norwalk, CT: Appleton-Century-Crofts; 1976.

Kent DL, Haynor DR, Longstreth WT, Larson EB. The clinical efficacy of magnetic resonance imaging in neuroimaging. Ann Intern Med. 1994;120:856-71.

Maldjian C, Mesgarzadeh TJ. Diagnostic and Therapeutic Features of Facet and Sacroiliac Joint Injection. Radiol Clin North Am. 1998;36:497-508.

Project on Osteopathic Principles Education. Glossary of Osteopathic Terminology. Chevy Chase, MD:The American Association of Osteopathic Colleges of America; 1982.

Slipman CW, Sterenfeld EB, Chou LH, Herzog R, Vresilovic E. The predictive value of provocative sacroiliac joint stress maneuvers in the diagnosis of sacroiliac joint syndrome. Arch Phys Med Rehabil. 1998;79:288-92.

Tan JC. Practical Manual of Physical Medicine and Rehabilitation. St. Louis: Mosby; 1998.

Tehranzadeh J. Discography 2000. Radiol Clin North Am. 1998;36:463-95.

SECTION II

ACUTE BACK PAIN

7

■　■　■

Acute Back Pain:
A Management Paradigm

Miles Colwell, MD

his chapter provides an overview for the evaluation and treatment of acute back pain (Figure 7-1). Acute low back pain is defined as posterior trunk pain below the level of the rib cage of less than 6 weeks duration. It is most often accompanied by achiness into the sacral region, buttock, and lower extremities. Most people do not even seek medical care for episodes of acute back pain because such episodes are often very brief. For those that do seek care from primary care physicians, 75-90% improve within 1 month (1,2). Based on symptoms, there are two main groups of acute low back pain: nonradiating and radiating. Radiating back pain is pain that radiates to below the knee and is frequently but not always the result of disk herniation. Low lumbar disk herniations are the most common cause, with the associated pain thus tending to radiate below the knee, but radiating back pain can also be secondary to foraminal stenosis, myofascial trigger point, muscle strain, and biomechanical dysfunctions. Causes such as facet arthropathy, sacroiliac dysfunction, or spondylolisthesis produce predominantly axial back pain with radiation into the buttock and thigh but rarely below the knee. The lifetime prevalence of herniated disks is 1-3% (3) and approximately half of patients with acute radiating low back pain (LBP) are better within 6 weeks (4,5). Furthermore, a large percentage of disk herniation will respond to nonsurgical intervention. With this knowledge, except in the cases of significant neurologic compromise, it is appropriate to provide conservative treatment.

Evaluation and Treatment

The initial office evaluation should include a focused history and examination to screen for "red flags" of serious disease or potentially serious

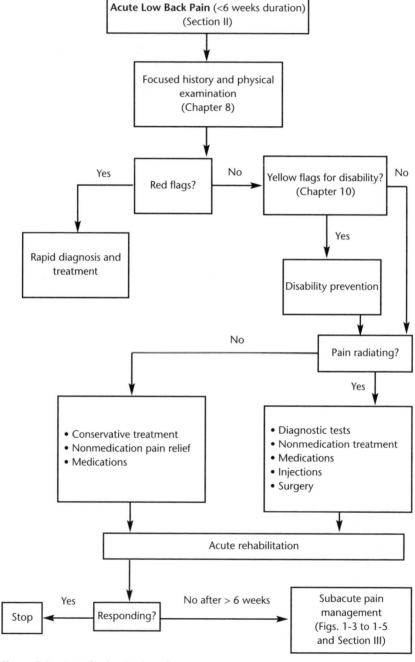

Figure 7-1   Acute back pain algorithm.

neurologic compromise and for "yellow flags" of high risk for chronicity or disability (see Chapters 8 to 10). The presence of red flags warrants further workup, diagnostics, and referrals as appropriate for rapid diagnosis and treatment of the underlying disease. Emergent imaging studies are indicated in the following clinical situations:

1. Suspicion of cauda equina syndrome: progressive weakness, new bowel or bladder dysfunction, or saddle anesthesia.
2. Suspicion of neoplastic spread.
3. Suspicion of neoplastic spread to the spine or spinal canal (e.g., suspected metastatic disease in the setting of a known malignancy).
4. Clinical suspicion of a spinal infection such as diskitis, osteomyelitis, or abscess in a patient at risk to develop such a process (e.g., immunocompromised patient).
5. Suspected noninfectious spinal inflammatory process (e.g., spondyloarthropathy).
6. The patient has acute trauma involving the spine. In these clinical situations, aggressive timely evaluation of the spine is necessary.

Pain inhibition, mild weakness, reflex asymmetry, and mild dermatomal sensory changes are not contraindications for conservative management but should be followed closely.

Ordering diagnostic tests for nonradiating acute low back pain has low yield and adds little to the initial treatment of minimizing rest, quick return to activity, and pain relief. Pharmacologic and nonmedication techniques such as icing and gradual stretching and patient reassurance are recommended (see Chapter 11). Pain radiating below the knee does not immediately need referral or diagnostics unless accompanied by clinical signs of greater than mild neurologic compromise, suspicion of active spondylolithesis, fracture, or red flags for infection, aneurysm, or tumor. If symptoms persist at 2 to 3 weeks without work disability, refer for physical therapy. At 2 to 3 weeks duration, if improvement is limited, work disability is present, and psychosocial risks are identified, referral to a specialist should be considered. In patients *without* yellow flags (e.g., psychosocial risks), on the other hand, referral to a specialist is necessary only after 4 to 6 weeks of treatment with no improvement. If progress is limited but no red or yellow flags are present, initiate acute rehabilitation. In the presence of radiating pain, injection therapy may need to be considered as an adjunct to comprehensive treatment, which includes pharmacotherapy and exercise (see Chapter 12, 13).

Resolution of Acute Back Pain

In the majority of cases, there is resolution of acute back pain by 6 weeks regardless of treatment. In cases that require limited physical therapy, the patient will usually be required to perform basic stretches and back-strengthening exercises. The patient should be encouraged to continue these on a regular basis. One rehabilitation tenet to share with all patients is to take every joint through its range of motion once a day; in other words, to perform the basic stretches *at least* several times a week (preferably every day). No data exist as to how long after symptom resolution people actually perform their home exercise program. For the generally active person, this may not be needed.

At 6 weeks, if progress is insufficient, proceed with subacute evaluation and management as outlined in the appropriate algorithms in Chapter 1 and in the chapters in Section III.

■   ■   ■

REFERENCES

1. **Coste J, Delecoeuillerie G, Cohen de Lara A, Le Parc JM, Paolaggi JB.** Clinical course and prognostic factors in acute low back pain: an inception cohort study in primary care practice. BMJ. 1994;308:577-80.

2. **Deyo RA, Phillips WR.** Low back pain. A primary care challenge. Spine. 1996;21:2826-32.

3. **Andersson GB.** The epidemiology of spinal disorders. In: Frymoyer JW, Ducker TB, et al., eds. The Adult Spine: Principles and Practice, 2nd ed. Philadelphia: Lippincott-Raven; 1997:93-141.

4. **Bush K, Cowan N, Katz D, Gishen P.** The natural history of sciatica associated with disc pathology: a prospective study with clinical and independent radiologic follow-up. Spine. 1992;17:1205-12.

5. **Saal JA, Saal JS, Herzog R.** The natural history of lumbar intervertebral disk extrusions treated nonoperatively. Spine. 1990;15:683-6.

8

■　■　■

Physical Examination
for Acute Back Pain

Ann Laidlaw, MD

A thorough yet focused physical examination can assist in the diagnosis of acute low back pain (i.e., the specific cause of the pain) and in selecting the appropriate treatment. Although a definitive diagnosis cannot be made in up to 85% of these patients, and no single test has a high degree of accuracy (1), the physical examination is a highly useful diagnostic tool, providing answers to these basic questions:

1. Is the pain reproduced in a specific anatomic structure?
2. Is there a serious systemic disorder?
3. Is there a neurologic deficit?
4. What is the extent and appropriateness of the patient's pain behavior?

General

Gait, Posture, and Tenderness

Observe the patient's gait. Almost all patients with acute low back pain will have a slow, deliberate gait, reduced range of motion, and a flattened lumbar lordosis. A Trendelenberg gait pattern indicates weakness of the gluteus medius and possible L5 nerve root involvement. Assess posture and note any deformities, scoliosis, and loss of the normal spinal curvatures (i.e., flattened lumbar lordosis or muscle asymmetry). Palpate the spine and paraspinal muscles for areas of local tenderness and muscle spasm or hypertonicity. Percussion tenderness of the spinous processes suggests involvement of the vertebral body, such as that seen in infection (i.e., vertebral osteomyelitis) or tumor. Patients with midline diskogenic pain, on the other hand, often have associated paraspinal muscle spasm but not percussion tenderness.

Mobility

Spinal range of motion testing may reproduce typical pain symptoms, help differentiate between mechanical and systemic disorders, and uncover functional magnification of symptoms. Mobility testing includes extension, forward flexion, lateral side bending, and rotation. When testing extension, the examiner should ensure that the patient's hips and knees are stabilized or pelvis blocked against the exam table, so that the extension moment is truly from the spine. In the acute situation, exact measurement is time-consuming and has limited diagnostic value (2). Instead, measure grossly; for example, fingertips are at knee level with forward flexion, trochanteric or knee level with standing sidebending.

Record production of typical pain symptoms. Increased pain with forward flexion suggests a diskogenic source of pain or a problem in the anterior column of the spine such as a compression fracture. Increased pain with extension suggests a pain source in the posterior elements of the spine (i.e., facet mediated or foraminal stenosis). Pain on extension, especially with rotation, suggests that the facets or less commonly a spondylolysis or spinous process are involved. Axial pain often suggests ligament tear. *Rotation* is performed while the examiner stabilizes the pelvis. If functional magnification is suspected, the patient should hold his or her arms at the sides while the examiner rotates the torso as a unit by rotating the pelvis. Because the shoulders and pelvis are in the same rotating plane, movement occurs through the hips and not the spine. A positive response of back pain indicates a psychogenic pain response per Waddell's signs. *Pattern of movement* may also be revealing. In patients with diskogenic pain, for example, forward flexion of the upper body may be performed at the hips, as if the patient were bending forward and around an obstacle in front of him or her. When returning from a forward flexed position, patients with mechanical back pain may fix the lumbar spine, flex the knees, and straighten through the hips to reduce movement in a painful segment.

The examination should include maneuvers to seek disorders that are not in the spine but can mimic spinal pain. These include hip range of motion in rotation to look for hip joint mobility and palpation of the greater trochanter to look for trochanteric bursitis.

Neuromuscular Testing

The neuromuscular examination includes testing of reflexes, muscle strength, sensation, and dural tension signs. A rapid screening examination emphasizes L5 and S1 reflexes, strength of ankle dorsiflexison, great toe extension, unipedal weight bearing heel raise, and sensory pin prick exam at the medial heel, dorsal foot, and lateral heel.

Reflexes

Muscle stretch reflexes are assessed for presence, absence, and symmetry. Minor asymmetry may be due to poor relaxation or variable percussion force with the reflex hammer. To ensure equivalent percussion"blows," the examiner may place a finger over the tendon to be tested and percuss through the monitoring finger briskly with the reflex hammer. Distracting the patient's focus may eliminate reflex asymmetry secondary to poor relaxation. Have them read a sign on the wall or isometrically attempt to pull their locked hands apart as you simultaneously tap the tendon. A valid test should show marked asymmetry with repeated testing. Many abnormalities may result in reflex changes. Remember to inquire about a history of reflex loss from previous herniated disk, diskectomy, nerve injury, or peripheral neuropathy. Reflexes may be graded as absent to brisk (Table 8-1).

Pathologic reflexes indicate an upper motor neuron lesion. Testing for Babinski's sign (plantar response) and clonus should be included in the routine examination of the back. In the lower extremities, the patellar reflex is L3/L4 innervation, the internal hamstring reflex is L5/S1, and the Achilles' reflex is S1/S2. The internal (medial) hamstring reflex is performed with the seated patient's knee bent to 90 degrees. Palpate the medial hamstring tendon just behind the knee with several fingers and then briskly percuss those fingers to initiate the reflex. Hamstring contraction is palpated by the fingers, and knee flexion may be observed. When prone, monitor the proximal hamstring tendon with several fingers just distal to the ischial tuberosity, place tension, and percuss as above. In the presence of complaints of bowel or bladder dysfunction, report of numbness or pain of the perianal region or perineum, the examiner should check anal wink reflex, sensation, and rectal sphincter tone. The anal wink reflex is S2-S4. Lightly scratching just lateral to the anus normally causes the sphincter to visibly tighten (wink).

Table 8-1   Reflex Grading

0	No response (note in record if you use reinforcement)
1 to 1+	Low normal (note in record if you use reinforcement)
2 to 2+	Average/normal
3 to 3+	Brisker than average but not necessarily abnormal
4 to 4+	Very brisk, often abnormal/pathologic, upper motor neuron disease, check for ankle clonus and movement of toes to plantar stimulation

Republished with permission from Cole AJ, Herring SA, eds. The Low Back Pain Handbook—A Practical Guide for the Primary Care Clinician. Hanley & Belfus: Philadelphia; 2002.

Strength Examination

There are many instructional texts describing manual muscle testing (2). The strength of each muscle is graded and recorded. The most commonly used scale is listed in Table 8-2.

The strength examination should overcome the strength of each screened muscle. Determination of a radiculopathy is more certain when two muscles supplied from different peripheral nerves, but the same root and corresponding reflex, are all abnormal. Repetitive strength testing improves the finding of weakness. For example, performing 10 unipedal heel raises is the way to test the ankle plantar flexors in a suspected S1 radiculopathy. Table 8-3 represents a sample strength examination with the corresponding myotomal innervation.

Table 8-2   Muscle Strength Grading

0	No movement
1	Palpable or visible contraction without joint motion
2	Full range of motion (ROM) with gravity eliminated
3	Full ROM against gravity
4	Full ROM against gravity and moderate resistance
5	Normal; full ROM against full resistance

Republished with permission from Cole AJ, Herring SA, eds. The Low Back Pain Handbook—A Practical Guide for the Primary Care Clinician. Hanley & Belfus: Philadelphia; 2002.

Table 8-3   Muscle Testing and Innervation

Position	Movement Tested	Innervation					
		L2	*L3*	*L4*	*L5*	*S1*	*S2-S4*
Seated	Hip flexion	X	X	X			
	Hip adduction	X	X				
	Knee extension	X	X	X			
	Ankle dorsiflexion			X	X		
	Great toe extension				X		
Standing on one leg	Ankle plantarflexion					X	
Side-lying	Hip abduction				X	X	
	Ankle evertors				X	X	
Prone	Hip extension				X	X	
	Knee flexion				X	X	
Rectal	Anal sphincter						X

Republished with permission from Cole AJ, Herring SA, eds. The Low Back Pain Handbook—A Practical Guide for the Primary Care Clinician. Hanley & Belfus: Philadelphia; 2002.

Sensory Examination

Patients distinguish differences in pinprick more accurately than differences in touch or temperature. Comparing pinprick sensitivity from side to side improves the sensitivity of the test. Only the most severe radiculopathy will prevent the patient from distinguishing sharp from dull. Additionally, sensory impairment from nerve root compression is most frequent in the distal extremes of the dermatomes (1). A rapid screening sensory examination for the L1 through S2 dermatomes as defined by the American Spinal Injury Association is presented in Table 8-4 (3).

Dural Tension Signs

When the normally mobile nerve root cannot move (e.g., due to disk herniation), pain results from stretching the nerve. Straight leg raising is useful for testing the lower lumbar nerve roots (L5, S1), where the majority of disk herniations occur. Most of the tension in the sciatic nerve roots (L5-S1) occurs when the leg is raised between 30 degrees and 70 degrees; a positive test reproduces the pain radiation below the knee. Straight leg raise is a sensitive test (72-97%) but nonspecific. Simultaneously adding ankle dorsiflexion and/or neck flexion may increase the sensitivity of the test. Crossed straight leg raise is positive when elevation of the contralateral aymptomatic leg elicits pain in the symptomatic leg. It is less sensitive but highly specific (85-100%) (4). Seated versus supine straight leg raising is helpful to confirm its presence. A significant difference between the two techniques should raise the examiners suspicion of psychological overlay.

Reverse straight leg raise (femoral stretch test L2, 3, 4) tests for tension of higher lumbar roots. It is performed with the patient prone while passively flexing the knee. Hip extension may add to its sensitivity. Neuropathic pain reproduced in the anterior thigh is a positive test.

Table 8-4   Lumbar Root Sensory Dermatomes

L1	Mid-anterior groin
L2	Mid-anterior thigh
L3	Medial femoral condyle
L4	Medial malleolus
L5	Dorsal foot at the third metatarsal phalangeal joint
S1	Lateral heel
S2	Popliteal fossa

From the American Spinal Injury Association. International Standards for Neurological Classification of Spinal Cord Injury. Chicago: American Spinal Injury Association; Revised 2000.American Spinal Injury Association. International Standards for Neurological Classification of Spinal Cord Injury. Chicago: American Spinal Injury Association; Revised 2000.

Common Sites of Referred Pain

Common sites of pain referred to the back include the hip and sacroiliac joints, as well as intra-abdominal, retroperitoneal, and vascular sources. The complete examination of back pain should include palpation of the abdomen, costovertebral angles, and peripheral pulses (2). Rectal examination is useful to gauge rectal tone and sensation, served by the lower sacral roots S2 to S4. It may also reveal an intrapelvic mass.

Pain Behavior

The examination includes evaluating for Gordon Waddell's five areas of non-organic pain (5). Presence of three or more of these signs suggests a psychogenic component to the patient's pain behavior (1). The Waddell signs are summarized in Table 8-5.

Presence of these signs does not mean that the patient is faking, just that there is likely a psychogenic component. This may be fear of movement, fear of pain, attempting to make sure they show the examiner they have pain, and acting out for secondary gain. The positive presence of Waddell's signs is a "yellow flag" that the patient is at risk for becoming chronically

---

Table 8-5   Waddell's Signs

1. *Overreaction* during the examination.
2. *Simulation* (pain reported with sham maneuvers). Positive when pain is reported with gentle axial compression over the head or with rotation of the pelvis and shoulder in the same plane so that no true spinal rotation occurs.
3. *Distraction* (less pain when attention is diverted). Test straight leg raising while the patient is seated on the pretense of performing a Babinski reflex or inspecting the feet. If there is no increase in pain behavior during this distracted maneuver, but a formalized straight leg raise test done while lying causes radiating pain, this non-physiologic response is a Waddell sign. As an added confirmation, when there is leg pain on the formal lying straight leg raise test, we sometimes plantarflex the foot when the limb is still raised, asking if there is an increase in pain, and then dorsiflex the leg, which in a patient with radiculopathy may indeed worsen symptoms. Patients who complain of pain increase on plantar flexion are likely not reporting on an organic source of pain.
4. *Nonanatomic* weakness or sensory loss. Positive when there is "ratchety" giveway on strength testing, nondermatomal sensory loss, or the entire extremity is weak or numb.
5. *Tenderness* (excess or widespread reaction). Reports of tenderness to superficial light touch or in non anatomic patterns. Skin rolling causes horrible pain. Mark areas of tenderness and examine later for reproducibility.

---

disabled. The presence of multiple Waddell signs during the exam may suggest the need for earlier referral to a multidisciplinary team for rehabilitation and is a relative contraindication to any surgical intervention.

Case Study 8-1

A 34-year-old male presents with low back pain since yesterday afternoon. He was lifting an anchor while on his boat, leaning over to the left side. When the anchor cleared the water, he felt a click and low back pain. When he awoke this morning, the pain radiated down his right leg to his foot. Pain is increased with sitting more than standing. Pain is also aggravated by sneezing and coughing.

Physical Examination

On inspection, there is lumbar paraspinal muscle spasm/fullness with loss of lordosis. The right internal hamstring reflex is diminished compared with the left side; patellar and Achilles' tendon reflexes are normal and symmetric. Strength is graded 5- for right great toe extension; otherwise full and symmetric. There is an equivocal decrease in pinprick sensation on the dorsal right foot. Right straight leg raising is positive for neuropathic pain along the posterolateral thigh, anterior lower leg, and dorsum of the foot at 45 degrees.

Discussion

This history is perfect for a disk herniation. This patient's posture (leaning over and twisted) and activity (force was away from his body) applied the greatest possible pressure to the lumbar disk.

The physical examination is consistent with an L5 radiculopathy. L5 is the most common radiculopathy because the nerve root can be compromised at the L4-L5 level by a central herniation or at the L5-S1 level by a posterolateral herniation. Internal hamstring reflex is L5/S1. Preservation of the ankle reflex (S1) on the same side suggests an L5 root lesion. Great toe extension is solidly L5. Comparing pinprick sensitivity from side to side improves the sensitivity of the test; however, the area of sensory loss is a poor predictor of the level of herniated disk. A positive straight leg test is sensitive and can be made more specific with a positive crossed straight leg test.

Key Points

- Percussion tenderness of the spinous process (+/- fever) suggests involvement of the vertebral body, such as that seen in infections or tumor.

- Spinal range of motion testing for purposes of reproducing the patient's pain symptoms can be helpful in determining the pain source. Alternatively, in the acute setting, test spinal range of motion grossly for reproduction of the patient's pain symptoms.
  —Increased pain with extension suggests a pain source in the posterior elements.
  —Increased pain with flexion suggests a diskogenic or anterior column pain source.
- Neuromuscular testing include reflexes, muscle strength, sensation, and dural tension signs.
- A rapid screening examination emphasizes L5 and S1 reflexes, strength of ankle dorsiflexison, great toe extension, unipedal weight bearing heel raise, and sensory pinprick exam at the medial heel, dorsal foot, and lateral heel.
- Presence of three or more Waddell's signs of non-organic pain suggests that there is likely a psychogenic component and serves as a "yellow flag" that the patient is at risk for becoming chronically disabled.

■   ■   ■

REFERENCES

1. **Deyo RA, Rainville J, Kent DL.** What can the history and physical examination tell us about low back pain? JAMA. 1992;268(6):760-65.
2. **Wiesel SW, Weinstein JN.** The Lumbar Spine. Philadelphia: WB Saunders; 1990.
3. **American Spinal Injury Association.** International Standards for Neurological Classification of Spinal Cord Injury. Chicago: American Spinal Injury Association; Revised 2000.
4. **Andersson G, Deyo RA.** History and physical examination in patients with herniated lumbar discs. Spine. 1996;21(24S):10-18S.
5. **Waddell, G, McCulloch JA, Kummel E, Verner RMO.** Nonorganic physical signs in low back pain. Spine. 1980; 5: 117-25.

9

■ ■ ■

When Low Back Pain Represents Severe Disease

James K. Richardson, MD

The proportion of patients seeking assistance from a physician for low back pain who actually have a malignant, infectious, or a rapidly progressive or potentially irreversible neurologic deficit is small. However, given the ubiquitous nature of back pain, the denominator in this proportion is large, so that the number of patients with such disorders is not trivial. The purpose of this chapter is to arm the physician with clues to identify that small fraction of patients with low back pain who have severe disease that requires rapid attention. Although physical examination and laboratory and imaging studies are of relevance in this discussion, the most important clues are generally elicited by the history (Table 9-1). These clues, termed "red flags," are relatively sensitive, but they are not often specific signs that there may be a dangerous pathology. For this reason, that most important of clinical skills—the physician's personal judgment—is what is paramount in detecting severe, underlying disorders in these patients.

Malignancy

The spine is much more frequently involved by metastatic disease than it is the site of primary tumors. Approximately 20% of all malignancies have spine involvement as the initial manifestation of the disease, with carcinoma of the lung, multiple myeloma, non-Hodgkin's lymphoma, carcinoma of unknown primary, and renal cell carcinoma being disproportionately represented (1). Colorectal and breast cancer are underrepresented in terms of their likelihood to initially manifest as spinal disease. The frequency with which low back pain represents a neoplastic process varies with the patient

Table 9-1   Red Flags for Serious Disease

	Cauda Equina	Fracture	Cancer	Infection
Progressive neurologic deficit	X			
Recent bowel or bladder dysfunction	X			
Saddle anesthesia	X			
Traumatic onset		X		
Steroid use history		X		X
Women age > 50		X	X	
Men age > 50			X	
Male with diffuse osteoporosis or compression fracture			X	
Cancer history			X	
Insidious onset			X	X
No relief at bedtime or worsens when supine			X	X
Constitutional symptoms (e.g., fever, weight loss)			X	X
History UTI/other infection				X
IV drug use				X
Immune suppression				X
Previous surgery				X

population considered. In one large series of outpatients at a walk-in clinic, only 13 of 1975 patients, or less than 1%, had a malignant cause of back pain (2). In another series of patients over 50 years of age referred to an orthopedic surgeon, 3.8% had cancer underlying their back pain (3). Clearly, these frequencies are insufficient to warrant imaging studies or laboratory tests on all patients. Fortunately, features have been identified, often termed "red flags," which allow stratification of patients with back pain into low-risk and high-risk populations (2). Table 9-2 lists important keys in diagnosing malignancy in the spine.

Before we go on to discuss this stratification, a reasonable question to ask, given the ominous prognosis of spinal malignancy, is, do we have anything to offer these patients by making this diagnosis-and after making this diagnosis? Aside from a knowledge and understanding of their prognosis, with which the patient can better make decisions for themselves and loved ones, the answer is a qualified "yes." The vast majority (96%) of patients who develop neurologic compromise due to spinal malignancy initially present with pain (4). Importantly, radiation and surgical stabilization procedures have been demonstrated to be effective in maintaining or improving neurologic function and decreasing pain. Early diagnosis and less neurologic deficit have been linked to better functional outcome (5). Mean survival time after surgery has been found to be greater than 1 year (6). Furthermore, many of the tumors are potentially responsive to relatively

Table 9-2   Keys to Diagnosing Malignant Low Back Pain

Malignancy	Infection		Cauda Equina Syndrome
	Vertebral Osteomyelitis	Diskitis	
History			
Age >50, history of CA No improvement at 4 weeks Worse at night	Mild pain, variable constitutional symptoms Recent infection, medical/dental procedure, or IV drug use common	Severe pain, variable constitutional symptoms, usually recent spinal procedure	Pain, saddle numbness, urinary retention or incontinence
Physical examination			
Maybe percussion tenderness Focus on neurologic	Fever often, but not invariable. Usually percussion tenderness	Fever infrequently, patient holds affected region still	Decreased perianal sensation/anal wink, decreased Achilles' reflexes
Screening lab (for patients with any of above historical risk factors)			
ESR, UA, lumbar spine x-ray	ESR, lumbar spine x-ray	ESR	Postvoid residual urine volume >100 ml
Imaging study			
MRI/bone scan for all patients with CA history, and others with any screening lab abnormality	MRI/bone scan	MRI	MRI and emergent surgical consultation

benign chemotherapeutic modalities such as steroids and/or hormonal manipulations. These features suggest that there is the potential for maintaining or improving quality of life among patients with spinal malignancies, even those who are frail.

History

For the most part, traditional historical features regarding pain such as location and quality are minimally helpful in determining who has a spinal malignancy. This is likely due to the variety of locations in which tumors may develop and the resultant heterogeneity of the pain. However, it should be kept in mind that most benign musculoskeletal causes of back pain are in the lumbar and cervical regions, because of the greater biomechanical demands and motion in these areas; therefore, prominent pain in a location outside of these areas should raise suspicion. In primary care populations, duration of pain has been found to be helpful in identifying spinal malignancy. Back pain due to cancer tends to be unrelenting. Unrelenting pain of greater than 4 weeks duration that is in some way disabling, despite treatment, is consistent with a malignant diagnosis. One of the most humble pieces of the patient history-age-is also one of the most helpful. In every case series reported, malignant causes of back pain were significantly more frequent among patients over age 50. For this reason, it is extremely important to remember that anyone over 50 should be considered at increased risk for a nonmusculoskeletal cause of back pain. Not surprisingly, a history of cancer has been demonstrated to be a marker for spinal malignancy. In the author's experience, this obvious piece of history may be minimized or ignored by patient and/or referring physicians-possibly for emotional reasons. Unexplained weight loss is not encountered frequently, but when it is part of the back pain history, then a neoplastic source of back pain should be considered. Night pain has been emphasized as a feature of malignant back pain. This may at first seem a nonspecific historical feature given the frequency with which benign back pain leads to disordered sleep. However, in the author's experience, pain due to malignancy does not just persist at night but actually accelerates significantly. The patient often gives a history of getting up to walk around or sleep sitting up in a chair to relieve the pain. This is decidedly different from musculoskeletal pain, which, although often persistent at night, usually is less intense. Pain on lying down, conversely, is somewhat worrisome. A history of progressive neurologic deficit is consistent with a malignant cause of pain given that most, but not all, benign causes of neurologic deficit tend to remit over time.

Physical Examination

Percussion tenderness over the spinous processes is thought to occur more frequently among patients with malignant spinal pain. However, other maneuvers that reproduce the patient's pain, commonly helpful in making musculoskeletal diagnoses, are not helpful in the diagnosis of spinal malignancy, most likely due to the heterogenous locations of spinal metastases. The neurologic examination is more useful in these patients. Asymmetries in tendon reflexes, strength, and sensation should be considered consistent with malignancy until proven otherwise given any of the above history. In addition to the patellar (L3/L4) and Achilles' reflexes (S1/S2), the internal hamstring reflex (L5/S1) can be obtained in most nonobese patients over the distal semimembranosis and semitendonosis tendons. Strength testing of hip flexion (L2, L3, L4) while the patient is sitting is sometimes difficult or unreliable, as the iliopsoas muscle originates from the lumbar spinous processes, and the resulting compression during muscle contraction invariably causes pain and a false suggestion of weakness. Thigh adduction (L2, L3) tests the same root level and is usually less aggravating. In addition, it is recommended that plantar flexion (L5, S1) strength be tested, if possible, with the patient standing. It is not possible to test this powerful muscle manually, and so it is recommended that the patient be evaluated performing 10 unilateral heel raises on each side. The neurologic examination can be an important clue that something objective is happening to the nerve roots, but neurologic deficit is often not present at the time of presentation of spinal malignancy or infection.

Laboratory and Radiologic Studies

Detailed analyses regarding the best screening laboratory and radiologic examinations have been performed, which take into account cost as well as diagnostic accuracy (7). Initial screens include lumbar spine radiographs and erythrocyte sedimentation rate (ESR). Patients with one or more of the historical risk factors, and either an abnormal lumbar spine film or an ESR >50, deserve an imaging study. The imaging study of choice is usually magnetic resonance imaging (MRI), but bone scan is also an effective, if overly sensitive, imaging study in patients over 50 years old. MRI is particularly useful if extraspinal involvement is suspected (8). Computed tomography (CT) scan detects most dangerous causes of back pain but can miss soft tissue changes from tumor and infection, so it is a second choice to MRI, used when MRI is not available within the urgent time frame. It should be remembered that bone scan is insensitive to myeloma due to the inhibition of osteoblasts associated with that disease. A worthy variation on this strategy is to weight more heavily any history of cancer and image all such patients with MRI/bone scan without bothering to assess lumbar x-rays or ESR. The author also advocates that urinalysis be included given the tendency for renal cell carcinoma to involve the spine.

Case Study 9-1

A 53-year-old male was referred for evaluation of back pain. The pain was in the low thoracic and high lumbar regions and had been gradually worsening for about 2 months. He could describe no inciting event or unusual activity that might have precipitated the pain. The pain did not radiate. Activity did not worsen his pain and often improved it. He was able to continue his work as an accountant. The pain was significantly worse at night and usually awakened him around 3:00 or 4:00 a.m. At times he was able to fall back asleep in a chair by sleeping more upright. He denied any history of cancer, and his weight was unchanged. Other constitutional symptoms were absent. His neurologic examination was normal, but paraspinal muscle spasm and percussion tenderness over the spinous processes in the low thoracic and high lumbar regions were present. His ESR was 78; urinalysis was unremarkable and a plain film of the thoracolumbar spine demonstrated lytic lesions. Further search of his medical records from an outside hospital revealed that he had undergone removal of a melanoma 6 years previously without the recommended follow-up.

Discussion

This case demonstrates many of the hallmarks of malignant back pain. The patient's pain had no clear inciting event; however, it is just as common for patients to ascribe such pain to some activity that, when scrutinized, would not be expected to lead to 2 months of pain. The patient was over 50 years old and pain was present, but tolerable, during the day and considerably worse at night after a few hours of sleep. This acceleration of pain after lying down for several hours is characteristic of malignant pain (benign pain syndromes often interfere with sleep, but the pain rarely increases at night). As can be the case, due to poor patient education or emotional minimizing, the patient did not feel that his cancer history was significant.

Infection

Back pain as a manifestation of infectious disease is less common than malignancy. However, like malignancy, spine infection can lead to neurologic compromise, either radiculopathy or myelopathy, which is usually treatable and/or preventable. Infection can be grossly divided into vertebral osteomyelitis, often with secondary infectious diskitis, and the more rare isolated diskitis.

Vertebral Osteomyelitis

History
Patients with vertebral osteomyelitis usually experience a dull, continuous pain that is typically not as disabling as malignancy or acute benign pain. There are unfortunately no discriminating features of the pain in terms of location or aggravating/alleviating factors that allow the physician to suspect vertebral osteomyelitis. Night pain is usually not a prominent feature as is often the case for malignancy. Fever, chills, malaise, night sweats, anorexia, and weight loss are commonly, but not universally, associated with osteomyelitis. A case series of six patients emphasized that osteomyelitis can mimic compression fracture (9). It should be kept in mind that most musculoskeletal sources of pain are lumbar and cervical and so pain in the thoracic region should heighten suspicion.

Because vertebral osteomyelitis is usually a blood-borne infection rather than a primary spinal infection, the most important history involves questions that will identify risk factors for infection. Risk factors can be divided into those that suppress the immune system and those that introduce bacteria into the bloodstream. Common clinical conditions associated with the suppression of the immune system include diabetes mellitus, sickle cell anemia, renal failure, history of organ transplantation, HIV/AIDS, history of malignancy and connective tissue diseases. An antecedent history of infection (in particular cellulitis, burns, genitourinary infection, endocarditis, and pneumonia), medical procedure (dental, gastrointenstinal, genitourinary, intravenous catheter), or intravenous drug usage are common risk factors for introducing bacteria into the bloodstream. Finally, because tuberculosis of the spine is common in the Third World, recent immigrants should also be considered at increased risk for vertebral osteomyelitis.

Physical Examination

An elevated temperature may suggest infection; however, about half of patients with pyogenic osteomyelitis and the majority of patients with tuberculosis osteomyelitis are afebrile (10). Localized tenderness of the spinous processes to percussion appears to be present commonly in infectious causes of back pain; however, the frequency in which percussion tenderness is present in musculoskeletal causes of back pain limits the finding's specificity (11).

Laboratory and Radiologic Examination

Appropriate laboratory studies for detecting osteomyelitis include spine radiographs, complete blood count, and ESR. Absolute abnormalities of white blood cell count, neutrophil count, or ESR according to the local laboratory values (or age-adjusted values for ESR) may be present, but with a high index of suspicion, borderline changes may be sufficient to take further steps. As was the case with maligancy, historical risk factors should lead to screening laboratory studies, which when positive should lead to imaging study. Imaging will then likely demonstrate destruction of the disk and perhaps bone margins with soft tissue mass.

Isolated Diskitis

Diskitis not associated with other spinal infection is uncommon. When isolated diskitis does occur, there is usually a history of an antecedent invasive procedure involving the spine. The procedure is most often surgical, but spinal anesthesia or multiple attempts at lumbar puncture can also lead to diskitis. Given the disk's relatively avascular nature, such a procedure is usually necessary to lead to infection. However, diskitis without such a history does occur, usually older patients over 50 years old, often with chronic disease such as diabetes mellitus (12).

By all accounts, the pain from diskitis is at least moderate and often intense. The patient endeavors to hold himself as still as possible because motion markedly increases the pain. After a spinal procedure, this is often simply interpreted as a failure of the procedure to reduce pain. However, the pain due to diskitis persists and increases over time if untreated. The pain is not known to have a radicular component and so is confined to the back. The lumbar spine is involved more than other regions. Systemic signs such as fever are usually mild or absent.

If there is historical suspicion, appropriate screening laboratories include ESR and complete blood count. The former is often difficult to interpret postoperatively, as the procedure itself increases the ESR. Therefore, it should be kept in mind that the postoperative ESR peaks on days 3 to 5 and declines significantly by postoperative week 2 and is back to baseline by week 4 (13). If either screening lab is positive, MRI has been found to be the most effective imaging study (14).

Cauda Equina Syndrome

Cauda equina syndrome, a bilateral sacral polyradiculopathy, is among the most feared of complications among patients presenting with low back pain. The syndrome results when the sacral roots, which lie in the midline in close proximity to one another, are compromised. The syndrome is caused by external compression of the cauda equina, most often by a herniated disk, and also by tumor, epidural hematoma or abscess, and trauma. Although the syndrome is not usually life-threatening, the compromised quality of life that results from the syndrome-bowel/bladder incontinence, lower extremity weakness, and sexual dysfunction-renders it "malignant" regardless the cause. Fortunately, cauda equina syndrome is rare, with a prevalence suggested to be 0.04% among patients with low back pain (11). This is likely due to the midline location of the posterior longitudinal ligament in the lumbar region, which reinforces the posterior annulus of the lumbar disk, making central herniation less likely.

History

In addition to low back pain, the patient commonly reports pain and dysesthesia into the lower extremities and the perineal regions. Most patients report some combination of urinary retention/incontinence, bowel incontinence, and/or sexual dysfunction. Urinary retention or incontinence is the most consistently reported concern. Symptoms develop relatively rapidly-for most patients in less than 24 hours. In the case where a lumbar disk herniation is leading to cauda equina syndrome, symptoms may be preceded by typical activities associated with disk injuries such as heavy/repetitive lifting and/or prolonged sitting such as a long plane flight. Cauda equina syndrome can also be caused by neoplasm, which tends to be primary in younger patients and metastatic in patients over 50 (15).

Physical Examination

Decreased Achilles' reflexes are common but not universal. In addition, this finding is less helpful among older patients and patients with diabetes mellitus who commonly do not have Achilles' reflexes prior to the onset of back or lower extremity pain. Urinary retention, as evidenced by a postvoiding residual bladder volume of >100 mL, is highly sensitive for cauda equina syndrome (11). Decreased sensation over the perianal region and medial buttocks is common, as is decreased anal sphincter tone. Anal wink reflex, a visible contraction of the anal sphincter that occurs with scratching the perianal region with a pin, is often absent or diminished. Plantar flexor weakness may be present and should be detected by asking the patient to perform 10 unilateral toe raises, if pain allows, using the upper extremities for balance as needed.

Imaging and Therapy

Given a back pain history that includes urinary retention or incontinence, particularly if coupled with a postvoiding residual urinary volume of >100 mL, urgent imaging is indicated. MRI is the study of choice. A recent study, which echoes previous work, underscores the urgency of the situation by strongly correlating neurologic recovery with emergent surgical decompression (16). For optimal outcome, it appears that decompression should occur within 24 to 48 hours.

Case Study 9-2

A 56-year-old male presented to the inpatient rehabilitation unit after surgical therapy at another hospital for cauda equina syndrome. He was well until 2 weeks prior to admission when, on a Friday, he assisted his wife in rearranging furniture in their home. He experienced a "popping" sensation in his low back during this activity and had low back pain that evening. During the night, his pain increased and began to radiate into his perineum and lower extremities. In the morning, he had trouble initiating his urine stream. He sought medical attention in the local emergency department on the next day, a Saturday. His neurologic examination was said to be unremarkable. A postvoiding residual urine volume was not checked. He was given acetaminophen and codeine and asked to follow up with his primary care physician. His pain worsened during the day and the next night. He continued to have difficulty with urinary retention but not incontinence. He felt weak walking but could still climb stairs with effort. He returned to the emergency room Sunday morning and was found to have absent Achilles' reflexes, decreased perianal sensation, and a postvoiding residual volume of 450 mLs of urine. MRI revealed a large, centrally located disk fragment at L5/S1. As it was the weekend, he did not undergo surgical decompression until Monday mid-day.

Discussion

This patient's cauda equina syndrome evolved over time. The initial inability to recognize the syndrome was likely due to the fact that the neurologic examination of the lower extremities was normal. However, perianal sensation, anal wink, and a postvoiding residual volume were not assessed. The next day the syndrome was unmistakable but surgery was not performed. This despite the fact that the number of hours prior to decompression of a cauda equina syndrome has repeatedly been shown to be the primary factor affecting prognosis. It was this patient's bad fortune to become injured on a weekend. During his rehabilitation stay, the patient progressed well from a functional standpoint due to his upper extremity strength, his overall excellent health, and support from his wife. Six years later, he ambulates household distances with a walker and braces and uses a wheelchair in the community. He performs intermittent catheterization to empty his bladder. He and his wife travel extensively in their large, modified motor coach, which they paid for from the proceeds of their successful malpractice litigation.

■   ■   ■

Key Points

- Malignancy as a cause of back pain is rare but should be considered if the patient is over 50, has had no improvement after 4 weeks, has increased pain at night, or has a history of cancer.
- An appropriate screen for patients with a history suggestive of malignancy includes an ESR, urinalysis, and plain radiograph; if any of the screens are abnormal, MRI or bone scan is indicated.
- Vertebral osteomyelitis is often only mildly painful and, except in cases of major trauma or surgery, is blood borne. Constitutional symptoms are variable.
- Risk factors for osteomyelitis include recent recovery from infectious disease, dental or medical procedures, or a history of intravenous drug abuse. Patients with these risk factors should be evaluated with a complete blood count, ESR, and plain radiographs.
- Diskitis is moderately to intensely painful and usually follows an invasive procedure such as lumbar puncture or spinal surgery/anesthesia.
- ESR is helpful in making the diagnosis of diskitis, keeping in mind that the elevation due to surgery is mostly reversed after 2 weeks, and MRI is the imaging study of choice.
- Cauda equina syndrome may occur due to benign or malignant processes. In either case, urinary retention, as identified by a postvoiding residual volume of >100 mL, is common. Good prognosis is inversely related to the time from symptom onset to surgical decompression. Thus diagnosis precipitates a true surgical emergency.

■   ■   ■

REFERENCES

1. **Schiff D, O'Neill BP, Suman VJ.** Spinal epidural metastasis as the initial manifestation of malignancy: clinical features and diagnostic approach. Neurology. 1997;49:452-56.

2. **Deyo RA, Diehl AK.** Cancer as a cause of back pain: frequency, clinical presentation and diagnostic strategies. J Gen Intern Med. 1988;3:230-8.

3. **Fernbach JC, Langer F, Gross AE.** The significance of low back pain in older adults. Can Med Assoc. 1976;115:898-900.

4. **Schmidt R, Markovchick V.** J Emerg Med. 1992;10:189-99.

5. **Daw HA, Markman M.** Epidural spinal cord compression in cancer patients: diagnosis and management. Cleve Clin J Med 2000;67(7):501-4.

6. **Wise JJ, Fischgrund JS, Herkowitz HN, Montgomery D, Kurz LT.** Complication, survival rates, and risk factors of surgery for metastatic disease of the spine. Spine. 1999;24:1943-51.

7. **Joines JD, McNutt RA, Carey TS, Deyo RA, Rouhani R.** Finding cancer in primary care outpatients with low back pain: a comparison of diagnostic strategies. J Gen Intern Med. 2001;16(1):14-23.

8. **Jacobson AF.** Musculoskeletal pain as an indicator of occult malignancy: yield of bone scintigraphy. Arch Intern Med 1997;157:105-09.

9. **McHenry MC, Duchesneau PM, Keys TF, Rehm SJ, Boumphrey FRS.** Vertebral osteomyelitis presenting as spinal compression fracture. Arch Intern Med 1988;148:417-23.

10. **Della-Giustina DA.** Emergency department evaluation and treatment of back pain. Emerg Med Clin North Am. 1999;17(4):877-93.

11. **Deyo RA, Rainville J, Kent DL.** What can the history and physical examination tell us about low back pain? JAMA. 1992;268(6):760-65.

12. **Kornberg M.** Erythrocyte sedimentation rate following lumbar discectomy. Spine. 1986;11(7):766-7.

13. **Honan M, White WG, Eisenberg GM.** Spontaneous infectious discitis in adults. Am J Med. 1996;100(1):85-89.

14. **Modic MT, Pavlicek W, Weinstein MA, Boumphrey F, Ngo F, Hardy R, Duchesneau PM.** Magnetic resonance imaging of intervertebral disk disease: clinical and pulse sequence considerations. Radiology. 1984;152:103-111.

15. **Wippold FJ, Smirniotopoulos JG, Pilgram TK.** Lesions of cauda equina: a clinical and pathology review from the Armed Forces Institute of Pathology. Clin Neurol Neurosurg. 1997;99(4):229-34.

16. **Shapiro S.** Medical realities of cauda equina syndrome secondary to lumbar disc herniation. Spine. 2000;25:1668-79.

10

■ ■ ■

Yellow Flags:
Predicting Disability

Irene A. Young, MD

The majority of acute low back pain episodes will resolve with little to no medical intervention. However, a small minority of acute low back pain sufferers will go on to become chronic low back pain patients (1). Predicting which patients are at high risk for future disability allows for early medical intervention. Primary care practitioners see the majority of low back pain presentations, and only a select few require referral to specialists. Primary care physicians therefore play a unique role in identifying potential problems at an early stage and executing treatment strategies to obtain optimal outcomes (2). Recognizing these risk factors for disability is essential.

Disability implies the inability to perform certain tasks. This can mean anything from inability to throw a baseball to the inability to get out of bed. For back pain, the most studied and arguably the most important aspect of disability is the inability to work. This is because work disability is costly to employers and insurers, not just the patient. However, it is a big mistake to ignore nonwork disability. Older people may become unable to perform basic activities of daily living. Caregivers who do not have formal employment may have crucial societal roles that are impaired by back pain. Even among people with traditional work disability, the motivating factor to get better may be more their bowling game than the boring job on the assembly line. The risk factors for work disability are fairly well-known. These items, termed "yellow flags," should never be missed in the initial evaluation of a back pain patient.

Yellow Flags: The Three Types
of Risk Factors for Disability

The concept of "red flags" as signs of serious disease has been extended to the idea of "yellow flags" that indicate psychosocial barriers to recovery (6).

Yellow flags highlight the need for further investigation of cognitive and behavioral aspects of an acute low back pain presentation. The presence of either red or yellow flags should lead to appropriate medical or psychosocial evaluation (3,4). For many acute back pain presentations, these issues need to be addressed early so the risk of long-term disability and work loss can be reduced.

Yellow flags are composed of 1) physical, 2) individual, and 3) psychological factors that together have the greatest influence on low back pain and disability. Low back pain in the workplace was originally believed to be solely based on the physical load borne at work. More recently, psychosocial and individual factors have been studied and are believed to play a more significant role. The mechanism or pathway by which these factors influence low back pain is far from clear (5-8).

Case Study 10-1

A 37-year-old female postal worker pulled a heavy box off a shelf while at work. She presents to a primary care office 3 weeks after her injury complaining of severe low back and left leg pain. This is her third work-related injury in the past 5 years. She is divorced with little social support. She is overweight, smokes, and does not exercise on a regular basis. Past medical history is significant for fibromyalgia and hypertension. Clinically, she is an anxious female with marked pain behavior on examination. She appears quite fearful with any motion, but neurologic examination is intact and no dural tension signs are appreciated. Workup, including lumbar spine magnetic resonance imaging and bone scan, is normal. She fails in a course of manual physical therapy, with the therapist reporting that compliance with a home exercise program may be a problem. She has been unable to return to work because she is fearful that she will reinjure herself.

Discussion

From the first interaction, her physician should have been aware of multiple yellow flags. From a personal and public health standpoint, detection and remedy of yellow flags is by far the most important thing a physician can do in the management of back pain. It is important for the attending physician to provide an expectation that she will return to work and normal activity. The physician should encourage her that pain can be controlled and that a normal active working life can be maintained. Frequent follow-up while out of work is crucial. Psychological intervention might be suggested early on if she appears to have psychological yellow flags. The physician should try to keep the patient active and at work if even for a small portion of the day. Consider reasonable requests for job modification. If the barriers to return to work seem substantial and overwhelming to the physician, then a very early referral to a physical medicine and rehabilitation specialist, even at 2-3 weeks, may be best. More typically, such a referral is made if there is not substantial progress by the subacute phase (at 6 weeks).

Physical Factors

Physical workplace factors are believed to influence the risk of low back pain by exceeding the biomechanical limits of the spine (8). Lab studies have found that increases in the load magnitude handled and dynamic and non-neutral postures (e.g., bending and twisting) can increase the loads imposed on the spinal structures. Several studies have noted that there is an association between lifting or forceful movements (e.g., pushing and pulling) and low back pain risk, whereas other studies found an increased risk with sedentary work. Therefore, association between the mechanical load on the spine and risk of low back pain does not appear to be linear (3). Physical and occupational risk factors are discussed in more detail in Chapter 2.

Individual Factors

Low back pain is also influenced by individual factors, and many studies have tried to discern which factors place someone at greatest susceptibility for disability. Individual factors studied include age, sex, education, marital status, posture, anthropometry, muscle strength, physical fitness, spine mobility, and smoking. Personal aspects of the pain itself and early management by others are yellow flags. These include an emotionally traumatic onset of pain, early personal belief that there will be chronic disability, disagreement with previous caregivers about the diagnosis, and the length of time already off of work.

Life experience dictates much of the person's belief about the relationship between physical and emotional pain and between pain and disability. Research has shown that an emotionally unpleasant childhood (alcoholic parent, death of a parent, difficult divorce, physical or sexual abuse), multiple divorces or never being married, a spouse who is either punishing or too supportive of disability, are important. The workplace experience has predictable effects: disability is more likely in persons who are new to the job or close to retirement. A job that is too physically or cognitively challenging (or one that is too boring, for an overqualified worker), any previous time on disability leave from work for any medical reason, and failure to get along with the supervisor are risk factors. General economic decline in the community, risk of layoff, and issues such as potential military duty all decrease motivation to return to work. On the other hand, single working mothers or self-employed workers are typically highly motivated to return to work.

Individual yellow flags thought to play the greatest role in predicting future disability include the presence of radiating leg pain, a higher than normal body mass index, low educational level, multiple marriages, tobacco use, past hospitalizations and prior low back compensation claims (8,9). In a given individual, a compilation of these yellow flags may contribute to produce the onset of low back symptoms (6).

Psychological Factors

Psychological factors including anger, fear, depression, anxiety, avoidance, stress, sense of entitlement, and somatization play a significant role in the patient's coping with an acute onset of low back pain. Alcohol and drug abuse are factors, probably due to the previous social dysfunction that they had caused at work, the poor coping ability of the patient, and the actual intoxication interfering with compliance and understanding. Much less commonly, classic somatoform disorders of hysteria and hypochondriasis are found. There is strong evidence from the literature for the role of psychological distress/depressive mood in the transition from acute to chronic low back pain (9,10). A recent comprehensive review suggest that psychological factors play an important role in the transition to chronicity in low back pain and may contribute at least as much as clinical factors (2). These findings constitute a strong indication for the development of clinical interventions to identify and target psychological factors.

Yellow Flags as Predictors of Chronicity

Yellow flags, as opposed to spinal pathology, are now recognized as the best predictors of chronicity (6). Many of the learned behaviors in chronic low back pain have their root in the first few weeks of pain onset. A confounding factor is the contributing psychosocial factors may confound the matter in a worker who perceives the onset of pain to be work-related (11). Workers' compensation plays a complex role and may serve as a deterrent to successful return to the workforce. One study found a lack of contributing effect of individual and physical factors and demonstrated the potential importance of psychosocial variables such as job dissatisfaction in the injured worker (6,12).

Using the History and Physical Examination to Identify Yellow Flags

During the history and physical examination, it is very important to obtain information that can help in identifying patients at high risk of disability. In the history, it is important to document previous injuries or other work-related claims. Patients with multiple work-related claims have failed in the vocational arena and will likely require special attention from their treating physician. Job satisfaction has also been shown to play a key factor in return to work. Litigation and the use of the services of an attorney are other predictors of disability. The clinician should note comorbid illnesses such as depression, anxiety, and fibromyalgia and a social history that suggests multiple failed relationships or substance abuse.

During the examination, it is important to note a patient's response to questions that may suggest a sense of entitlement, fear, stress, anxiety, or depression. The Waddell signs or physical examination evidence for "nonphysiological" pain behavior are important predictors of future trouble (Table 10-1).

Identifying which patients stand a greater chance of future disability and initiating early intervention is crucial. Barriers to their recovery need to be addressed quickly just as one would work up red flags. There are effective strategies for helping a patient at risk of chronic disability or work loss. Work restrictions are helpful by allowing the patient to return to work and a semblance of a normal schedule. Counseling and antidepressant usage in patients with numerous psychological issues is often overlooked and is crucial. If the patient's low back pain is not getting better and complex barriers are noted, consider an early referral to a specialist dealing with occupational low back pain or a multidisciplinary team.

The person's ability and interest in taking on the problem head on, sometimes termed "self-efficacy" or "internal locus of control," is an important factor in success. An unskilled physician interaction typically imposes an external locus of control ("I'm the doctor, do what I say"). More experienced clinicians will recognize the reality that they are neither the expert on the patient's level of pain nor the person's work activity. They will ask questions like "What do you think we should do with work restrictions?" This may be one of the most modifiable yellow flags.

Table 10-1   Exam Findings Associated with Poor Resolution of Back Pain and Risk for Chronic Pain and Disability (Waddell Signs)

- Overreaction and significant pain behavior during examination
- Nonanatomic sensory and motor findings
- Reports of low back pain with axial loading by light to moderate pushing on the shoulders or head
- Reports of low back pain during rotation of the spine en bloc (shoulders and pelvis kept in alignment)
- Inconsistent reports of pain with straight leg raising in the seated vs. supine position
- Pain with superficial palpation

■   ■   ■

Recommendations

- All patients with low back pain should be screened for yellow flags.
- Document previous injuries or work-related claims.
- When taking the history, note if the patient has a low educational level, a history of multiple marriages, tobacco use, substance abuse, or job dissatisfaction.
- Screen for psychological factors such as anger, fear, depression, anxiety, avoidance, high level of stress, sense of entitlement, and somatization.
- Patients who appear to be at risk for chronic disability should be followed closely.
- Barriers to recovery should be addressed aggressively.
- If recovery does not occur within 6 weeks, the patient should be referred to a specialist with a rehabilitation team.

■   ■   ■

Key Points

- Physical workplace yellow flags (i.e., risk factors for disability) include jobs that require repetitive heavy lifting and twisting that place high biomechanical loads onto the spine.
- Individual factors to be aware of include radiating leg pain, a higher than normal body mass index, low educational level, multiple marriages, tobacco use, past hospitalizations, and prior low back compensation claims.
- Psychological factors include anger, depression, anxiety, fear, stress, and a sense of entitlement.
- Promote self-efficacy and early return to work with modifications. Consider early referral to a spine specialist or multidisciplinary team in these patients if recovery does not occur within 6 weeks.
- The presence of yellow flags, rather than detection of spinal disease itself, is the best predictor of chronic pain.
- Promote active participation in problem solving regarding treatment and return to work.
- Consider referral to a physical medicine and rehabilitation specialist or physiatrist very early (2-3 weeks) if yellow flags are overwhelming, otherwise if there is no progress at 6 weeks.
- Identifying the presence of yellow flags is by far more important than the diagnosis of a specific spinal disorder in the prevention of future pain and disability.

■   ■   ■

REFERENCES

1. **Truchon M.** Determinants of chronic disability related to low back pain: towards an integrative biopsychosocial model. Disabil Rehabil. 2001;23(17):758-67.

2. **Frymoyer JW.** Predicting disability from low back pain. Clin Orthop. 1992;279:101-9.

3. **Spitzer WO, et al.** Scientific approach to the assessment and management of activity-related spinal disorders: a monograph for clinicians. Report of the Quebec Task Force on Spinal Disorders. Spine. 1987;12:1.

4. **Cats-Baril WL, Frymoyer JW.** Identifying patients at risk of becoming disabled because of low back pain. The Vermont Rehabilitation Engineering Center Predictive Model. Spine. 1991;16(6):605-7.

5. **Pincus T, Burton AK, Vogel S, Field AP.** A systematic review of psychological factors as predictors of chronic/disability in prospective cohorts of low back pain. Spine. 2002;27(5):E109-120.

6. **Kendall NA.** Psychological approaches to the prevention of chronic pain: the low back paradigm. Balliere's Clin Rheumatol. 1999;13(3):545-54.

7. **Marras WS.** The influence of psychological stress, gender, and personality on mechanical loading of the lumbar spine. Spine. 2002;25(23):3045-54.

8. **Kerr MS.** Biomechanical and psychosocial risk factors for low back pain at work. Am J Public Health. 2001;91(7):1069-75.

9. **Fransen M, Woodward M, Norton R, Coggan C, Dawe M, Sheridan N.** Risk factors associated with the transition from acute to chronic occupational back pain. Spine. 2002;27(1):92-8.

10. **Fritz JM, George SZ, Delitto A.** The role of fear-avoidance beliefs in acute low back pain: relationships with current and future disability and work status. Pain. 2001;94:7-15.

11. **Lehmann TR.** Predicting long-term disability in low back injured workers presenting to a spine consultant. Spine. 1993;18(8):1103-12.

12. **Williams RA, Pruitt SD, Doctor JN, Epping-Jordan JE, Wahlgren DR, Grant I, et al.** The contribution of job satisfaction to the transition from acute to chronic low back pain. Arch Phys Med Rehabil. 1998;79:368-73.

■   ■   ■

KEY REFERENCES

Kendall NA. Psychological approaches to the prevention of chronic pain: the low back paradigm. Balliere's Clin Rheumatol. 1999;13(3):545-54.
A satisfactory guideline to the Yellow Flag theory and to approaches for dealing with patients at high risk for disability.

11

■ ■ ■

Acute Nonradiating
Low Back Pain

Anita S.W. Craig, DO

cute nonradiating low back pain is defined as pain of less than 6 weeks duration, located in the posterior trunk, anywhere between the lower ribcage and the gluteal folds. This is opposed to radiating pain, which involves some pain down into the leg, usually posteriorly into the calf or foot. Most people do not seek medical care for episodes of acute nonradiating back pain because they are often very brief. For those persons who do seek care from primary care physicians, from 75 to 90% improve within 1 month (1,2).

History and Physical Examination

Because most episodes of acute back pain are self-limited, the goal at initial presentation is to conduct a focused evaluation to screen efficiently for any potentially serious causes (see Chapter 9) and to identify patients who may be at higher risk to progress on to chronic pain (for yellow flags, see Chapter 10). This chapter de-emphasizes the specific anatomic diagnosis. Aside from red flags, the specific anatomic diagnosis is seldom important in the management of acute back pain. Most patients get better on their own or with a little encouragement to stay active. Psychosocial factors are often more important in predicting and treating those who do not get better. Although a physician skilled in manual or manipulative therapy may improve pain (but not function) quicker with a specific treatment plan, the cost-effectiveness of very early referral to specific manual therapy is questionable. It is only in the subacute phase that anatomic lesions are subjected to anatomically specific treatments. A back pain questionnaire is often helpful in assessing red flags for serious illness and yellow flags for prolonged disability (Table 9-1 and Table 11-1) (3).

The physical examination (described in Chapter 8) is performed with special attention to spinal and pelvic girdle symmetry, posture, and spinal and lower extremity flexibility. Palpation can assess for both bony and soft tissue tenderness, hypertonicity, and spasm. Abdominal palpation and auscultation are performed for suspicion of possible abdominal process, such as aortic aneurysm. The hip joint should also be checked, particularly for complaints of buttock, hip region, or groin pain. Neurologic examination of the lower extremities is done; however, findings are rare in nonradiating pain.

Patients with history or physical exam findings that are serious may warrant earlier diagnostic testing. Waddell signs (Table 8-5) are associated with patients having a poor response to treatment, and prolonged symptoms and disability. Patients with significant history of psychosocial factors, and multiple Waddell signs noted during physical examination, may need earlier referral for multidisciplinary intervention to forestall progression on to chronic pain behavior. Although much is said about these two categories of patients, the vast majority of patients presenting to the primary care physician's office with back pain are quite self-limited and do not require workup beyond a good history and physical examination.

Table 11-1   Risk Factors for Chronic Disability

Clinical factors
- Previous episodes of back pain
- Multiple previous musculoskeletal complaints
- Hysteria or hypochodriasis
- Alcohol, drugs, cigarettes
- Waddell signs

Pain experience
- Rates pain as severe
- Blames others for pain
- Legal issues or compensation

Premorbid factors
- Rates job as physically demanding
- Patient believes he or she will not be working in 6 months
- Not getting along with supervisors
- Near retirement
- Spouse too supportive
- Unmarried or have been married multiple times
- Low socioeconomic status
- Troubled childhood (abuse, parental death, alcohol, difficult divorce)

Adapted from Acute Low Back Pain, Guidelines for Clinical Care. The University of Michigan Medical Center, Ann Arbor, Michigan. 1997.

Diagnostic Testing

Unless there are red flags, diagnostic testing is rarely indicated in acute nonradiating back pain. The findings on imaging studies are very poorly associated with symptoms, and many causes of back pain are not identified on imaging studies (5). This is true for both plain radiographs, computed tomography (CT), and magnetic resonance imaging (MRI) studies. The poor association of symptoms with findings on the imaging studies can be particularly troublesome to efficient treatment. Many patients may mistakenly believe that the noted finding on their spinal radiograph or MRI is the "cause" of their pain, even when the health care provider explains that it is likely an incidental, age appropriate, or inconsequential finding. This can create significant barriers in their treatment. Disk degeneration is a prime example of this. A third of patients under the age of 30 will demonstrate evidence of disk degeneration on spinal films, 60% between 40 and 60 years old, and virtually all above the age of 60 (6). Similar findings have been found for osteophytes and facet joint arthritis (7).

Patients may come with expectations for studies; however, education regarding the proper role for imaging usually suffices. Imaging should only be considered for those with red flags. Other studies, such as laboratory studies, are appropriate if the history or physical examination suggests an infectious, inflammatory, or neoplastic cause. Electromyography is not indicated for acute nonradiating low back pain both due to a lack of radiating symptoms that would suggest neurologic involvement and because electodiagnostic findings of denervation are not seen in the first several weeks of clinical onset.

Treatment

Initial treatment consists of medication and nonmedication means of pain control, judicious activity limitation, and patient education. Medications should be used with careful consideration, starting with NSAIDs or acetaminophen, and with limited use of muscle relaxants and opioids. On subsequent visits, addition of appropriate physical therapy may be indicated. If pain and disability continues beyond 4-6 weeks, particularly if there are psychosocial risk factors for chronic disability, consider referral to a nonsurgical spine specialist or multidisciplinary spine rehabilitation program.

Nonpharmacologic Pain Control

Initial modalities that the patient can employ in acute pain include such measures as local icing or heat and gentle self-stretching. Ice may bring temporary pain relief, decrease spasm, and have some local anti-inflammatory effect. Ice should be applied for 20 minutes at a time as needed. Heat may also be effective for muscle relaxation. Patients often ask which is better; however, in absence of true inflammation, such as an acutely inflamed joint (which is not an issue for back pain), either can be effective and is strictly based on patient preference. Some simple stretches may be given to the patient to initiate as tolerated. Once more comfortable, some practitioners recommend icing, as there is some research indicating icing combined with stretching will provide a longer duration of the muscle lengthening

Pharmacologic Pain Control

Several classes of medications have been used in the acute phase. These include nonsteroidal anti-inflammatory drugs (NSAIDs), acetaminophen, "muscle relaxants," opiate analgesics, and antidepressants (particularly the tricyclic class). Although Chapter 13 deals with the specific medications and doses, a few paragraphs on medication strategy for acute back pain are warranted.

Acetaminophen and NSAIDs are generally the first choice for pain relief. NSAIDs are typically prescribed, but care must be given due to the potential for gastrointestinal (GI) side effects. Various types of NSAIDs are equally as effective, and the choice should be based on side-effect profile and practitioner experience (8). Although not studied in acute back pain, acetaminophen has been found to be equally effective as NSAIDs in other musculoskeletal disorders (9) and therefore should be considered, particularly in patients with contraindications for NSAID use.

The so-called muscle relaxants, such as cyclobenzaprine, diazepam, and carisoprodol, actually do not have any direct effect on skeletal muscles but rather act through central mechanisms. These medications can cause significant drowsiness, which may limit their use. Although studies have shown benefit when compared to placebo, they have not been shown to be more efficacious than NSAIDS (8). Diazepam should be used with particular caution due to its abuse potential, particularly in patients with substance abuse histories. Cyclobenzaprine may have some additive effect with analgesic use in moderate to severe acute pain, but use should be limited to short term and bedtime due to its significant sedation. Patients should be advised not to drive or use heavy equipment while taking these medications.

Opioids have not been shown to be more effective than NSAIDs for acute back pain during controlled studies (8). Significant side effects, including constipation, sedation, possible dependence, and potential for abuse, warrant extreme caution in prescribing these medications. If narcotics are prescribed for acute back pain, it should be for very short duration and be used on a time-based schedule, not on an as-needed basis. These medications should not be used in acute pain for patients with a history of prior or current substance abuse.

Activity Limitation

Bed rest had long been prescribed for acute low back pain; however, it has fallen out of favor after being shown to prolong rather than shorten disability. Studies have shown that patients who are not placed on bed rest return to work sooner and have better outcomes (8,10). The patient should be advised to maintain usual activities as tolerated. Low-impact activities such as walking should be encouraged. In the acute period, high-impact activities and very heavy lifting should be limited. Prolonged sitting or standing may be poorly tolerated, therefore frequent posture changes should be encouraged.

Work disability is a troublesome issue. The length of time off work is correlated with risk of long-term disability and therefore should be minimized. Work activity limitations should be minimized; however, due respect should be paid to those jobs that involve unusually high physical demands. Although participation in even these jobs seldom places a patient with nonradiating pain at any risk for permanent orthopedic or neurologic impairment, the pain related to job performance may outweigh the risk of becoming disabled by being put on restrictions. Work restrictions should be as specific as possible, and the patient should be an active participant in formulating realistic restrictions that address the patient's specific work situation (see Chapter 27). Communication with the employer regarding limited duties or hours may be helpful in keeping a patient at some level of work. Good communication with the employer may also facilitate better worker/supervisor relationships, a key factor in preventing long-term disability (11).

Patient Education

The role of patient education in acute nonradiating back pain may be very significant; however, the effectiveness of educational interventions, particularly between patient and physician, can be difficult to measure. In a study by Thomas, patients with a variety of problems without specific diagnosis improved more quickly when given a specific diagnosis, timeline, and positive reassurances than those given nonspecific answers and no prognostication (12). This would suggest that giving patients specific education and positive reassurance of the generally benign nature of most acute back pain may lead to more rapid recovery and better patient satisfaction. Studies showing better satisfaction among patients receiving chiropractic care (13) may be partly due to this phenomenon, as these patients are generally given very specific labels for their back problems. Difficulty arises in patients who do not have the expected resolution of their back pain. If they continue to be told that their pain should get better and it is not, they may develop mistrust, fear of misdiagnosis, and develop pain behaviors to "prove" their pain is legitimate.

Table 11-2   Educational Points

- Benign course of acute nonradiating back pain
- No evidence on history and physical examination of dangerous process or nerve damage
- Diagnostic testing not useful in acute stage
- Adverse effects of prolonged bed rest, and encouragement of return to usual activities
- Stress nonmedication pain management modalities
- Review risks and side effects of any prescribed medication
- If work restrictions are necessary, make restrictions specific and time limited

The literature is conflicting on the role and exact approach for education (and arguably there is no one approach appropriate for every patient and every physician). Common sense and experience suggests that good patient education can only help, if not with actual length of symptoms, at least with forging a good relationship between patient and physician. Education of the patient with acute nonradiating back pain should include expectation of quick resolution of back pain, methods of pain control, encouragement for resumption of normal activities within reason, the negative effects of prolonged bedrest, reassurances about the lack of red flags, instruction on simple exercises in the acute phase, and a general outline of other treatment measures if symptoms persist (Table 11-2). The latter may be helpful for those that ultimately proceed into the subacute or chronic phase. Other appropriate areas of education may also include rationale for not ordering diagnostic tests in the acute phase (especially if the patient presents with expectation for them), when such testing may be appropriate, and work issues, particularly for patients with physically demanding occupations.

Physical Therapy

If there is no improvement in symptoms within 2 weeks, it would be appropriate to consider referral to physical therapy. Specific therapeutic exercise and manual manipulation may be effective in speeding recovery and increasing patient satisfaction (13). In addition to specific exercises, the therapist can also introduce general back strengthening and aerobic conditioning exercises. The therapist has an important role in patient education. The use of passive modalities, such as ice, heat, ultrasound, and electrical stimulation, should be used on a very limited basis and not make up a significant portion of the therapeutic intervention. Being familiar with the local therapists and facilities is essential to ensure that the patient works with skilled physical therapists and thus optimizes his or her treatment. The therapist should provide detailed progress reports and be willing to confer when necessary on challenging patients. The more specifically written the therapy prescription, the more likely the appropriate treatment will be delivered.

Injections

Injections are not considered in most cases of acute nonradiating back pain. Toward the end of the acute phase or if a patient's problem is quite severe, some physicians may try injection treatment. There is a wide array of therapeutic injections available. Spinal injections, such as epidurals and facet joint injections, do not have a role in acute, nonradiating back pain (14). Injections to bursae, such as the trochanteric and ischial, may be indicated if supported by specific physical exam findings. Occasionally, sacroiliac joint injections may be used in the acute phase if a detailed examination suggests this joint to be the primary pain generator. In true axial low back pain, trigger point injections have been advocated by some. There may be a role for trigger point injections if appropriate trigger points are identified and the patient's pain is not improving after a few weeks. Typically, the patient should be engaged in physical therapy while receiving these injections, as active stretching of the injected area must occur to maximize the benefits of the injection (15,16).

Case Study 11-1

A 32-year-old woman, who works as an engineer, presents with complaint of 1-day history of back pain. She states she was raking leaves for most of the day. She bent over to pick up her 2-year-old son and felt a severe pain in the right low back that brought her to her knees. Her husband assisted her to the couch where she has pretty much stayed until presentation to her family physician. She denies any radiation of her pain into the buttocks or lower extremity. On physical examination, she appears in some distress, is unable to straighten fully to an upright position, and changes position on the table with difficulty. Acute spasm is noted in the paraspinal muscles, with nonradiating tenderness to palpation. Guarding is noted with movement. Neurologic examination is intact.

The patient is informed that she has no neurologic deficits and will likely note improvement in a few days. She is instructed to apply ice frequently and is given some gentle stretches to do. It is advised that bedrest be minimized and that the patient get up frequently to move about. Prescriptions are written for ibuprofen and cyclobenzaprine to take at night. Barring any side effects, it is recommended that the ibuprofen be taken on a regular basis for several days. She is advised to return to work, change positions frequently, and continue with periodic icing and stretching. No imaging studies are ordered.

At 2 weeks, follow-up exam reveals improved posture and less active muscle spasm, but there remains decreased range of motion and continued report of pain. Physical therapy is ordered, with emphasis on McKenzie exercises and manual mobilization. The patient has complete resolution of her symptoms within a month.

Case Study 11-2

A 35-year-old gentleman presents with 1-day history of back pain. He states it began after working. He recently began a new job in a small manufacturing facility making auto parts. His job entails moving parts weighing up to 75 pounds. When asked about opportunities for restricted duties, he states that his supervisor is not very accommodating and he does not get along well with him. The patient has a history of substance abuse, including illicit drug use, but denies current use. Physical examination demonstrates only guarding and hypertonicity of the lumbar paraspinal muscles and significant pain behavior. He has pain to very superficial palpation of the lumbar paraspinal muscles. Neurologic examination revealed giveway weakness.

The patient is educated on the natural history of back pain and advised to resume normal household activities. The patient is given a prescription for NSAIDs and is instructed on ice and stretching. Limited restrictions are recommended for work; however, the patient states he cannot return to work with any restrictions. This is confirmed by the employer. The patient is therefore kept off of work, and follow-up is arranged in 2 days. At that time, the patient states his pain is the same in spite of recommended measures for pain control. Cyclobenzaprine is added; narcotic medication is not used due to the patient's substance abuse history. At 1-week follow-up he continues to report the same level of pain, and significant pain behavior is noted. At 2 weeks, he is referred to physical therapy. When he makes minimal improvement with 2 weeks of therapy and remains disabled from work, he is referred to a local nonsurgical spine specialist for further management due to the number of yellow flags present.

This patient represents one with significant yellow flags for disability. These include poor job satisfaction, a physically demanding job, prior history of substance abuse, and physical exam findings of excessive pain behavior and Waddell signs. Without the yellow flags, one may have treated 4 to 6 weeks before referral to the specialist or multidisciplinary treatment team.

Follow-up

If the pain does not resolve, the patient should be seen in a week for follow-up, particularly if there are activity restrictions or risk factors for disability. If a patient is off work, it would be appropriate to see the patient in 2-3 days. Physical therapy may be initiated if there is no improvement in 1-2 weeks, emphasizing therapeutic exercise such as the McKenzie technique and manual therapy. Medications may be adjusted as appropriate. If there is no improvement in 4 weeks, plain radiographs may be considered. If pain and disability continues to 6 weeks, particularly in at-risk patients (e.g., those with severe pain or those with important Yellow Flags for chronic disability), consider referral to a nonsurgical spine specialist or a multidisciplinary spine rehabilitation program. Patients with Yellow Flags for risk of chronicity may require referral to a specialist sooner, within 4 weeks.

Conclusion

The bad news is that acute back pain is an extremely common problem seen by the primary care physician. The good news is that it is generally self-limiting and with a simple paradigm can be easily and effectively managed in a cost-effective manner. In the vast majority of cases, good patient education and reassurance is all that is required. Being able to identify early those who are at risk for progression to chronic pain and disability is a key to planning early intervention.

■   ■   ■

Recommendations

- At the initial visit, perform a detailed history and physical examination to evaluate for any red flags suggesting dangerous underlying disorders and for yellow flags suggesting risk for chronicity of pain.
- The first choice of medication is usually NSAIDs or acetaminophen.
- Muscle relaxants should be limited to short-term use. Narcotics should likewise be used only for the short term and on a time-based schedule rather than an as-needed schedule; they are not recommended for those with a history of substance abuse.
- During the initial visit, patient education should be emphasized.
- Activity limitation should be minimized, and return to normal activity should be encouraged.
- If pain does not resolve within 1 week, the patient should be seen for follow-up. If the patient is unable to work due to pain, he or she should be seen even sooner—within 2 to 3 days.
- If patient's pain is not resolving within 1 to 2 weeks, physical therapy should be initiated.

- If yellow flags are present and pain does not resolve within 4 weeks, the patient should be referred to a nonsurgical spine specialist or to multidisciplinary treatment.
- If there are no yellow flags but pain does not resolve within 6 weeks, the patient should be referred to a nonsurgical spine specialist or to multidisciplinary treatment.
- If there is no improvement in 4 weeks, plain radiographs may be considered.

Key Points

- Most episodes of acute back pain are self-limited.
- At initial presentation, a focused evaluation should be conducted to screen for any potentially serious causes and to identify patients who may be at higher risk to progress to chronic pain.
- Diagnostic testing is rarely indicated in acute nonradiating low back pain.
- Initial management consists of nonmedication modalities, limited use of medication, and early return to activity.
- Patient education may lead to faster recovery and better patient satisfaction.

REFERENCES

1. **Coste J, Delecoeuillerie G, Cohen de Lara A, Le Parc JM, Paolaggi JB.** Clinical course and prognostic factors in acute low back pain: an inception cohort study in primary care practice. BMJ. 1994;308:577-80.

2. **Deyo RA, Phillips WR.** Low back pain. A primary care challenge. Spine. 1996;21:2826-32.

3. **Haig AJ, Standiford C, Alvarez D, Graziano G, Harrison RV, Popadopoulos S, Tremper A.** Acute Low Back Pain. University of Michigan Health System Guidelines for Clinical Care. 1997, University of Michigan Health System; 1997. Update pending 2002. http://www.med.umich.edu/i/oca/practiceguides/back/back.pdf

4. **Waddell G, McCulloch JA, Kummel E, Venner RM.** Nonorganic physical signs in low back pain. Spine. 1980;5:117-25.

5. **Van Tulder MW, Assendelft WJ, Koes BW, Bouter LM.** Spinal radiographic findings and nonspecific low back pain. A systematic review of observational studies. Spine. 1997;22:427-34.

6. **Powell MC, Wilson M, Szypryt P, Symonds EM, Worthington BS.** Prevalence of lumbar disc degeneration observed by magnetic resonance in symptomless women. Lancet. 1986;2:1366-7.

7. **Atlas SJ, Deyo RA.** Evaluating and managing acute low back pain in the primary care setting. JGIM. 2001;16:120-31.

8. **Van Tulder MW, Koes BW, Bouter LM.** Conservative treatment of acute and chronic nonspecific low back pain. A systematic review of randomized controlled trials of the most common interventions. Spine. 1997;22:2128-56.

9. **Bradley JD, Brandt KD, Katz BP, Kalasinski LA, Ryan SI.** Comparison of an antiinflammatory dose of ibuprofen, and analgesic dose of ibuprofen, and acetaminophen in the treatment of patients with low back pain. N Engl J Med. 1991;325:87-91.

10. **Malmivaara A, Hakkinen U, Aro T, Heinrichs ML, Koskenniemi L, Kuosma E, Lappi S, et al.** The treatment of acute low back pain-bed rest, exercises, or ordinary activity? N Engl J Med. 1995;332:351-5.

11. **Deyo RA, Diehl AK.** Psychosocial predictors of disability in patients with low back pain. J Rheumatol. 1988;15:1557-64.

12. **Thomas KB.** General practice consultations: is there any point in being positive? Br Med J (Clin Res). 1987;294:1200-2.

13. **Cary TS, Garrett J, Jackman A, et al.** The outcomes and costs of care for acute low back pain among patients seen by primary care practitioners, chiropractors, and orthopedic surgeons. N Engl J Med. 1995;333:913-7.

14. **Bigos S, Bowyer O, Braen G, et al.** Acute Low Back Problems in Adults. Clinical Practice Guideline No. 14, AHCPR Publication No. 95-0642. Rockville, MD: Agency for Health Care Policy and Research, Public Health Service, U.S. Department of Health and Human Services; December 1994.

15. **Kraus H.** Clinical treatment of back and neck pain. New York: McGraw-Hill; 1970.

16. **Rachlin ES.** Myofascial Pain and Fibromyalgia: Trigger Point Management. St. Louis: Mosby; 1994:48.

12

■ ■ ■

Acute Radiating Low Back Pain

J. Steven Schultz, MD

A cute radiating low back pain (LBP), also referred to as sciatica, is a common problem encountered by the primary care physician. Strictly defined, sciatica is pain or paresthesia that radiates beyond the knee. It is important to remember that sciatica is a symptom, not a diagnosis, thus the underlying cause and pathophysiology must be understood to guide appropriate treatment. Approximately half of patients with acute radiating LBP are better within 6 weeks, and 86-96% will improve with nonoperative treatment (1,2). However, the resolution of pain does not guarantee that the underlying pathologic process has resolved. Inflammation related to disk herniation or biomechanical causes of impingement of the lateral recess can recur. Accordingly, rehabilitation of patients with acute sciatica should begin early and continue beyond symptom resolution. Such an approach significantly decreases the risk of recurrent episodes of LBP and minimizes the risk of chronic disability.

Etiology

The most common cause of radiating LBP in patients under the age of 60 is herniated nucleus pulposus (HNP). With HNP, the herniation compresses and inflames the spinal nerves. The lifetime incidence of developing HNP after age 35 is 5%. Ninety percent of symptomatic disk herniations occur at L4-L5 and L5-S1. Patients over the age of 60 are more likely to experience radiculopathy from degenerative lumbar stenosis. Aside from red flags, (cancer, infection, fracture), the other mechanical causes of radiating pain, such as spondylolisthesis and facet joint cyst, are uncommon and treated the same as disk herniation in the first weeks. Rarer causes, such as herpes zoster, and diabetic or vasculitic radiculitis, have atypical presentation.

Table 12-1   Frequency of Radiculopathy by Root Level

Root Level	Frequency
L2-3	1%
L4	4%
L5	47%
S1	49%

Reprinted with permission from Leonard J, Schultz J. Radiculopathy: a quality assurance review. Muscle Nerve. 1991;14:890.

Regardless of the structural cause, the vast majority of radiculopathies involve the L5 and S1 roots (Table 12-1).

Nerve root irritation occurs from compression within the neural canal and inflammation caused by release of biochemical mediators such as phospholipase A2 and cytokines from the nucleus pulposis (4,5). Anatomic factors that determine if an HNP will become symptomatic include the type of herniation (contained, extruded, or sequestered) and the capacity of the spinal canal.

Epidural hematoma and tumor are uncommon causes of radiculopathy. The differential diagnosis for unilateral radicular pain includes lumbosacral plexopathy, sciatic nerve injury, and peroneal and tibial neuropathy in the leg.

Case Study 12-1

A 61-year-old previously healthy male engineer developed sudden onset of low back and radiating left leg pain after a slip and fall. Over the next 2 days, his pain increased and he developed numbness and tingling into the left foot and great toe. He saw his primary care physician on day 5 at which time he stated his pain was exacerbated by sitting and alleviated by standing or lying supine. He denied bladder or bowel dysfunction and there were no constitutional symptoms. His examination at that time was normal except for diminished reflexes on the left. Ibuprofen and hydrocodone were prescribed. Magnetic resonance imaging (MRI) was also ordered at the initial visit, which demonstrated an HNP at L4-5 on the left with compression of the L5 root. At follow-up 2 weeks later, there was no improvement; he was referred for physical therapy, and consultation with a spine specialist was obtained.

By the time he was seen by the spine specialist on day 30, his pain was 95% better with mild residual numbness in the left foot. He had resumed all activities including work and golf. His examination demonstrated a depressed left medial hamstring reflex but otherwise was normal. He was advised to continue his home exercise and activities as tolerated. No other treatment was recommended.

Discussion

This case highlights two important aspects of acute HNP with radiculopathy: overuse of MRI and the highly favorable prognosis. This patient presented with stereotypic features of diskogenic back pain and L5 radiculopathy. There was no clinical suspicion of cauda equina lesion or dangerous pathology. Thus, obtaining an MRI at the initial visit was unnecessary, as it did not affect treatment or clinical decision making. This is consistent with studies demonstrating that up to 66% of advanced neurodiagnostic imaging studies obtained for LBP are inappropriate or unnecessary (10).

Clinical Features

The most consistent clinical feature of lumbosacral radiculopathy is the presence of leg pain of equal or greater severity than LBP. The nature of the pain may be highly variable, from painful dysesthesia to a dull ache. Other causes of LBP, such as facet arthropathy, sacroiliac dysfunction, or spondylolisthesis, produce predominantly axial back pain with radiation into the buttock and thigh but rarely below the knee. Patients with paracentral HNP typically complain of significant sitting intolerance, owing to the elevated intradiskal pressure associated with the flexed position. Additionally, these patients may complain of increased pain with bending, riding in a car, cough, valsalva, or donning shoes and socks. In contrast, patients with radiculopathy secondary to spinal stenosis or HNP into a stenotic neuroforamen are most symptomatic when standing, walking, or lying prone due narrowing of the neuroforamina that occurs upon extending the lumbar spine. Compression of nerve roots alone will produce paresthesias but not pain. It appears that there must also be inflammation of nerve tissue in order to experience radicular pain.

Diagnostic Tests

Unless there is a high index of suspicion of tumor, infection, or cauda equina lesion, diagnostic studies are not indicated in the first 4 weeks. The diagnosis of lumbar disk herniation and radiculopathy is based on clinical history and physical examination, and the results of diagnostic testing will not alter the initial management. If, however, there is no improvement after 4 weeks of treatment, then diagnostic studies should be performed to guide further treatment.

Radiographs

Plain radiographs are generally not helpful in the evaluation of patients with radiating LBP. Radiographs have a relatively low specificity and sensitivity, and their use as a routine screening study is not justified.

Magnetic Resonance Imaging

Magnetic resonance imaging (MRI) is the study of choice in the evaluation of lumbar spine disorders and should be the initial diagnostic test in patients with radiating LBP of at least 4 weeks duration (6). It is unsurpassed in its ability to delineate lesions involving soft tissue, disk, and the neural elements. The primary utility of MRI is to exclude serious pathology and define structural lesions amenable to interventional or surgical treatment. Thus, MRI should be obtained to guide medical decision-making rather than simply to confirm the diagnosis of HNP. The incidence of asymptomatic disk protrusion on MRI is 30-40% (7). MRI can also miss up to 10% of clinically relevant low lumbar disks and up to 50% of surgically proven high lumbar disk herniations. Consequently, the findings on imaging studies must be interpreted in the context of the clinical picture.

Electromyography

Electromyography (EMG) is unique in its ability to determine the physiologic significance of structural lesions found on imaging studies. It is not helpful in the initial evaluation of patients with radiating LBP, as the full spectrum of electrodiagnostic abnormalities is not evident until symptoms have been present for at least 3 weeks. Electrodiagnostic evaluation should be performed in patients with greater than 4 weeks of radiating LBP unresponsive to treatment and in whom MRI is nondiagnostic or does not correlate with the clinical findings. EMG has a very low false positive rate and can differentiate root lesions from other neurologic conditions that can masquerade as lumbosacral radiculopathy, such as plexopathy, sciatic nerve injury, or peroneal neuropathy at the knee. Moreover, EMG can determine the severity of axon loss and access for reinnervation, thereby assisting in medical decision-making and prognosis.

CT/CT Myelography

The advent of MRI has relegated computerized tomography (CT) to a secondary role in the evaluation of patients with suspected radiculopathy. CT may be helpful in patients with radiculopathy from bony canal stenosis and when MRI is contraindicated, such as in patients with retained metal fragments or severe claustrophobia. Myelography has largely been supplanted by MRI as well. One advantage myelography has over MRI is its ability to assess dynamic lesions in the lumbar spine (6), however, the diagnostic yield must be weighed against the invasive nature of the procedure and associated morbidity. CT myelography is more accurate than MRI in assessing the severity of spinal stenosis, although MRI can detect the presence of stenosis as well. CT myelography is occasionally used by spine surgeons as an adjunctive study in selected patients to assist in presurgical planning.

Case Study 12-2

A 31-year-old healthy female was referred to a spine center with a 4-week history of low back and right leg pain with paresthesias in the foot. There was no history of bladder or bowel involvement. She was employed as an administrative assistant and had been off work since the onset of pain. Her examination demonstrated positive seated and supine straight leg raise on the right. Strength, sensation, and reflexes were normal. Diagnostic impression was diskogenic pain and right L5 radiculopathy.

Rofecoxib, hydrocortisone, nortriptyline, and physical therapy were prescribed. She noted worsening radicular symptoms after 4 weeks of treatment and an MRI was obtained, demonstrating a paracentral HNP at L4-5. She underwent a right L5-S1 transforaminal epidural steroid injection that resulted in dramatic pain relief. She continued with physical therapy and had complete resolution of symptoms by 8 weeks.

Discussion

This case illustrates the efficacy of epidural steroid injections in shortening the pain control phase of treatment. She had disabling leg pain after 4 weeks of treatment and her progress in physical therapy was limited. The findings on MRI were used to plan appropriate interventional treatment. Improvement in radicular symptoms facilitated participation in an active therapy program and subsequently led to recovery.

Treatment

The cornerstones of treatment of the patient with radicular LBP are early intervention, relative rest, medications, and an active exercise program. Patients often have an expectation that an MRI or other diagnostic test is necessary at the initial visit. It is therefore important for the clinician to educate the patient that, based on his or her clinical presentation, the most likely diagnosis is HNP and the results of diagnostic studies will not alter the initial management. Reassurance regarding the favorable prognosis is also provided. Treatment is divided into the pain control phase, exercise phase, and maintenance phase.

Pain Control Phase

The pain control phase is initiated as early as possible to allow efficient progression to the more active and participatory exercise phase. Treatment begins with the prescription of relative rest and activity modification. Short periods of bed rest are occasionally necessary in severe cases but should not exceed 3 days (8). Patients are instructed to rest in a position of comfort and apply ice or heat to control muscle spasm. Extension exercises, such as prone press-ups, may be helpful in alleviating pain by decreasing dural tension. Exacerbation of leg pain with extension suggests the presence of spinal stenosis or disk extrusion into the neuroforamen; in this case, extension exercises should be abandoned. Pelvic traction, ultrasound, massage, and transcutaneous electrical stimulation are often used in the pain control stage of treatment. Time off work is minimized to reduce the risk of chronic disability. Contrary to popular belief, the rare progression to cauda equina syndrome has not been associated with increased activity once a disk herniation has occurred. It is preferable to impose specific activity restrictions, thereby allowing the employer opportunity to find modified work for the patient (Table 12-2). Work restrictions should be time-limited and liberalized as recovery progresses.

Nonsteroidal anti-inflammatory drugs (NSAIDs) are used in this phase to control pain and chemically mediated inflammation. These provide adequate analgesia in the majority of patients and should be considered as a first-line drug. No studies have demonstrated the efficacy of one NSAID over another in acute radiculopathy. Thus, the decision about which drug to prescribe is based on prior experience, side-effect profile, and cost. NSAIDs are prescribed on a time-contingent basis and in sufficient doses to achieve an anti-inflammatory effect. For patients with severe pain, narcotic analgesics are appropriate. The risk of addiction and abuse of these medications is low in patients with a defined pathoanatomic source of pain. Muscle relaxants should be used sparingly. All are central nervous system depressants and have no direct effect on muscle tone.

Cyclobenzaprine has tricyclic properties and is often beneficial for sleep restoration, although long-term use is discouraged. Antidepressants, such as amitriptyline, doxepin, and trazodone are also used in patients with disturbed sleep and may alleviate neuropathic pain (see also Chapter 29). The rationale for oral corticosteroids in the treatment of acute radiculopathy is well established (4,5). These medications have proved successful in many patients; however, the optimal dose and duration of administration are not clear. There has never been a controlled trial comparing injection of

---

Table 12-2   Common Short-Term Work Restrictions In Patients with HNP*

- No lifting more than 20 pounds
- No repetitive bending
- No repetitive twisting
- No stooping
- Sit-stand at will

* Must be individualized for each patient based on pain tolerance and specific job demands.

cortisone into the epidural space with oral steroid use, but it is the impression of many clinicians that oral steroids are less effective, and the potential for side effects is greater.

If the patient has not had sufficient relief of pain to participate in an active exercise program after 4 weeks of treatment, then an MRI should be obtained. Appropriate interventional treatment with epidural steroid injections can then be tailored to the specific type and level of HNP. Epidural steroids are used to shorten the pain control phase and such administration is performed as an adjunct to comprehensive treatment, rather than in isolation. They are most effective in alleviating leg pain in patients with dural tension signs on physical examination. Epidural steroid injections should be performed by an experienced practitioner under fluoroscopic guidance to insure accurate localization and delivery of medication.

Exercise Phase

Once adequate pain control is achieved, physical therapy is prescribed, and the emphasis changes to restoring proper biomechanics and increasing flexibility and strength of musculoligamentous structures. McKenzie exercises, commonly thought of as "extension" exercises, are often employed in an effort to centralize the pain, although there is no scientific evidence that these cause migration of nuclear material. Stretching and conditioning of large muscle groups is emphasized, especially the paraspinals, iliopsoas, hamstrings, hip rotators, and quadriceps. A dynamic stabilization program is undertaken to minimize further microtrauma to the motion segment and potentially slow the degenerative cascade (9). This is accomplished through strengthening of the spinal extensor group and abdominal musculature. When progress plateaus, formal therapy is discontinued and the patient continues with an independent home exercise program. Activity and work restrictions are liberalized accordingly.

Maintenance Phase

In the maintenance phase, patients are encouraged to assume responsibility for their own back care. The importance of continuing a home exercise program on a long-term basis is emphasized. Back school, instruction in proper body mechanics, and workplace redesign decrease recurrence in industrial settings. Smoking cessation is also recommended, as there appears to be a dose-response relationship between smoking and HNP.

When to Refer

Depending on the comfort level of the individual practitioner, acute lumbar radiculopathy can be successfully managed by the primary care physician. Failure of the patient to progress at any stage (e.g., no change in pain or disability over the course of 2 weeks or more) should prompt a referral to a spine specialist to plan appropriate interventional procedures, guide rehabilitative efforts, and manage disability. Patients with cauda equina lesions or progressive weakness require prompt surgical consultation; however, static motor deficits can be managed nonoperatively (2). Additionally, surgical management is appropriate in patients with clearly defined structural pathology who have failed at least 2 months of aggressive rehabilitation, including medications, physical therapy, and epidural steroid injections. In some patients with severe, debilitating pain, operative intervention is undertaken earlier.

Recommendations

- Pain control should be initiated as soon as possible. Relative rest, extension exercises, and analgesics such as NSAIDs should be employed during this early phase of treatment.
- For patients with severe pain, pain control may necessitate narcotic analgesics and short periods of bedrest (not to exceed 3 days).
- For patients with severe pain and dural tension signs, a burst prednisone 60 mg daily for 5 days may be considered.
- When pain control has been achieved, physical therapy and an attendant exercise program should be started.
- Once progress plateaus, physical therapy is discontinued and the patient should be encouraged to assume responsibility for his or her own back care. Activity and work restrictions should be modified to reflect the improvement.
- If the patient has not had at least a 50% reduction in pain after 4 weeks, MRI should be performed and referral to a spine specialist considered.
- If the MRI confirms the diagnosis of HNP, then a trial of epidural steroids is recommended.
- If MRI is nondiagnostic, electrodiagnostic studies should be done to exclude other neurologic conditions that mimic radiculopathy.
- Patients with a progressive motor deficit or intractable leg pain after 2 months of nonoperative care should be referred for surgical evaluation.

Key Points

- Radiating LBP is usually due to HNP resulting in L5 or S1 radiculopathy.
- Diagnostic studies are rarely indicated in the initial 4 weeks.

- MRI is the study of choice in the evaluation of patients with radiating LBP. MRI should be used to rule out serious disease and to define structural lesions that are amenable to treatment and should not be used solely to confirm a diagnosis of HNP.
- The vast majority of patients with acute HNP recover with nonoperative treatment. Such treatment consists of relative rest, medications, and an exercise program.
- Surgical consultation is indicated for patients with cauda equina lesions, progressive weakness, and failure of nonoperative care

■   ■   ■

REFERENCES

1. **Bush K, Cowan N, Katz D, Gishen P.** The natural history of sciatica associated with disc pathology: a prospective study with clinical and independent radiologic follow-up. Spine. 1992;17:1205-12.
2. **Saal JS, Franson RC, Dobrow R, Saal JA, White AH, Goldthwaite N.** The natural history of lumbar intervertebral disk extrusions treated nonoperatively. Spine. 1990;15:683-6.
3. **Leonard J, Schultz J.** Radiculopathy: a quality assurance review. Muscle Nerve. 1991;14:890.
4. **Saal JS, Transon R, Dobrow R, et al.** High levels of inflammatory phospholipase A2 activity in lumbar disc herniations. Spine. 1990;15:674-8.
5. **Gordon S, Weinstein J.** A review of basic science issues in low back pain. Phys Med Rehabil Clin North Am. 1998;9(2):323-42.
6. **Mink JH, Deutsch AL, Goldstein TB, Bray R, Pashman R, Armstrong II, et al.** Spinal imaging and intervention: 1998. Phys Med Rehabil Clin North Am. 1998;9(2):343-80.
7. **Jensen MC, Brant-Zawadzki MN, Obuchowski N, Modic MT, Malkasian D, Ross JS.** Magnetic resonance imaging of the lumbar spine in people without back pain. N Engl J Med. 1994;331:69-73.
8. **Deyo R, Diehl A, Rosenthal M.** How many days of bedrest for acute low back pain? A randomized clinical trial. N Engl J Med. 1986;315:1064-70.
9. **Saal JA.** Dynamic muscular stabilization in the nonoperative treatment of lumbar pain syndromes. Orthop Rev. 1990;19:691-700.
10. **Schroth WS, Schectman JM, Elinsky EG, Panagides JC.** Utilization of medical services for the treatment of acute low back pain: Conformance with clinical guidelines. J Gen Intern Med. 1992;7:486-91.

■   ■   ■

KEY REFERENCES

Andersson GB, Brown MD, Dvorak J, Herzog RJ, Kambin P, Malter A, et al. Consensus summary on the diagnosis and treatment of lumbar disc herniation. Spine. 1996;24S:75S-78S.

Bogduk N. Clinical Anatomy of the Lumbar Spine and Sacrum, 3rd ed. Edinburgh: Churchill Livingstone; 1997.

A comprehensive review of functional anatomy, biomechanics, and pathophysiology of lumbar spine disorders.

Weber H. Lumbar disc herniation: a controlled prospective study with ten years of observation. Spine. 1983;8:131-40.

Volvo award-winning study demonstrating no difference in long-term outcome between surgically and nonsurgically treated patients with HNP.

13

■ ■ ■

Medications for the Management of Acute and Subacute Back Pain and Medications for Injection Techniques

Nancy E. Wirth, MD

Medications are often used for treatment of pain, even though many patients treated for pain do not have a specific pathoanatomic diagnosis (1). The symptoms that are treated by these medications, without necessarily affecting the anatomic lesion, include inflammation, muscle spasm, and central pain perception. This chapter will provide a succinct review of the literature, pharmacology, and dosing of the most commonly used medications for the treatment of acute and subacute back pain.

There is controversy over which medication regimen works best. One recent study of initial visit prescription of medication for back pain in primary care showed that 69% of patients were given nonsteroidal anti-inflammatory drugs (NSAIDs), most commonly ibuprofen, 35% muscle relaxants, and 12% narcotics. Those who received medications reported less severe symptoms at follow-up than those who did not receive medication. A regimen in which two medications were prescribed (as opposed to single-drug therapy) was used in 34% of patients based on the nature and severity of the pain and impaired functioning. In this study, the best outcomes were noted with a combination of NSAIDs and a muscle relaxant (2). However, other studies did not find this combination to be more effective than single-drug therapy (3). Drug therapy on a scheduled basis, rather than as needed, is believed to result in improved symptom relief (4).

The Agency for Health Care Policy and Research has issued medication guidelines for patients with acute low back pain (5,6). Initially, acetaminophen or an NSAID is recommended. A time-limited prescription of narcotics (less than 2 weeks) and/or muscle relaxants is optional. The agency recommended against opioids for greater than 2 weeks and also recommended not using phenylbutazone, oral steroids, colchicine, and antidepressants.

Medications for Management of Acute and Subacute Back Pain

Nonsteroidal Anti-Inflammatory Drugs

Most nonsteroidal anti-inflammatory drugs (NSAIDs) are effective against mild to moderate pain, and all, with the exception of acetaminophen, provide some degree of anti-inflammatory action. Unlike opioids, they change only pain perception and not other sensory modalities.

Mechanism of Action

The best-known mechanism of action of NSAIDs is inhibition of prostaglandin (PG) synthesis (7). Fatty acid cyclooxygenase (COX) catalyzes the synthesis of prostaglandins from arachadonic acid. First formed is PGG2, which is unstable, then PGH2. Isomerases, which vary depending on the tissue type, convert PGH2 to PGD2, PGI2, PGE2, and PGI2 alpha. The biological effects of prostaglandins depend on the tissue type and amount of PG produced. NSAIDs share as a mechanism the inhibition of COX catalysis. There are two isoenzymes of COX. COX-1 maintains physiologic functions including the gastrointestinal (GI) mucosal barrier, renal hemodynamics, and platelet aggregation. COX-1 is also found in T cells, as well as most normal tissues and cells (5). COX-2 is constitutionally present in the brain, endothelial cells of arteries, veins, and intraglomerular podocytes. Some of its functions include assisting with the renal regulation of sodium, response to water deprivation, and spinal cord response to pain. COX-2 also occurs in macrophages and monocytes and is rapidly upregulated in inflammatory processes, with a 10- to 80-fold increase in stimulation of monocytes, synovial cells, and fibroblasts (1). Once prostaglandins are formed, NSAIDs do not affect the pain caused by direct action of PGs, but rather act via the indirect mechanism of inhibition of synthesis of further prostaglandins. NSAIDs may also have other mechanisms of pain relief, such as a role in the inhibition of certain types of endothelial activation that leads to leukocyte adhesion during an inflammatory reaction.

Side Effects, Toxicity, and Contraindications

NSAID side effects and toxicity occur usually because of COX-1 inhibition in the kidneys, stomach, and platelets (7). Gastrointestinal side effects are also secondary to the molecular structure of NSAIDs, which are weak organic acids that can cause a back diffusion of acid into the mucosa, resulting in mucosal breaks. Inhibition of COX-1 in the kidneys leads to vasoconstriction and renal insufficiency in some patients, usually those with reduced intravascular volume (5). Preferential or selective COX-2 inhibitors, including nabumetone, etololac, and meloxicam, are not free of gastrointestinal side effects, and at anti-inflammatory dosages tend to lose their specificity. Literature tends to support that the specific COX-2 inhibitors, celecoxib and rofecoxib, may have fewer GI side effects compared with other NSAIDs, but there has certainly been serious GI bleeding reportedly associated with the drugs (8-10).* When side effects of NSAIDs occur, it tends to be within the first week of therapy. Although there are numerous potential side effects to NSAIDs, contraindications, aside from allergy, are relative. Celecoxib* has a cross-reactivity to sulfa drug allergy. NSAIDs typically should not be used with coumadin or heparin treatment, severe bleeding disorders, or in persons with active GI ulcer disease. Certain NSAIDS are renal toxic or hepatotoxic, making their use undesirable in persons with severe liver or kidney disease.

Efficacy

An extensive review of studies using oral NSAIDs for treatment of back pain symptoms showed somewhat mixed results in terms of comparison of NSAIDs over simple analgesics, such as acetaminophen (3,4). NSAIDs are believed to be superior to placebo. There did not appear to be a significant advantage, in terms of pain relief, of one particular NSAID over another; all appeared to be about equal in effectiveness. One study found that for severe acute pain, a single IM dose of ketorolac had the same efficacy as a single IM dose of meperidine, but with fewer side effects than meperidine (5). A study comparing acetaminophen-codeine versus oral ketorolac showed similar results (6). NSAIDs are found to be less effective for radicular pain than when used for musculoskeletal pain.

Dosage and General Recommendations

There are currently many NSAIDs from which to choose (a representative sampling is included in Table 13-1). There can be a wide variation of response between individuals to a particular NSAID (7). Therefore, if one agent does not give benefit, another drug should be tried. It is not necessary to change chemical families. Combination therapy with a second NSAID does not give additional relief and is best avoided. It is often useful to begin with salsalate or acetaminophen, then progress to nonacetylated

---

* N.B. See footnote to Table 13-1.

Table 13-1   Medications for Low Back Pain (Nonradiating and Radiating)

Class	NSAID Generic Name	Brand Name	Typical Oral Dose (mg)	Comments
Carbolic acids	Aspirin	Multiple	325-650 TID-QID	Tinnitus, salicylism
	Salsalate	Disalcid	1500 BID	Lower GI effect/ renal risk
	Choline magnesium trisalicylate	Trilisate, Tricosal	1500 BID	Lower GI effect/ renal risk
	Diflunisal	Dolobid	500-1000 followed by 250-500 BID-TID	Lower GI effect/ renal risk
Acetic acids	Diclofenac	Cataflam, Voltaren	100-200/24 h, in divided doses	Greater risk for liver disease
	Etodolac	Lodine	200-400 q 6-8 h, maximum 1000/24 h	Low GI effect
	Indomethacin	Indocin	Starting 25-50, up to 50 TID	Risk of headaches Avoid in renal disease
	Sulindac	Clinoril	150-200 BID	
	Tolmetin	Tolectin	400 TID	
	Ketorolac	Toradol Acular	10 QID (see text)	
Proprionic acids	Ibuprofen	Advil, Motrin, Nuprin	400 q 4-6 h, max. 3200/24 h	Aseptic meningitis
	Fenoprofen	Nalfon	600 TID	
	Flurbiprofen	Ansaid	200-300/day in divided doses	
	Ketoprofen	Orudis	75 TID	
	Naproxen	Naprosyn, Anaprox	250-500 BID	Avoid in renal disease
	Oxaprozin	Daypro	1200 q AM	
Enolic acids (Oxicams)	Piroxicam	Feldene	20 q D or 10 BID	Peak concentrations after 2 weeks therapy
Naphthylkanones	Nabumetone	Relafen	1000 q D	Low gastric irritation (comparable to using Etodolac)
Diaryl substituted furanone	Rofecoxib*	Vioxx*	12.5 up to 50 q D	Does not inhibit platelets
Diaryl substituted pyrazole	Celecoxib*	Celebrex*	400 initial, then 200 BID	Does not inhibit platelets

* There is ongoing controversy concerning potential cardiovascular side effects of the COX-2 inhibitors. Do not prescribe unless deemed safe by the latest safety, efficacy, and prescribing data bulletins from the governmental review boards and pharmaceutical reports. *Editor's Note:* Vioxx was withdrawn by its manufacturer from the U.S. and worldwide markets in November 2004.

salicylates or ibuprofen at the lowest anti-inflammatory dose, with increases in the dosage based on clinical response. Maximum anti-inflammatory doses are typically reached at about 2 weeks, and initial prescriptions should be limited to that time (4). For cost containment, if more than one NSAID works, the least costly should be chosen. The dosages and information shown in Table 13-1 are considered general recommendations, and as with any medication, a dosage should be individualized to the lowest effective dose.

Salicylates

Salicylates are commonly prescribed. This group of drugs includes aspirin, salsalate (Disalcid), choline salicylate (Arthropan), magnesium salicylate (Magan), diflunisal (Dolobid), and choline and magnesium salicylate combined (Trilisate). Peak levels occur at about 1 hour after oral ingestion.

Aspirin modifies COX-1 and -2 irreversibly; therefore, the duration of action is dependent on the turnover rate of cyclooxygenase in the various tissues and cells. If renal impairment is present or at risk, salsalate (Disalcid) is the least expensive, relatively renal sparing agent. They can stimulate nausea and vomiting centrally and tend to stimulate respiration, as well as cause acid-base changes (7). Toxic doses of most of these drugs results in salicylism. They can cause hepatic injury, usually when given in high doses, and should be used cautiously in the presence of liver disease. In those with aspirin sensitivity and asthma, generally they react when other NSAIDs are given. Nonacetylated salicylates and acetaminophen may be less likely to produce the reaction. A recent study showed that rofecoxib (Vioxx)* may be safe to give in aspirin-sensitive patients (11). Diflunisal (Dolobid), when compared to aspirin, is more potent, has no auditory side effects, and fewer GI effects.

Indole and Indene Acetic Acid Derivatives

Indole and indene acetic acid derivatives include indomethacin, sulindac, and etodolac (7). Indomethacin (Indocin) usage is often limited by side effects. It is an effective anti-inflammatory and analgesic, with 10-40 times the potency of aspirin. Twenty percent of patients discontinue usage because of side effects, including gastrointestinal and CNS; the most common CNS side effect is severe headache. Sulindac (Clinoril) is a prodrug; its sulfide metabolite is 500 times more potent than sulindac. There is a high rate of GI toxicity. It has a somewhat renal-sparing effect that is dose dependent. Etidolac (Lodine) is now available in a sustained-release form that can be given once daily. It has relatively low gastric toxicity when compared with nonselective COX inhibitors.

Heteroaryl- and Phenyl-Acetic Acid Derivatives

Tolmentin (Tolectin) achieves a peak plasma concentration at 20-60 minutes (7). It is given in divided doses, with a maximum dose of 2 g/day. Ketorolac (Toradol) has a high analgesic effect, with only moderate anti-inflammatory action. It can be used both orally and parenterally and can be as effective as opioids (12,13). Oral dosage ranges from 5 to 20 mg/dose, with a 24-hour limit of 40 mg, and is intended for a 5-day maximum use because of high

---

* N.B. See footnote to Table 13-1.

GI toxicity, which is present even with parenteral injections. Diclofenac (Cataflam, Voltarin) is a potent anti-inflammatory agent available in intermediate-, delayed-, and extended-release forms. It can cause elevated aminotransferase levels, which are usually reversible. Aminotransferase levels should be monitored in the first 8 weeks of therapy.

Propionic Acid Derivatives
Ibuprofen (Motrin, Advil, Nuprin) was the first member of this group (7). Naproxen (Naprosyn, Anaprox) has a 14-hour half-life, which can double in the geriatric population. Ketoprofen (Orudis) is another commonly used drug in this class. It can cause elevations in creatinine and fluid retention, most commonly in the elderly. Oxaprozin (Daypro) is administered once daily, an advantage if compliance with taking multiple doses is an issue.

Oxicams
Piroxicam (Feldene) is an effective anti-inflammatory agent in the enolic acid family with analgesic properties (7). It has a long half-life of 50 hours. Because of the long half-life, it does not reach a maximal therapeutic effect until about 2 weeks, making it not as useful for acute pain as other drugs. Nambumetone (Relafen) is a prodrug, which is converted in the liver to its active metabolite. It is sometimes tolerated better than other NSAIDs.

Selective COX-2 Inhibitors (Coxibs)
This is the newest category of NSAIDs. These drugs have fewer gastrointestinal side effects than other NSAIDs (8-10). Selective COX-2 inhibitors decrease endothelial prostaglandin production without a concomitant inhibition of platelet thromboxane production, which may predispose to thrombosis. These medications do not provide improved pain relief when compared with other NSAIDs. Rofecoxib (Vioxx)* is a diaryl-substituted furanone that has a half-life of about 17 hours. There is no alteration of plasma levels in the presence of renal insufficiency, but it can cause hypertension and fluid retention in these patients (7). Celecoxib (Celebrex) is another selective COX-2 inhibitor and is a diaryl-substituted pyrazole. In renal insufficiency, plasma levels will be significantly lower than in those with normal renal function. However, in hepatic dysfunction, the plasma concentration may be increased up to 180%. Celecoxib should not be given to patients with a known allergy to sulfonamides (14).*

Aminophenol Derivatives
Acetaminophen, a p-aminophenol derivative, is an analgesic that is available as an over-the-counter product or in combination with various narcotic

---

* N.B. See footnote to Table 13-1.

agents. There are few reported studies using trials of acetaminophen alone for back pain, although it is commonly recommended (4). It has fewer side effects than NSAIDs, and its analgesic properties are similar to aspirin (7). However, acetaminophen has only very weak anti-inflammatory action. Peak serum levels are reached about 30-60 minutes after ingestion. A single dose ranges from 325 to 1000 mg, with a recommended 24-hour limit of 4 g. Hepatotoxicity is the main toxic effect, generally at high dosages. Alcoholics may suffer hepatotoxicity, even when within the therapeutic range of dosing.

Opioid Analgesics

Opioid analgesics are most typically prescribed when the patient presents with symptoms of acute severe or intractable pain. All opioids, with the exception of tramadol, are controlled substances.

Mechanism of Action

Several opioid receptor isoforms have been found, with the most well-known being mu, delta, and kappa (15). Most of the clinically used opioids are relatively selective for mu receptors, which is where their effects are demonstrated. Mu receptor agonists all have analgesic action. Stimulation of mu opioid receptors results in a number of effects, including analgesia, mood changes, and changes in cardiovascular and gastrointestinal systems. Delta agonists do not cross the blood-brain barrier and are not clinically useful as oral medications. Kappa receptor agonists can produce analgesia or be anti-analgesic, with less respiratory inhibition but more dysphoria and psychomimetic effects. Mixed agonist-antagonist drugs have been shown to produce the same degree of side effects as agonist drugs and may have a ceiling effect on the amount of analgesia produced. Opioids work best for patients with noiciceptive pain, rather than neuropathic pain, as they act to inhibit the transmission of nociceptive signals from the spinal cord and activate descending pain control circuits in the midbrain.

Side Effects and Toxicity

Side effects include euphoria, tranquility, dose-dependent respiratory depression, orthostatic hypotension, increase in the external urethral sphincter tone, increased bladder volume, inhibition of the voiding reflex, nausea, vomiting, and dizziness. Gastrointestinal effects include prolongation of gastric emptying time, slowing of peristalsis and digestion in the large and small intestines, and increased anal sphincter tone, all leading to severe constipation. In patients with coronary artery disease, a decrease in oxygen consumption, left ventricular end-diastolic pressure, and cardiac work is seen.

Precautions and Contraindications

Opioids should be used with caution for patients with coronary artery disease, cor pulmonale, and liver disease (15). In the presence of renal disease, be aware that the half-life of the active metabolites increases and may result in toxicity. The depressant effects of opioids may be prolonged and increased by tricyclic antidepressants, monoamine oxidase (MAO) inhibitors, and phenothiazines. Antihistamines, tricyclics, and some phenothiazines enhance the analgesic effects of opioids. Severe reactions can occur with giving meperidine or tramadol to patients taking MAO inhibitors.

Absorption, Distribution, and Excretion

Most opioids are well absorbed from the GI tract and have varying degrees of hepatic metabolism via a first-pass effect (15). In the presence of liver disease, plasma levels of opioids may be markedly increased. Opioids and their metabolites are excreted by glomerular filtration.

Efficacy

Opioids are effective in the management of acute back pain, but at typically prescribed doses are not clearly better than NSAIDs. Side effects are common in short-term use. They have not been shown to change the prognosis or speed return to function.

Dosage and General Recommendations

Opioids should be used occasionally for acute pain, for instance if NSAIDs and physical interventions do not suffiently relieve the pain or if the initial presentation is of excruciating pain. Except in extreme circumstances (e.g., a patient awaiting surgery), they should be discontinued after a few weeks at the latest. In subacute pain, initiation of opioid treatment should be done cautiously for worsening pain, with an end point in mind (e.g., an injection, surgery, physical therapy, or healing of a fracture) but may be appropriate occasionally. Table 13-2 provides recommended dosages of the more commonly prescribed opiods for acute and subacute pain. It is recommended that prescriptions be written as time limited, usually for 1 to 2 weeks (4). Additive or synergistic effects can be seen if they are given along with an NSAID or acetaminophen, thus reducing the dosage and side effects of the opioid (15). The most consistent analgesic levels are provided with scheduled dosing. Information on more regulated narcotics (U.S. Drug Enforcement Agency schedule II narcotics) is detailed in Chapter 29.

Codeine

Codeine has less first-pass metabolism by the liver, with excretion of inactive metabolites by the kidneys (15). It is converted to morphine in vivo. The half-life in plasma is 2-4 hours. Ten percent of the white population has the inability to convert codeine to morphine. Thirty milligrams of codeine is equivalent to 325-600 mg aspirin. If the two are combined (or codeine with acetaminophen), the effects can be synergistic.

Table 13-2   Commonly Used Opioids for Acute and Subacute Back Pain

Drug Name	Trade Name	Typical Dosage (mg)
Codeine	Various, with or without acetaminophen	15-60 codeine, max. 360/24 h (max. acetaminophen 4000/24 h)
Meperidine	Demerol	50-100 orally every 3-4 h (see text; *not* for long-term use)
Propoxyphene hydrochloride	Darvon (65 mg) Darvon Compound 65 (65 mg + 389 mg ASA + 32 mg caffeine)	65 propoxyphene HCl q 4 h, max. 390/24 h
Propoxyphene napsylate	Darvon N (100 mg) Darvocet N 50 (50 mg + 325 mg acetaminophen) Darvocet N 100 (100 mg + 650 mg acetaminophen)	100 napsylate q 4 h, max. 600/24 h
Tramadol	Ultram (50 mg)	50-100 q 4-6 h, max. 12 tabs/24 h
	Ultracet (37.5 mg + 325 mg acetaminophen)	2 tabs q 4-6 h, max. 8 tabs/24 h
Hydrocodone	Vicodin (5 mg + 500 mg acetaminophen)	1-2 tabs q 4-6 h, max. 8 tabs/24 h
	Vicodin ES (7.5 mg + 750 mg acetaminophen)	1 tab q 4-6 h, max. 5 tabs/24 h
	Vicodin HP (10 mg + 660 mg acetaminophen)	1 tab q 4-6 h, max. 6 tabs/24 h
	Vicoprofen (7.5 mg + 200 mg ibuprofen)	1 tab q 4-6 h, max. 5 tabs/24 h

Meperidine

Meperidine (Demerol) has actions similar to morphine but with less constipation (15). Peak concentrations are seen at 1-2 hours with oral administration. With liver disease, the bioavailability rises from 50% to 80%. Prolonged dosing can result in accumulation of the CNS toxic metabolite, normeperidine, which excites the CNS; therefore, it is not the drug of choice for oral dosing. It can be given parenterally to the patient with severe acute pain.

Propoxyphene Hydrochloride or Napsylate

Propoxyphene hydrochloride (Darvon) or napsylate (Darvon-N, Darvocet-N) is an opioid similar in side-effect profile to codeine but with less mu opioid receptor selectivity (15). Propoxyphene is one half to two thirds as potent as codeine. Combining propoxyphene with aspirin or acetaminophen produces enhanced analgesia. Peak plasma levels are reached at 1-2 hours, with a half-life of 6-12 hours, with the half-life of its metabolite, norpropoxyphene, of 30 hours.

Tramadol

Tramadol (Ultram) is a fairly recently developed synthetic codeine analog that acts centrally to inhibit the reuptake of norepinephrine and serotonin as well as having weak agonist binding activity to mu opioid receptors (16-18). It has been shown to provide some relief of back pain versus placebo and when compared to NSAIDS. The potency is 1/5 to 1/20 that of morphine. It is 95-100% orally absorbed, with 30% first-pass metabolism. Peak concentrations are found at 2 hours. However, there is a high rate of discontinuance because of side effects, most commonly nausea, vomiting, dizziness, lightheadedness, headache, and somnolence. One advantage is that tramadol has little effect on respiration. Abrupt stoppage of tramadol may result in withdrawal symptoms (19). Analgesia begins at 1 hour after the dose, peaks at 2 to 3 hours, with the duration of analgesia being about 6 hours.

Hydrocodone Bitartrate

Hydrocodone bitartrate is a semisynthetic hydrogenated-ketone derivative of codeine (10). It has analgesic and antitussive effects, with actions qualitatively similar to codeine. It is found in preparations with aspirin, acetaminophen, and ibuprofen.

Muscle Relaxants

These drugs act centrally and are used for acute muscular spasms, such as those caused by local trauma or inflammation. The mechanism of action of many of these agents is not known. There may be blocking of spinal or supraspinal interneurons and/or a sedative effect leading to muscle relaxation (20). All of these medications may impair physical and mental abilities for tasks requiring concentration or physical coordination secondary to their sedation properties. Side-effect profiles are common and include sedation, nausea, dizziness, lightheadness, and anticholengeric effects (21). Table 13-3 gives recommended dosages of several agents.

Cyclobenzaprine (Flexeril), which is chemically related to the tricyclic antidepressants, is a commonly used muscle relaxant that is active at the brainstem reticular formation and the spinal cord (20). There have been studies reporting that when spasm is a clear factor in acute back pain, the combination of an analgesic, plus cyclobenzaprine, showed modest superiority in pain relief when compared to taking the analgesic or cyclobenzaprine alone (22,23). There is a high incidence of side effects, with drowsiness being reported most commonly, as well as dry mouth. It has anticholinergic action and should be given with caution in patients with urinary retention or angle closure glaucoma. Cyclobenzaprine should not be given in conjunction with MAO inhibitors (21). The efficacy appears to be the greatest in the first few days of onset of pain.

Table 13-3   Muscle Relaxants for Acute and Subacute Back Pain

Drug Name	Onset of Action	Duration of Action	Dose
Cyclobenzaprine (Flexeril)	1 h	12-24 h	10-60 mg/day in divided doses
Carisoprodol (Soma) Soma compound (with or without caffeine)	30 min	4-6 h	350 mg q 3-4 h (Soma) 1-2 tabs QID (Soma compound)
Diazepam (Valium)			2-10 mg TID-QID
Mexalatone*	1 h	4-6 h	800 mg TID-QID
Methocarbamol (Robaxin)	30 min	4 h	1.5 g QID, initially†
Orphenadrine (Norflex Extended Release)			100 mg BID (Norflex)
Norgesic (25 mg + 385 mg ASA + 30 mg caffeine)			25-50 mg TID-QID (Norgesic/
Norgesic Forte (50 mg + 770 mg ASA + 60 mg caffeine)			Norgesic Forte)

*Can cause hepatotoxicity.
†Maintenance dosing: 1 g QID, 750 mg q 4 h, or 1.5 g TID.

Carisoprodol (Soma) is a precursor of meprobamate that is metabolized by the liver and excreted in the urine (21). Dosages may need to be reduced for patients with hepatic or renal failure (20). Occasionally, an idiosyncratic reaction of profound weakness, dizziness, ataxia, dysarthria, and visual and cognitive changes can be seen after the first dose. This event lasts several hours.

Diazepam (Valium) acts in the reticular formation and enhances GABA-mediated presynaptic inhibition at the spinal cord level (20,21). Because of addiction and abuse potential, it is a controlled substance, and prescriptions should be written for a time-limited period. Significant respiratory depression can be a side effect.

Orphenadrine (Norflex, Norgesic) acts on interneuronal activity in the brainstem reticular formation and also has analgesic activity (20,21). Some of the formulations contain sulfites. The main side effects are anticholenergic in nature, and because of this, it is contraindicated in those with angle closure glaucoma and should be used cautiously in those with cardiac disease. A typical oral dose is 100 mg twice daily.

Medications for Injection Techniques

Increasingly, the effective management of subacute pain syndromes involves injection of therapeutic agents directly into the pain generator site. Medications are used for injection into the spinal canal, facet and sacroiliac joints, and muscle areas.

Steroidal Anti-inflammatory Agents

Injectable corticosteroids are used for intra-articular and epidural injections. Glucocorticoids inhibit COX-2-mediated prostaglandin synthesis and can impair cell-mediated and immunologic responses (24). The theorized mechanism of action is that they stabilize membranes, inhibit neuropeptide synthesis and action, decrease inflammation and edema around the nerve root, and block nociceptor C-fiber conduction. Only suspensions are used, as soluble preparations are rapidly cleared from the spinal canal during epidural procedures and cause side effects such as seizures and segmental hyperalgesia (25). When using these agents for epidural injection, concern has been raised over the possible neurotoxicity of the preservatives, including benzyl alcohol, benzalkonium chloride, and polyethylene glycol (26).

Methylprednisolone acetate (MPA) is the most commonly used agent for epidural injection (26). It is a 6-alpha-methycorticosteroid with 10 times the anti-inflammatory activity of cortisol, with mild mineralocorticoid effects (20). Multidose vials contain benzyl alcohol and 1-ml vials contain myristyl-gamma-picolinium chloride, and both contain polyethylene glycol (26). Examples of typical doses would be 80 mg for an epidural, 20-40 mg for a facet joint, and 40 mg for a sacroiliac joint injection (24,25,27).

Triamcinolone acetonide is a 16-alpha-dehydroxycorticoid derivative with 40 times the anti-inflammatory action of cortisone and virtually no mineralocorticoid effects (20). Fifty milligrams is a common dosage for epidural injection and 2-6 mg for a sacroiliac joint injection (24,25,27).

Betamethasone is a synthetic steroid ester suspension with equal parts of the sodium phosphate and acetate forms in an aqueous suspension. It is a 16-methycorticosteroid with 20 times the potency of cortisol. Of the steroids mentioned, it has the strongest glucocorticoid and anti-inflammatory activity (20). The disodium phosphate form is miscible in water, therefore having a more rapid onset of action compared to the insoluble acetate form, which is longer acting.

Prednisolone is a 1,2-dehydrocorticosteroid that has glucocorticoid activity and minimal mineralocorticoid action and 4 to 5 times the anti-inflammatory action of cortisone (20).

Local Anesthetics

Local anesthetics are used alone, as a test dose, or in combination with a long-acting steroid for joint, epidural, and other spine injections. Local anesthetic agents used for trigger point injections include bupivacaine 0.25%; 0.5% mepivacaine; 0.5%, 1%, and 4% lidocaine, procaine; and 1.5% lignocaine (lidocaine) (28).

Mepivacaine hydrochloride is an amide-type local anesthetic with a more rapid onset of action and longer duration of action compared to lidocaine, with a duration of action of 115-150 minutes. Preservative-free mepivacaine is available for epidural injection in concentrations of 1%, 1.5%, and 2% (17).

Lidocaine hydrochloride is a highly soluble amide-type local anesthetic with a rapid onset of action and a duration of action of about 100 minutes. Preservative-free preparations of 1-2%, without epinephrine, are used for epidural injections, with volumes of 2-3 cc for each level blocked. Some preparations contain sodium metabisulfite, which may cause allergic reactions. Parenteral preparations of 0.5% to 4.0% are available (17).

Bupivacaine hydrochloride has the longest duration of action, with an onset of 4-17 minutes and duration of action of 3 to 7 hours. Some preparations contain sulfates. Concentrations of 0.25% or 0.5% are typically used for epidural injection (17).

▦   ▦   ▦

REFERENCES

1. **Curatolo M, Bogduk N.** Pharmocologic pain treatment of musculoskeletal disorders: current perspectives and future prospects. Clin J Pain. 2001;17:25-32.

2. **Cherkin DC, Wheeler KJ, Barlow W, Deyo RA.** Medication use for low back pain in primary care. Spine. 1998;23:607-14.

3. **Van Tulder MW, Scholten RJ, Koes BW, Deyo RA.** Nonsteroidal anti-inflammatory drugs for low back pain. A systematic review within the framework of the Cochrane Collaboration Back Review Group. Spine. 2000;25:2501-13.

4. **Deyo, R.** Drug therapy for back pain. Which drugs help which patients? Spine. 1996;21:2840-49.

5. **Osiri M, Moreland L.** Specific cyclooxygenase 2 inhibitors: a new choice of nonsteroidal anti-inflammatory drug therapy. Arthritis Care Res. 1999;12:351-60.

6. **Bigos S, Bowyer O, Braen G, et al.** Acute low back problems in adults. Clinical Practice Guideline No. 14, AHCPR Publication No. 95-0642. Agency for Health Care Policy and Research, Public Health Service, U.S. Department of Health and Human Services; December 1994.

7. **Robert L II, Morrow J.** Analgesic-antipyretic and antiinflammatory and drugs employed in the treatment of gout. In: Wonsiewicz MJ, Morriss JM; eds. Goodman and Gilman's The Pharmacological Basis of Therapeutics, 10th ed. New York: McGraw-Hill; 2001.

8. **McMurray RW, Hardy KJ.** COX-2 inhibitors: today and tomorrow. Am J Med Sci. 2002;323: 181-9.

9. **Foral PA, Wilson AF, Nystrom DD.** Gastrointestinal bleeds associated with rofecoxib. Pharmacotherapy. 2000;22(3):384-6.

10. **Nissen D; ed.** 2003 Mosby's Drug Consult. St. Louis, MO: Mosby; 2003.

11. **Stevenson DD, Simon RA.** Lack of cross-reactivity between rofecoxib and aspirin in aspirin-sensitive patients with asthma. J Allergy Clin Immunol. 2001;108:47-51.

12. **Veenema K., Leahey N, Schneider S.** Ketorolac versus medperidine: ED treatment of severe musculoskeletal low back pain. J Emerg Med 2000;18:404-7.

13. **Innes GD, Croskerry P, Worthington J, Beveridge R, Jones D.** Ketorolac versus acetaminophen-codeine in the emergency department treatment of acute low back pain. J Emerg Med. 1998;16:549-56.

14. **Sifton DW, ed.** 2003 Physicians' Desk Reference. Montvale, NJ: Thompson PDR; 2003.

15. **Gutstein H, Akil H.** Opiod analgesics. In: Wonsiewicz MJ, Morriss JM, eds. Goodman and Gilman's The Pharmacological Basis of Therapeutics, 10th ed. New York: McGraw-Hill; 2001.

16. **McEvoy GK, et al., eds.** AHFS Drug Information 2003. Bethesda, MD: American Society of Health System Pharmacists, Inc.; 2003.

17. **Shipton EA.** Tramadol-present and future. Anesth Intensive Care 2000;28:363-74.

18. **Schnitzer TJ, Gray WL, Paster RZ, Kamin M.** Efficacy of tramadol in treatment of chronic low back pain. J Rheumatol. 2000;27:772-8.

29. **McGuire JL, ed.** Pharmaceuticals. New York: Wiley-VCH; 2000.

20. **Burnham TH, ed.** Drug Facts and Comparisons, 2003 ed. St. Louis, MO: Wolters Kluwer.

21. **Basmajian J.** Acute back pain and spasm. A controlled multicenter trial of combined analgesic and antispasm agents. Arch Phys Med Rehabil. 1989;438-9.

22. **Browning R, Jackson J, O'Malley P.** Cyclobenzaprine and back pain. A meta-analysis. Arch Intern Med. 2001;161:1613-20.

23. **Papagelopoulos PJ, Petrou HG, Triantafyllidis PG, Vlamis JA, Psomas-Pasalis M, Korres DS, Stamos KG.** Treatment of lumbosacral radicular pain with epidural steroid injections. Orthopedics. 2001;24:145-9.

24. **Weiskopf R.** Treatment of lumbosacral radiculopathy with epidural steroids. Anesthesiology. 1999;91:1937-41.

25. **Nelson D, Landau WM.** Intraspinal steroids: history, efficacy, accidentality, and controversy with review of United States Food and Drug Administration reports. J Neurol Neurosurg Psychiatry. 2001;70:433-43.

26. **Maldjian C, Mesgarzedeh M, Tehranzadeh J.** Diagnostic and therapeutic features of facet and sacroiliac joint injection. Radiol Clin North Am. 1998;35:497-508.

27. **Cummings T, White A.** Needling therapies in the management of myofascial trigger point pain: a systematic review. Arch Phys Med Rehabil. 2001;82:986-92.

14

■ ■ ■

Acute Rehabilitation
of Low Back Pain

Wing K. Chang, MD

As has been stated in the previous chapters, the majority (90%) of low back pain (LBP) cases resolve without medical attention in 6-12 weeks. Forty to fifty percent of patients are symptom-free within 1 week, and 75% with sciatica symptoms have relief of pain at 6 weeks. Out of these, only a small percentage are optimal surgical candidates. The rest usually receive "nonoperative" or "conservative" treatment. Knowing this, focusing on rehabilitation of the patient with acute, less than 6 weeks, LBP is extremely crucial. It has been shown that prompt assessment and initiation of treatment decreased time loss and the rate of back injury (1). A well coordinated and successful rehabilitation program strives to achieve several goals: 1) prevent the pain syndrome from evolving into a subacute or even a chronic one, 2) maximize conservative management, 3) determine optimal surgical candidates, 4) identify and minimize risk factors for poor surgical outcome by aggressively treating to ensure a more favorable surgical outcome, and 5) to reduce future disability, whether surgery is undertaken or not, as one of the proven risk factors for future disability from LBP is a previous history of LBP or low back surgery (2). A rehabilitation program is most successful when specific goals are set and agreed upon from the very beginning (Table 14-1).

Education

Back School

Back school is individual or group education on back pain care in which various aspects are discussed: back anatomy, pathophysiology, body

Table 14-1   Goals of Acute Spinal Rehabilitation

- Education and protection of injured tissue.
- Control of pain and reduction of inflammation.
- Early mobilization and physiologic loading of joint and soft-tissue structures.
- Implementation of therapeutic exercises.
- Restore full, pain-free range of motion (ROM) of the injured and the adjacent segments as well as the entire kinetic chain (i.e., other spinal, hip/shoulder girdle, and lower/upper extremity structures that influence the spine). Optimize strength, endurance, and coordination of the neuromuscular system affecting the spine.
- Return to normal activity.
- Prevention of further injury and recurrences.

Republished with permission from Weinstein SM, Herring SA, Cole AJ. Chapter 57. Rehabilitation of the patient with spinal pain. In: DeLisa JA, Gans BM, eds. Rehabilitation Medicine: Principles and Practice, 3rd ed. Philadelphia: Lippincott-Raven Publishers,1998:1439-47.

mechanics, ergonomics, exercises, and psychological aspects. The aim of the course is to increase pain tolerance, improve function, and prevention of future recurrence. In a study done comparing three groups of patients with acute LBP in an industrial setting (group I, back school; group II, physiotherapy; group III, placebo), the back school group on average returned to work 6 days earlier than the other two groups (3). A later study showed that patients going through a "mini back school" returned to work earlier and had fewer recurrences. These patients were managed successfully with an approach that included a clinical examination combined with educational information about the nature of the problem. The information was provided in a manner designed to reduce fear and give them reason and permission to resume light activity (4).

Rest

How Many Days of Rest?

The deleterious affects of prolonged bed rest may include but are not limited to decreased muscle strength, loss of flexibility, lower cardiovascular fitness, increased spinal segmental stiffness, and possible depression. Therefore, it has been established and advocated that no more than 2 days of bed rest is recommended for patients with nonspecific LBP (5). In general, if there is no specific structural pathology, it is advised that the patient observe a short period of "relative rest" then resume and continue ordinary activities (6). Activity or exercise is then advanced as tolerated guided by the patient's symptoms of pain. This approach is taken in order to avoid the deleterious affects of immobility and to return the patient to normal daily activities as early as possible.

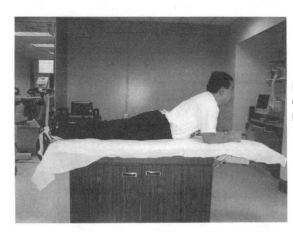

Figure 14-1   Example of extension bias exercise: prone on elbows.

Therapeutic Exercise

Introduction

The main goal of exercise for acute LBP is restoration of function, which most often also results in pain control. Once fracture or neurologic compromise is ruled out, having a definitive diagnostic cause is not an absolute in order to begin an exercise program. Strengthening is not as important in the acute setting because such loss should be small at this stage. A proper and effective exercise program may be individually tailored after a dynamic assessment of the patient. One approach often used is to determine which direction of spinal motion either increases or reduces pain. An extension bias, flexion bias, or a neutral spine dynamic lumbar stabilization exercise program is undertaken depending on which spinal motion centralizes LBP (i.e., less radicular pain) or does not exacerbate LBP. A general aerobic conditioning program can complement the specific spine-directed exercises. These exercises are usually initiated via one-to-one supervision or in a class setting with a skilled spine-trained physical therapist.

Extension Bias Exercises

Extension exercises are commonly advocated for LBP with disk pathology causing radicular symptoms. With spinal extension motion, this pain is either reduced or centralized according to the disk pathology. It is theorized that extension exercises reduce intradiskal pressure, allow anterior migration of the nucleus pulposus, and decrease tension on the spinal nerve root. Prior to performing extension exercises, it is important to remember to correct any spinal segmental lateral shifts. Examples of extension exercises are prone position with a pillow support under the stomach, an unsupported prone position, a pillow support under the chest, and prone on elbows (Figure 14-1). Contraindications to extension exercises include spinal segmental hypermobility or instability, large or uncontained herniated disk, bilateral neurologic symptoms, significant increase in LBP unless associated with concomitant reduction in radicular pain, and increase in radicular sensory symptoms.

Flexion Bias Exercises

Flexion exercises are commonly used for posterior spinal column pain that may be reduced or centralized in a flexed spine position. The concept is that spine flexion reduces the posterior facet joint reactive force and provides a stretch of the paraspinal muscles, ligamentous, and myofascial structures. Flexion exercises are usually better tolerated in patients with central disk herniations, facet-mediated pain, and foraminal stenosis. Common flexion bias exercises include pelvic tilts, single knee to chest (Figure 14-2), double knee to chest, and crunches. In addition, a flexed spine position may be incorporated in the cardiovascular fitness training such as a stationary bike or a stair-stepper program. Contraindications to flexion exercises include spinal segmental hypermobility, spinal instability, or aggravation of radicular pain. Increasing LBP is a relative contraindication.

Neutral Spine Dynamic Stabilization Exercises

This position provides the greatest functional stability, decreasing tension on ligaments and spinal neural elements while allowing a more balanced segmental force distribution between the disk and facet joints. The neutral spine position tends to be the least painful and most biomechanically advantageous position, thus is typically the initial training position. Patients

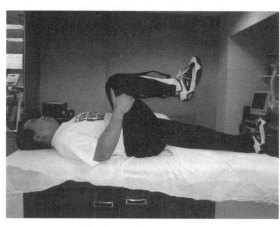

Figure 14-2   Example of flexion bias exercise: single knee to chest.

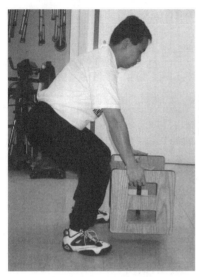

Figure 14-3 Example of neutral spine dynamic stabilization exercise: lifting while maintaining a neutral spine position.

are taught to maintain a neutral spine position during dynamic stabilization exercises simulating various activities such as lifting, bending, pushing, and pulling (Figure 14-3). Contraindications to neutral spine exercises include spinal segmental hypermobility, instability, and radicular pain. An increase in LBP is a relative contraindication.

Cardiovascular Conditioning

General aerobic training may help decrease acute pain by elevating systemic endorphin levels, promote tissue healing, increase endurance, and improve coordinated activity of the neuromuscular system. It has been shown that firefighters with superior cardiovascular fitness experienced the least number of back injuries at work (7). When an episode of back pain did occur, the days off from work was significantly less than their peers of similar age who were less cardiovascularly fit (8). This is not conclusive evidence that superior cardiovascular fitness alone prevents LBP or even shortens the recovery time. However, it is thought that those who are cardiovascularly fit likely have increased flexibility, strength, and endurance. These associated factors may be protective against LBP and reduce the rate of deconditioning after a back injury. Cardiovascular exercises may include the use of stationary bicycles, ski machines, stair climbers, treadmills, and aquatic-based exercises. Barring cardiac limitations, to be effective these should be used at an intensity that is at least 70% of the age-predicted maximum heart rate, for a duration of at least 15 minutes continuously, and a frequency of 3-5 times a week.

Manual Techniques

An array of manual therapy techniques may be undertaken in the hands of a skilled physical therapist, including myofascial release, spinal segmental mobilization or manipulation, strain/counter-strain techniques, muscle energy techniques, acupressure, massage, proprioceptive neuromuscular facilitation (PNF) techniques, and stretching. The details of each of the above techniques are explained in Chapter 24. The main goal of manual therapy is to correct any preexisting or resultant biomechanical restrictions or dysfunction. This will in addition afford pain relief to a significant extent. In general, manual therapy, particularly manipulations, is beneficial in a select population. The patient population that will most likely respond to manipulation is the population with acute LBP usually less than 1-month duration with either minor or absent neurologic or radicular symptoms (9).

Adjunctive Treatment

Adjunctive treatment usually alludes to physical modalities in the form of superficial or deep heating and cooling modalities. It is strongly stressed that these treatments not be used in isolation but as intended, for acute pain management in concert with a comprehensive rehabilitation program. Examples of these include superficial cold (i.e., ice packs), superficial heat (i.e., heating pads, hydrocollator, whirlpool baths), deep heat (i.e., ultrasound), electrical stimulation, and transcutaneous electrical nerve stimulation (TENS). Mechanical traction may also be included in this section as an adjunctive treatment and other reversible causes often is not used in the treatment of acute lumbar spine pain. The above-mentioned treatments are all passive treatments in that they require no patient initiative or participation. Used judiciously, they can be an effective supplemental tool. In rehabilitation programs that are based predominantly on these treatments, one must be careful not to inadvertently create dependent, passive patients who want to be "fixed" versus active participants in their own recovery. Such situations potentially result in a delay or no return to work.

Bracing

Bracing in the setting of acute LBP usually refers to lumbosacral corsets or belts. Biomechanically, a corset does not provide sufficient support to truly stabilize the bony spine. However, it does serve as a proprioceptive feedback for the patient to avoid spinal motions that may cause or exacerbate their pain. In addition, it may provide some pain relief with soft tissue warmth, a sense of support, less fear of movement, and in theory may compress soft tissues, elongate the trunk, and thus decrease intradiskal pressure. A few studies show that when judiciously used in combination with a back school program, back bracing can decrease work days lost and accelerate recovery from low back injuries (10). Many practitioners avoid the use of back braces. If they are used, however, it is recommended that back braces be worn only during working hours (no more than 8 hours a day) to minimize the potential risk of dependence on the brace, muscle atrophy, impaired muscle firing, and poor proprioceptive control. Once the acute pain period has resolved, patients should be weaned off their braces as soon as possible.

Work Restrictions/Return to Activity

Return to work or preinjury activities is the ultimate goal of a successful rehabilitation program. Only 50% of injured workers return to work after 6 months of disability, 25% after 1 year of disability, and 0% at >2 years of disability. These statistics suggest that the initial period, the first 6 weeks, is crucial in returning patients to work. Although there is little literature to support specific work restrictions for any spinal disorder, early return to work correlates with better outcomes. It is clear that occupations that involve heavy lifting, repetitive bending, twisting, and seated vibration are risk factors for LBP. When considering work restrictions, the clinician must weigh the decision on the demands of the job as well as the patient's concordant subjective and objective findings of spinal pain generators. If work excuse or restrictions are given, a time limit should be set, and a timeline for future milestones should be agreed on. Multidisciplinary evaluations may document physical abilities, but other reversible causes for limited performance, including deconditioning or psychosocial factors, must be considered.

Case Study 14-1

A 45-year-old male who is an automobile assembly-line worker presents with a 2-week chief complaint of lower back spasms with associated sharp shooting pain radiating down the right lateral leg region that started while driving home from work. He denies focal weakness, numbness, bowel/bladder or sexual dysfunction. No other pertinent associated manifestations are noted. This is his first episode of back pain. Past medical history is negative. On physical examination, lumbosacral motion in flexion reproduced his pain, hypertonicity is noted in the right lower lumbar paraspinal musculature, and straight leg raise creates a positive neural tension sign reproducing concordant pain into the right lateral leg. The neurologic examination is otherwise negative.

A provisional diagnosis of right L5 radiculopathy is made, most likely due to a focal right lateral L5-S1 disk herniation. The patient was

reassured of the good prognosis that about one half of the patient population with this diagnosis recover spontaneously within 6 weeks. He
was then started on a nonsteroidal anti-inflammatory medication to
take continuously for the next 2 weeks, started on an extension bias
physical therapy program, and was given time off from work for 2
weeks but encouraged to continue activities of daily living. At his 2-
week follow-up, he experienced minor improvement but not significant
enough to return to work as an automobile factory assembly-line worker
involving repetitive bending and twisting. An MRI of the lumbosacral
spine was done at that time and showed an extraforaminal right L5-S1
focal disk herniation with minor compression on the exiting right L5
spinal nerve root. To expedite pain relief and to facilitate physical therapeutic exercises, a right L5-S1 transforaminal epidural steroid injection
was performed under fluoroscopy. Two weeks after the injection, with a
continued extension bias physical therapy program, the patient had significant relief and was medically cleared to return to work. Exam revealed resolution of the muscle hypertonicity, mild neural tension at end
range, and no pain with spinal flexion. With aggressive treatment, his
time off from activity was limited to less than 6 weeks, and as such he
did not develop any risk factors for chronic disability.

■   ■   ■

Recommendations

- Patients should be educated about their condition and reassured about
  the positive prognosis.
- Relative rest, a time-contingent pain medication schedule (preferably
  non-opioid), a progressive therapeutic exercise program in concert with
  physical modalities, and proper body mechanics with postural training
  should be instituted acutely.
- The patient should be encouraged to maintain usual activities with an
  ultimate functional goal of returning to work or key life activities within
  6 weeks of injury.
- Close follow-up visits, weekly if possible, may be warranted.
- If no significant improvement is noted at about the 2-week follow-up
  visit, a more aggressive diagnostic approach (e.g., MRI, EMG) or therapeutic approach (selective spine injections, manipulations, or even a
  spine surgical referral) may be undertaken.
- Risk factors (physical and psychosocial) for chronic disability should be
  sought at each office visit and, if present, aggressively and appropriately

addressed. A multidisciplinary team approach may be best suited to assess and treat these issues further.

▦   ▦   ▦

Key Points

- Educate patient about condition and reassure about good prognosis.
- Give permission to take pain medications to control the acute pain on a time-contingent basis.
- Encourage resuming activities of daily living despite the pain.
- After 2 weeks, if needed, be aggressive with initiating treatment, especially physical therapeutics, and with diagnostic testing, in that order of importance.
- Employ other aggressive pain control treatments (e.g., therapeutic spine injections) when needed to facilitate physical therapy.
- Identify physical and psychosocial barriers to success and address them aggressively.
- Aim to return patient to work or key life activities in 6 weeks or less.

▦   ▦   ▦

REFERENCES

1. **Nadler SF, Stitik TP, Malanga GA.** Optimizing outcome in the injured worker with low back pain. Crit Rev Phys Med Rehabil Med. 1999;11:139-69.
2. **Rosen NB, Hoffberg HJ.** Conservative management of low back pain. Phys Med Rehabil Clin N Am. 1998;9(2):viii, 391-410.
3. **Bergquist-Ullman M, Larsson U.** Acute low back pain in industry. A controlled prospective study with special reference to therapy and confounding factors. Acta Orthop Scand. 1977;170:1-117.
4. **Indahl A, Haldorsen EH, Holm S, Reikeras O, Ursin H.** Five-year follow-up study of a controlled clinical trial using mobilization and an informative approach to low back pain. Spine. 1998;23(23):2625-30.
5. **Deyo RA, Diehl AK, Rosenthal M.** How many days of bed rest for acute low back pain? A randomized clinical trial. N Engl J Med. 1986;315(17):1064-70.
6. **Malmivaara A, Hakkinen U, Aro T, Heinrichs ML, Koskenniemi L, Kuosma E, et al.** The treatment of acute low back pain-bed rest, exercises, or ordinary activity? N Engl J Med. 1995;332(6):351-5.
7. **Cady LD, Bischoff DP, O'Connell ER, Thomas PC, Allan JH.** Strength and fitness and subsequent back injury in firefighters. J Occup Med. 1979;21:269-72.

8. **Cady LD, Thomas PC, Karwasky RJ.** Program for increasing health and physical fitness of firefighters. J Occup Med. 1985;27:110-14.

9. **Agency for Health Care Policy and Research (AHCPR).** Clinical Practice Guidelines No. 14. Rockville MD: U.S. Department of Health and Human Services, Public Health Service; 1994.

10. **Walsh NE, Schwartz RK.** The influence of prophylactic orthoses on abdominal strength and low back injury in the workplace. Am J Phys Med Rehabil. 1990;69(5):245-50.

KEY REFERENCES

Agency for Health Care Policy and Research (AHCPR). Clinical Practice Guidelines No. 14. Rockville MD: U.S. Department of Health and Human Services, Public Health Service; 1994.

This reference is a research evidence-based guideline approach to the care and treatment of acute low back pain. It was developed by the Agency for Health Care Policy and Research (AHCPR). It contains the "nuts and bolts" of the care of acute low back pain. It is available online at http://www.guideline.gov.

Saal JA, Saal JS. Physical rehabilitation of low back pain. In Frymoyer JW; ed. The Adult Spine: Principles and Practice, 2nd ed. Philadelphia: Lippincott-Raven; 1997:1805-20.

Arguably, the most comprehensive standard text in spine care. Referenced by spine specialists everywhere. This chapter covers the rehabilitation aspects of low back pain extremely well.

Weinstein SM, Herring SA, Cole AJ. Rehabilitation of the patient with spinal pain. In: DeLisa JA, Gans BM; eds. Rehabilitation Medicine: Principles and Practice, 3rd ed. Philadelphia: Lippincott-Raven; 1998:1423-52.

One of the standard texts referenced by rehabilitation medicine specialists. This chapter gives a great overview of caring for patients with spinal pain.

SECTION III

SUBACUTE BACK PAIN

15

■ ■ ■

Subacute Back Pain

Miles Colwell, MD

ubacute back pain is technically defined as back pain lasting greater than 6 weeks and not longer than 12 weeks. After 12 weeks it is considered chronic. At the subacute level, the odds of spontaneous improvement are less and the chances increase that the patient has a specific treatable lesion such as nerve root irritation, muscle injury, muscle imbalance, or biomechanical lesion. The patient has not yet reached the point where he or she has picked up the habits and comorbidities of chronic back pain and disability. It is at this level where the "diagnose, treat, cure" physician should be in a comfort zone. Guided by symptoms and physical exam findings, this is the time where diagnostic tests have more utility. Patients should not leave this time frame without either a diagnosis or substantial comfort that no dangerous or specifically treatable pathology exists. This is especially true if there is work or lifestyle disability associated with the pain. Aside from treatment to abate symptoms, efforts should focus on getting the client back into functional activities. The use of highly technical and skilled physical therapists with specialized physical therapy interventions, referral for injections, and surgery make the most sense here. Physical examination techniques beyond the basic ones taught in medical school come into play. In this phase, the physician must begin to reckon with the fact that there is not just pain, but often disability. Simple and more comprehensive rehabilitation measures are important to maintain function.

The detailed history and physical examination should give the clinician sufficient information to focus the potential etiology of symptoms and findings into one of three categories: neurogenic, structural, or myofascial (Figure 15-1). Neurogenic refers to symptoms and exam findings consistent with nerve or nervous system involvement. Structural will be those etiologies related to dysfunction of the body framework such as skeletal malrotations, restrictions to movement, and bone pathology such as arthritis, stress fracture, and inflammation. Myofascial pain refers to pain and tenderness in

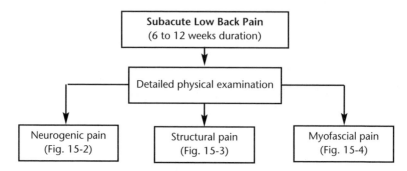

Figure 15-1   Critical decision points in subacute low back pain.

the muscle and their fascial components. Possible etiologies of myofascial pain include systemic diagnoses such as rheumatologic diseases, metabolic imbalances, endocrine dysfunction, and medication side effects. Other etiologies are overuse syndromes, emotional stress, and fibromyalgia.

Subacute History

For the patient presenting for the first time with subacute pain, the acute history is reviewed to rule out Red Flags for serious causes of back pain. Progressive neurologic deficit, bowel or bladder dysfunction, or saddle anesthesia warrant prompt diagnostic testing and imaging. Trauma, age >50 years, insidious onset, pain worse when supine or at night, diffuse osteoporosis, fever, chills, night sweats, weight loss, relatively recent history of infection, surgery, concurrent medical disease such as HIV, immunosupresssion, steroid use, and IV drug use are indicators for further medical workup if not already done (see Chapter 9 and Table 15-1).

Time should be dedicated to reviewing functional history as well as screening for any Yellow Flags indicating heightened risk for chronic disability (see Chapter 10). Depending on the examining clinician's time constraints and level of experience, referral to a specialist may be made at this stage to deal with the more involved back pain case.

Subacute rehabilitation should focus on resolving functional limitations once the patient is able to tolerate therapy. If pain and/or dysfunction is too severe to fully participate in therapy, diagnostic testing should be completed and appropriate interventions initiated. Injection therapy to treat or further rule in or rule out radiculopathy, nerve root inflammation, facet mediated pain, or central or foraminal stenosis can be used. If testing does not reveal a significant systemic, neurologic, or severe structural cause for pain, patient reassurance, medication adjustments, and comprehensive therapy should begin. Case coordination and efficient treatment becomes crucial if activity limitations remain at 6 weeks, referral to a comprehensive back pain specialist such as a physiatrist or a multidisciplinary clinic is recommended.

Subacute Physical Exam

Whereas the acute physical examination has a simple goal of detecting dangerous causes of pain, at the subacute stage a specific diagnosis should be made, if possible. Thus, the subacute physical exam should combine detailed elements of a neurologic and structural exam. The proposed structural exam will screen for skeletal and myofascial symmetry, muscle firing, muscle length, leg length, as well as the alignment and mobility of individual vertebrae, the sacrum, the hemi pelvis, hip, and rib cage. Most clinicians are familiar with the neurologic components of sensation, reflexes,

Table 15-1   Differential Diagnosis of Back Pain

Systemic Causes	Structural Causes	Local Pathology That Mimics Radiating Low Back Pain
Aortic aneurysm	Tumor	Osteoarthritis of the hip
Aortic atherosclerosis	Disk space infection	Aseptic necrosis of the
Renal infection	Epidural abscess	femoral head
Renal calculi	Fractures	Sciatic nerve injury due to
Peritonitis	Osteoporosis with fracture	pressure, stretch, or
Tumors	Disk herniation	piriformismuscle entrapment
Subacute bacterial	Internal disk disruption	
endocarditis	Spinal stenosis	Cyclic radiating low back pain:
Metabolic disorders:	Spondylolisthesis	endometriosis on the sciatic
Porphyria	Failed back surgery	nerve of sacral plexus
Sickle cell disease	Biomechanical dysfunctions	Intrapelvic masses:
Renal osteodystrophy	Sacroiliac joint dysfunction	Benign or malignant
Seronegative spondylitic	Facet joint syndrome	Peroneal (fibular) nerve
dysfunctions:	"Manipulable" lesions	entrapment at the fibular
Ankylosing spondylitis	Pelvic asymmetry	head
Reiter syndrome	Sacral malalignment	
Arthritis of ulcerative	Vertebral segmental	
colitis	dysfunction	
Psoriatic arthritis	Facet joint syndrome	
Other arthritis:	Pelvic tilt syndrome	
Diffuse idiopathic	Muscle imbalance:	
skeletalhyperostosis	Hypertonicity	
(DISH)	Weakness	
Schuerman epiphisitis	Overuse	
Rheumatoid arthritis	Fatigue	
(uncommon)	Shortening	
Connective tissue		
disorders:		
Marfan syndrome		
Ehlers-Danlos syndrome		
Myopathy		
Inflammatory radiculopathy		
Arachnoiditis		

Adapted from Table 3 (Differential Diagnosis of Back Pain) in Haig AJ, Standiford C, Alvarez D, Graziano G, Harrison V, Papadopoulos S, et al. Acute Low Back Pain. University of Michigan Health System Guidelines for Clinical Care. University of Michigan Health System; November 1997, updated April 2003. Available at http://cme.med.umich.edu/pdf/guideline/backpain03.pdf.

nerve root tension testing, and strength. Many will look for the basic structural elements of muscle spasm, general tightness, tenderness over bony prominences, and possibly leg length discrepancy. Some have the luxury of relying on skilled physical therapists to sort out and treat these details. In areas where physical therapy is more modality based with some stretching and strengthening, especially for the patient that has not fully responded to this and is in the subacute phase, a more detailed subacute examination by the physician team is recommended. Chapter 16 will provide a working summary and review of the subacute physical exam.

Subacute Neurogenic Pain

Subacute neurogenic pain most commonly suggests radiculopathy, usually from a disk herniation. The client will frequently report a component of burning pain, electric sensations, or numbness in a specific pattern. This combined with exam findings of exacerbating or eliciting neuropathic pain with stretch or compression maneuvers, sensory loss, dysethesia, abnormal reflexes, or true weakness warrants further evaluation and treatment via the neurogenic algorithm. The differential also includes foraminal stenosis, facet mediated pain, muscle trigger point referring as neuropathic pain, plexopathy, nerve stretch injury, idiopathic neuritis, and central nervous system lesions. Diagnostic tests can be used to confirm or refute a diagnosis. Symptoms, exam findings, and when needed positive versus negative test results lead toward the use of specific medications, physical therapy, injections, and surgery when needed. Figure 15-2 gives the algorithm for subacute neurogenic pain.

If there are one or more deficits on neurologic exam of diminished reflexes, weakness, sensory loss, or positive neural tension signs, magnetic resonance imaging (MRI) is recommended for confirmation of a lesion causing impingement. In the face of mild deficits, unclear true weakness versus pain inhibition, or a nonfocal multilevel presentation, electrodiagnosis (i.e., EMG) can be helpful to objectify the level of involvement. It can be used to confirm radiculopathy, peripheral nerve lesion, neuropathy, myopathy, or show changes suggestive of a central nervous system lesion. The data can also assist to rate the severity of involvement. The information can be used to guide the type and area of focus for diagnostic imaging. If reflexes are increased, plantar responses upward and neuropathic pain present, evaluate for myelopathy or other central lesion. Depending on the practitioner's level of expertise, treat accordingly or refer for specialist evaluation and treatment.

When the neurologic exam and diagnostics are consistent with radiculopathy, deficits are mild and the client can tolerate therapy, maximize medications, and consider an extension-based therapy program (as described for acute back pain; see Chapter 14). Recommended medications

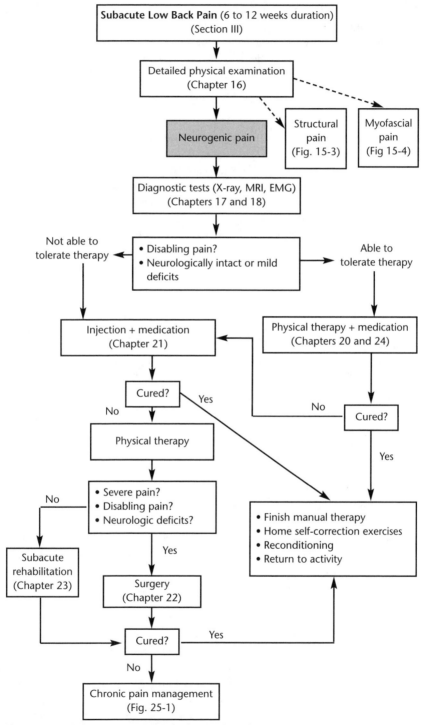

Figure 15-2   Subacute neurogenic back pain algorithm.

include an antiinflamatory, an agent for neuropathic pain such as low-dose tricyclic antidepressant or membrane stabilizer, and when necessary an additional analgesic (see Chapter 13). Often, the additional analgesic is only needed for comfort during sleep or as an adjunct to tolerate therapy. The majority of medication should dosed on a scheduled basis and not here and there as needed by symptoms. If symptoms are severe despite oral medications and the client cannot tolerate therapy, consider referal for injection therapy. Per algorithm, if this significantly helps, proceed to physical therapy, treat any secondary myofascial and structural lesions, finalize the home exercise program, and return to activity (see Chapters 12 and 23 for further details concerning return to activity after disk herniation). If not successful, refer for surgical evaluation and treatment (see Chapter 22).

If the neurologic exam is normal and neuropathic symptoms are set off by spinal extension that closes the foramen and loads the facets, plain x-rays with oblique views of the facets and foramen may be sufficient to confirm facet arthritis mediated pain or foramenal stenosis. If spondylolisthesis is present, this may be an incidental finding or an active pain generator. Flexion and extension x-rays can be obtained to assess stability. If x-rays show foraminal stenosis, MRI should be obtained to confirm the anatomy and rule out any other lesions prior to attempting transforaminal epidural or central epidural injection therapy. A three-phase bone scan or single photon emission computed tomography (SPECT) scan will rule in or out active bone inflammation or stress fracture as a possible pain generator. Several studies are reporting that MRI is useful to look for evidence of inflammatory changes in the pedicle as an indicator of which cases will procede to bony healing. If unclear and facet mediated pain is suspected, facet blocks can be done to clarify the diagnosis and treatment. Relatively mild symptoms may respond to medication and therapy. (This as well as facet joint pain will be covered later in this chapter under subacute structural pain.) Therapy is directed at releasing hip flexors, elongating paraspinal muscles, muscle firing, and stabilization. A flexion-based program is recommended. Bracing may first be used for a spondylolisthesis with active bone inflammation, followed by stabilization strengthening. Stretching of the paraspinal tissues across this level is minimized. When healing is complete, therapy should focus on strengthening and to maximize the segmental mobility above and below the involved level. If symptoms are moderate to severe, maximize medication and refer for injection therapy. If this minimizes symptoms, finalize physical therapy, home program, and return to activity. If not, and pain is significantly limiting, refer for surgical evaluation (see Chapter 22). If in the middle zone of not markedly better but not severe, proceed with subacute rehabilitation as described in Chapter 23.

If the neurologic exam is normal and spinal extension does not set off symptoms, be sure to look for myofascial trigger points. These can be treated with injection, needling, acupressure, acupuncture, stretching, neuroprobe, ultrasound, and myofascial release. When the primary trigger is located, injecting or needling the area can provide almost instantaneous release of this and corresponding satellite trigger point/tender nodules.

Subacute Structural Pain

Much is made of radiating versus nonradiating pain in the subacute phase. The vast majority of subacute back pain is not truly radiating or neuropathic. Achiness into the buttock, hip, and posterior thigh are very common with muscle imbalance and biomechanical lesions. Diagnostic tests are typically negative for nonradiating pain, but depending on symptoms, it may be important to rule out disease and reassure the patient and physician that nothing serious has been missed.

Here is where the physician focused on the "diagnose, treat, cure" role can easily become frustrated. Specialists have dedicated clinic time and have a number of tools to deal with this population. Implementation requires special physical examination skills, knowledge, collaboration with allied health professionals, and multidisciplinary procedures practiced and more efficiently used by the specialist.

To help the reader get a handle on subacute nonradiating pain, we further delineate it into myofascial versus structural or biomechanical. The concepts are somewhat intertwined, but the flow of patients through the process of care is distinctly different. People with pain that is reproducible on specific maneuvers that suggest pathology in a specific anatomical structure have mechanical pain. People whose pain is vague or generalized with fairly normal biomechanical exam are a bit more likely to have systemic disease or psychiatric overlay.

Subacute structural or myofascial pain is the kind of pain that "makes sense" to a clinician who is familiar with the anatomy of the spine. On exam, ligaments hurt when stretched, joints hurt when they are compressed, and muscle achiness is present when they are activated. With a detailed "manual physical examination," the clinician will have a comfort level with what the pain generator is. The decision will need to be made as to whether this is more biomechanical due to focal structural asymmetries, muscle imbalance and malalignments, or diffusely myofascial. If diffusely myofascial, rheumatologic, autoimmune, metabolic, endocrine, stress or overuse should be explored.

Severe musculoskeletal pain from joint or biomechanical dysfunctions may need a more aggressive approach, including various injection procedures (Figure 15-3). Less severe pain can initially be treated with a specialized group of physical therapy techniques known collectively as "manual therapy." If response is insufficient, the primary care physician has some skill-based questions to ask: Was this the right set of therapy techniques to use? Was the therapy technically well done? Do biomechanical asymmetries remain? Am I misreading the diagnosis? Is there a hidden factor causing

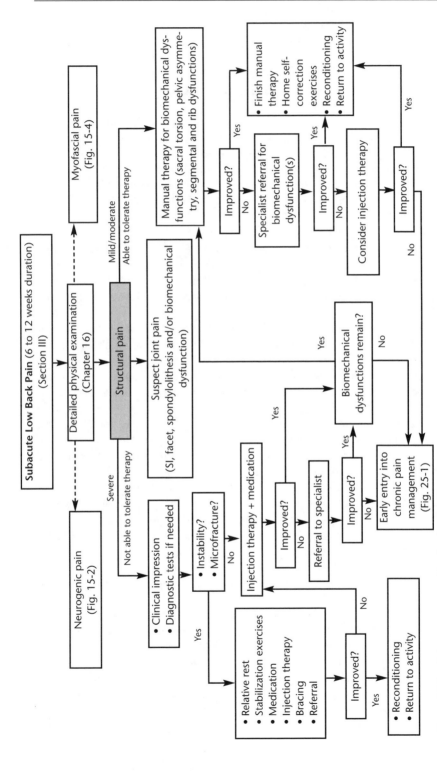

Figure 15-3   Subacute structural back pain algorithm.

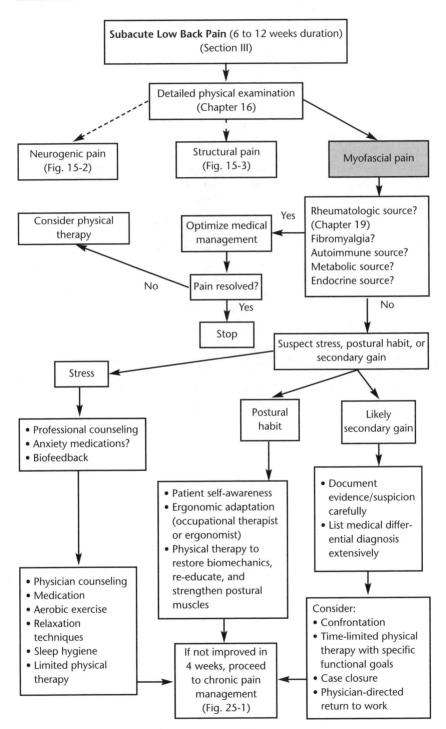

Figure 15-4   Subacute myofascial back pain algorithm.

disability? Depending on his or her experience, this may be where the physician refers the patient to a specialist.

Subacute Myofascial Pain

Subacute myofascial pain is troubling to the treating physician. This category encompasses diffuse tenderness or aching. Although there may be pain reproduction on exam, the main aspect of the pain does not seem to relate to a specific joint or ligament. Muscle strains always heal within weeks after an injury and should be significantly improved or resolved at this stage (Figure 15-4).

The first consideration is the possibility of generalized medical disease. A long list of medical and rheumatologic causes can be considered. Another consideration is psychosocial factors. Stress, depression, and anxiety can cause muscle tension and increase vigilance toward otherwise trivial discomfort. Severe psychiatric disease can present with bizarre or inconsistent pain behaviors. Finally, one must recognize the great social rewards for back pain disability. Often, people who are malingering (premeditated fictitious pain behavior) or exaggerating the pain that they really feel will present with more diffuse complaints. If present, these issues often will need to be dealt with first, sometimes simultaneously, before any real progress can be made. In the end, after all of these concerns are dealt with, many people with myofascial type pain of a nonsystemic disease etiology may still have hidden biomechanical asymmetries perpetuating a component of their pain and disability.

16

■ ■ ■

Subacute Back Pain: Physical Examination

Miles Colwell, MD

A t weeks 6 to 12, subacute back pain that is not spontaneously resolving warrants a more detailed physical exam than is performed for acute back pain to improve the clinician's ability to sort out neurogenic, structural, or myofascial pain. If no red flags are present, the clinician can then follow the appropriate treatment algorithm presented in Chapter 15. With practice, the exam can be accomplished in 10 minutes. Record keeping is most efficient with a manual medicine exam worksheet. This chapter presents the full screening exam, with an abbreviated version summarized in Appendix A for the busy clinician who only needs to know whether or not biomechanical lesions are present and will refer to a physician specialist or skilled physical therapist for more detailed evaluation and treatment. The subacute examination includes all aspects of the acute examination as outlined in Chapter 8. These include strength, reflexes, Waddell's nonorganic pain signs, and nerve root tension signs. This chapter will introduce some new components of the examination that are designed to determine a specific anatomical lesion.

The Manual Medicine Screening Exam

The manual medicine screening exam is used to look for structural asymmetries such as leg length discrepancy, malalignments of the musculoskeletal system, and muscle imbalances such as hypertonicity or impaired muscle firing. A "minicourse" in manual medicine follows to give the reader clarification of what is involved in the exam. With a little practice, it can be accomplished in 10 minutes, and clinicians should be able to answer the question yes or no as to the presence of manual lesions on the basis of examination findings. Attending an actual course will be necessary for those who wish to gain skills and proficiency beyond that. There are variations in terminology, depending on the person or discipline who wrote initial texts on the subject. The examination presented here is based on a system of nomenclature and exam techniques collected under the auspices of the Michigan State University College of Osteopathic Medicine and summarized by Philip E. Greenman (1-4).

At first, the manual exam may seem cumbersome and time consuming as the examiner becomes acquainted with the landmarks and techniques. For the clinician who sees many patients with back pain, learning this exam will improve diagnostic skills in the long run and will likely lead to improved treatment efficiency. Everyone has different ways of learning. Consider learning this exam in stages. One week, concentrate on the standing portions of the exam, and another week the seated. Then add the two together for a while. Proceed on to the seated portion and so forth, adding sections when familiar and able to be performed quickly enough.

The exam is frequently modified in the presence of pain behavior to first document sensation, reflexes, strength, seated straight leg raise, and possibly Waddell's nonorganic pain signs. Short of severe disk herniation or fracture, most patients should tolerate a comprehensive manual exam. Clinicians will figure out what sequence works best for them. We begin our discussion with the components of the standing exam, followed by seated, supine, side lying, prone, and contralateral side lying.

A. Standing

1. Gait and Posture

Observing posture gives important clues to areas needing further detailed exam. Observe for unleveling of shoulders, iliac crests, muscle fullness, and forward head tilt. Unleveling of the shoulders during standing may be related to asymmetric muscle hypertonicity, a restricted elevated first or second rib asymmetric muscle hypertonicity, or from lower in the body secondary to a short leg, pelvic asymmetry, or sacral torsion. Iliac crest height unleveling is usually from the latter three but can also be from asymmetric hypertonic paraspinal muscles, possibly perpetuated by rib cage dysfunction above. If not treated, the paraspinal asymmetry persists, maintaining a pelvic asymmetry and ongoing back pain. Kyphotic restriction of the thoracic spine leads to excessive forward head tilt, compensatory increased lumbar lordosis if the lumbar segments are flexible enough, and overuse of upper back muscles. The lower back muscle may become hypertonic or hypotonic with poor firing and endurance depending on the muscle firing substitution patterns.

Standing Flexion Test, Standing Stork Test

The standing flexion test, one-legged standing stork test, and seated flexion test are used to assess the relative joint glide of the sacroiliac joint. It is presumed that increased muscle and ligament tension across the joint can close compact the joint and limit the range and smoothness of motion. They are performed early in the exam because if restriction is present, the side of restriction is used to label the side of asymmetry for medial malleolus, anterior superior iliac spine (ASIS), pubic symphysis, ischial tuberosity, and sacral base exams.

2. *Standing Flexion Test*

The standing flexion test (Figure 16-1) is performed by hooking the examiners thumbs on the inferior slope of the posterior superior iliac spines (PSIS) and remainder of fingers and hand along the iliac crests and buttocks. Ask the patient to bend forward at the waist as if to touch their toes. The examiner maintains light pressure and follows the movement of the PSISs. If there is restriction to joint glide, the restricted side will be pulled anterior-superior by the movement of the trunk and the examiner's thumb, the restricted side will appear cephalad and is recorded as positive. If both thumbs remain symmetric (i.e., "appear level"), this indicates presumed normal bilateral joint glide and is recorded as negative. The examiner should be cautious, as this could also be bilateral equally restricted sacroiliac (SI) joint glide such that both PSISs traveled anterior-superior the same. The standing flexion test (Figure 16-1) should be used in conjunction with the one-legged stork test to avoid missing bilateral restriction to SI joint glide.

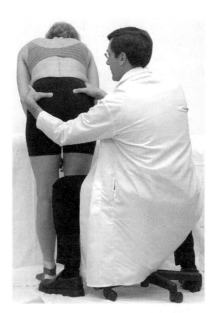

Figure 16-1 Standing flexion test. Right PSIS gliding superior, indicating right sacroiliac joint restrictions or possible hamstring tightness.

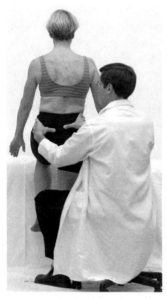

Figure 16-2 Standing stork test. Patient touches surface for balance, on command initiates left hip flexion to 90 degrees "as if doing a marching step." PSIS glides/rotates inferior, thumb appears to drop, indicates preserved SI joint movement. Lack of glide indicates restriction.

3. *Standing Stork Test*

   The standing stork test (Figure 16-2) can be used to confirm normal motion or bilateral restriction. Ask the patient to stand beside the exam table or a counter that they can touch with their hand for stability. This limits total body movement and makes it easier for the examiner to observe relative movement of the PSIS to a horizontal reference point of the examiner's contralateral thumb on the midportion of the sacrum. Ask the patient to initiate hip flexion on the side for which the examiner's thumb is monitoring the inferior slope of the PSIS. A negative (normal) test of motion is noted when there is inferior glide of the thumb relative to the midsacral reference point. If the monitoring thumb remains level or seems to travel cephalad, that side is recorded positive for SI joint restriction. Thumb placement is switched to monitor the contralateral PSIS, and the test is repeated initiating hip flexion on the other side. In the situation where both sides remain relatively stationary and do not drop inferiorly, there is bilateral restriction. This is how the one-legged stork test can differentiate bilateral restriction, whereas the standing stork test does not.

4. *Standing Side Bending Test*
5. *Standing Trunk Rotation Test*
6. *Standing Facet Loading/Foraminal Closure*

   Standing side bending can be used to evaluate for restricted segments of spine. Transition next to *standing trunk rotation* and if desired Waddell's modification of simultaneous trunk and pelvic rotation en bloc. The experienced clinician can also get a sense of sacral base glide if monitoring over the sacral bases during trunk rotation. Ask the patient to put their upper anterior thighs against the exam table or counter to stabilize their pelvis. *Standing facet loading/foraminal closing* can be accomplished by guiding the patient into spinal extension, rotation, and side bending (Figure 16-3). If this is painful, document the quality, location, and pattern of the pain and confirm if this is part of the main problem or additional.

Localized sharp to aching pain lateral to midline may be facet mediated. Similar pain with slight radiation into buttock or partially into the leg may also be referred pain from a facet joint. At times, the body co-operates and pain will refer in a dermatomal pattern indicating a level to consider a facet block. Pain that seems as if it might be neurogenic and radiates below the knee can still be facet mediated but has a higher likelihood of being nerve root irritation from true foraminal stenosis or possibly far lateral disk herniation into the foramen. Diagnostic imaging such as oblique x-rays, computed tomography (CT), or magnetic resonance imaging (MRI) can be used to confirm the clinical diagnosis.

B. Seated

7. *Seated Flexion Test*

The seated flexion test (Figure 16-4) is very similar to the standing flexion test assessing SI joint glide. The main difference is that the

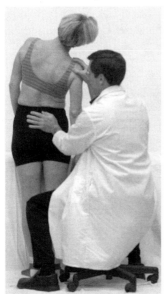

Figure 16-3   Standing facet loading/foraminal closure. Stabilize upper legs and pelvis against table; initiate ipsilateral spinal extension, rotation, and side bending.

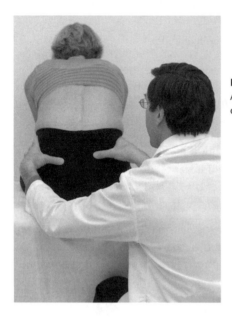

Figure 16-4   Seated flexion test. Asymmetric superior glide of PSIS indicates sacroiliac joint restriction.

hamstrings are on relative slack, as the hips and knees are flexed. The concept is that tight hamstrings tugging on their origin at the ischial tuberosity transmit the pull through the ligamentous connections across to the sacrum, thus close compacting the joint. This can lead to a false positive standing flexion test for local SI joint restriction. If the standing test is positive but the seated test negative, the SI joint glide is not restricted locally by joint or overlying fascia but secondarily only when the hamstrings are on tension. In this case, the hamstring tightness needs treatment, not the SI joint.

8. *Upper Extremity Screen*
9. *Passive Trunk Rotation (Seated)*
10. *Passive Trunk Side Bending (Seated)*

    If the patient lists upper back, neck, or shoulder discomfort, a quick screen of upper extremity range of motion can be accomplished by asking the patient to bring their hands up over head, palms facing together, then lower their arms and repeat, this time bringing the volar surface of their hands together over head. If asymmetry of motion and range are observed, further detailed exam is warranted. *Seated trunk side bending* and *passive trunk rotation* can be used to confirm restriction, asymmetry, or potential lack of effort noted during active standing trunk rotation and side bending (Figure 16-5).

11. *Cervical Spine Range of Motion (Seated)*

    Active cervical flexion, extension, side bending, and *rotation* can be observed to get a global sense of *cervical range of motion*. Note that

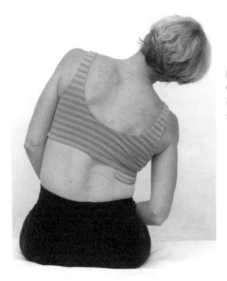

Figure 16-5 Seated side bending. Observe asymmetric location of skin creasing and decreased mid- to upper-thoracic spine side bending.

overall range may look good, and there can still be several tight achy hypomobile cervical segments. Painful relatively hypermobile segments may exist. (The term *relatively hypermobile* is used to describe individual vertebrae that on the supine cervical segmental exam move more than those above and below but on x-ray do not show movement during flexion and extension views.) A skilled therapist or specialized clinician who does this work daily would be able to offer an opinion whether stabilization strengthening is mainly needed or if the levels above and below need mobilization to allow the relatively hypermobile segment to normalize.

12. *Thoracic Spine Segmental Motion*

   Aside from referred pain secondary to arthritis, fracture, or medical condition, upper back achiness may be perpetuated by restrictions of individual thoracic spine segments, restrictions of groups of vertebrae, muscle hypertonicity, or rib cage dysfunction. Evaluate the alignment of the thoracic vertebrae in flexion and extension. While the patient is seated, ask them to slump or slouch forward into thoracic flexion then sit tall into *extension*. Monitor the tissue overlying the transverse processes. This is best done by moving lateral to medial with the examiner's thumbs maintaining anteriorly directed pressure as the thumbs roll into the gutter between the longissimus and multifidus muscles of the erector spinae muscles. Maintain equal pressure and compare the anterior to posterior position of the thumbs relative to each other. If one thumb appears to be relatively posterior, note the level, record the side and whether the spine is in extension or flexion.

To simplify a system of naming asymmetries that is consistent among clinicians, always note and record the side the thumb is posterior. Conceptually, if the asymmetry is maximized during spinal flexion, think of the asymmetric segment as not flexing forward on the side that the thumb is posterior. It is sticking in extension; call this an extended segment on that side. Example: if T4 right side is posterior during flexion, think of it as being extended, rotated, and side bent to the right. For record keeping, this can be labeled T4 ERS right.

During extension, if the right side of T6 is posterior, the concept is a bit different. Think of the facets going into extension and closing. If one of the facets cannot close but the contralateral facet can, the vertebrae will rotate toward the side that can extend into closure. The thumb monitoring the closing side will appear to be posterior. The opposite side does not close and stays relatively anterior or flexed. For record keeping, this vertebra is flexed, it will not go fully into extension and is rotated and side bent toward the side the thumb is posterior. The right thumb is posterior and the segment is named as being T6 FRS-right being flexed, rotated, and side bent to the right. The presumption is that the muscles and tissues are not allowing the vertebrae to move symmetrically.

If there is local corresponding deep muscle hypertonicity and tenderness, this is deemed a significant biomechanical dysfunction and should be treated. Scoliosis and group curves involve multiple levels and will be asymmetric during thoracic flexion and extension and thus do not fit the simplified naming noted above. In this case, just note the levels of involvement and which side is posterior. The therapist or consultant can further sort it out as needed.

13. *First Rib: Rule Out Superior Displacement*

Evaluating the relative position and travel of the first rib during inhalation and exhalation is the remaining exam technique recommended while the patient is seated (Figure 16-6). The examiner, from behind the patient, places their second and third fingers along the anterior border of the trapezius muscles. Applying posterior, inferior pressure, pull the trapezius back so that the fingers overlie the first rib. Hold steady pressure downward on this region and follow the travel of the rib during inhalation and exhalation. A common lesion is a superiorly subluxed first rib. The examiner will note it is superior at rest and during exhalation compared to the opposite side. It is beyond the scope of the screening exam to evaluate the second rib in detail, but be aware that tight muscles may hold it laterally flexed and thus keep the first rib from traveling inferioly. It may result in a first rib dysfunction that is seemingly resistant to treatment. This can perpetuate cervico-thoracic junction, neck, shoulder, and arm pain. If not already noted and treated, consider this in cases of such symptoms where imaging studies, diagnostics, and electromyography (EMG) are normal.

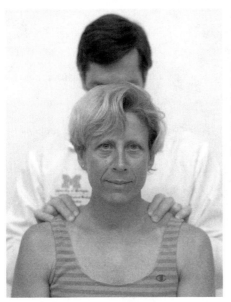

Figure 16-6   First rib evaluation. Examiner from behind patient reaches anterior to posterior to slide upper trapezius out of the way and places fingers over first rib. Observe for symmetry at rest and during motion as patient fully inhales then exhales.

C. Supine

The supine portion of the exam focuses on asymmetries of the pelvis, pubis, potential leg length discrepancies, hip mobility, pyriformis-gluteal muscle flexibility, straight leg raises, and rib glide. In an effort to have the patient lie straight on the table, ask them to bridge: "Lay on your back, bend your knees up, place you feet on the table, and lift your bottom briefly off the table and back down again. Now straighten your legs together back onto the table." The examiner can facilitate this by gently holding the dorsum of each foot and after the bridge, guide sliding the feet and both legs evenly back into extension onto the table.

14. Medial Malleolus Symmetry

15. Anterior Superior Iliac Spine Symmetry

The examiner now simultaneously hooks their thumbs under the inferior slope of the medial malleoli and from above looks down at the symmetry or asymmetry of the thumbs. If asymmetric, note which side is inferior or superior according to which side the standing flexion and one-legged stork tests were positive for restriction. Proceed now to the *anterior superior iliac spines (ASIS)* and simultaneously hook the thumbs under the inferior slope of the ASISs (Figure 16-7). Scan side-to-side for symmetry or asymmetry in a cephalad-caudal direction. Per standing flexion or stork test, record whether that side is superior or inferior.

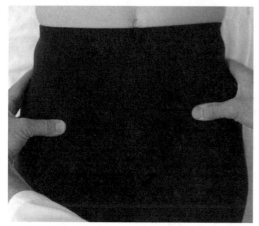

Figure 16-7   Anterior iliac spine symmetry (ASIS): right inferior. Examiner palpates inferior aspect of ASIS. Standing/seated flexion and one-legged stork test revealed right-sided restriction; thus right ASIS is recorded as inferior (not left ASIS superior).

16. Pubic Symphysis Symmetry

To check for pubic symphysis unleveling (Figure 16-8), the examiner takes the heel of their hand to begin palpating over the bladder region, proceeding inferiorly until one feels increased tension as the musculature begins to attach to the pubic rami. Stop and rotate your second and third fingers to the position over the pubic tubercle region. Ask the patient to breathe out to relax the abdominal muscles and then nearly simultaneously push the fingers posteriorly into the muscle and fascia followed by inferiorly on top of the pubic tubercle. Scan for symmetry or asymmetry in a cephalad-caudal direction. When unlevel, record the relative position of the ipsilateral side of the positive standing flexion or stork test. If asymmetries are present, measure leg length from hooking under the inferior slope of the ASIS to the inferior slope of the medial malleous.

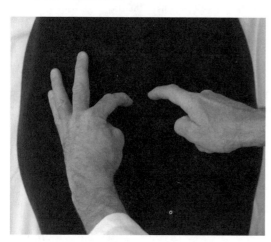

Figure 16-8   Pubic symphysis symmetry: right inferior. Standing/seated flexion and one-legged stork test positive on right for right-sided restriction; thus right pubic tubercle recorded as inferior.

17. *Lower Extremity Internal-External Rotation, Passive, 90/90 Hip and Knee Flexion*

18. *Straight Leg Raise (monitor ASIS for pelvic rotation)*

   Test straight leg raising now for hamstring length and the presence or absence of paresthesia. If nerve irritation is present, record the distribution and leg angle of onset. *Monitor the contralateral ASIS* to note the point at which the end stretch of the hamstring and pelvic rotation begins in compensation. While holding the leg, it is easy to position it in *90/90 hip and knee flexion,* then add *passive internal and external rotation* of the femur to look at hip range of motion.

19. *Pyriformis-Gluteal Muscle and Hip Capsule Flexibility*

20. *FABERE*

   Next proceed to passively ranging the femur and knee toward the patient's contralateral shoulder. This screens for pyriformis-gluteal muscle flexibility. If restriction is met, reach down and palpate the gluteal muscle. Is it tight in proportion to the overpressure being added through the femur toward the patient's contralateral shoulder? If it is not, the lack of range may be related to hip capsule restriction or hip arthritis. Now drop the femur into *flexion, abduction, and external rotation and extension (FABERE)* to load the hip. Further test for hip capsule restriction or consider obtaining an x-ray of the hip if clinically warranted.

21. *Rib Cage*

   The supine portion of exam is nearly done. Next assess rib travel during full inhalation and exhalation (Figure 16-9). With the second and third fingers, simultaneously palpate the corresponding bilateral ribs with steady pressure on the superior aspect along the anterior axillary line. Follow the ribs superior-inferior during deep breathing. Note if there is asymmetry of movement. Record the rib and side that is restricted in inhalation or exhalation. A key rib is determined by the therapist or clinician that is actually going to treat the dysfunction. If

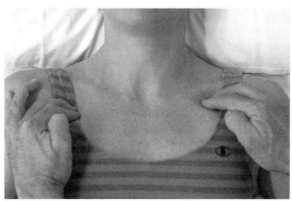

Figure 16-9 Rib evaluation. Left second rib exhalation restriction. Rib symmetry during full inhalation and exhalation. In this example, the patient's left second rib did not travel as far inferiorly as the right rib.

restriction is noted during exhalation, it is the lowest rib that does not move that is likely the key rib. An analogy is a multilevel parking garage with a stack of cars waiting to exit because the lowest car at the street has not left and is holding everyone up. Similarly, for an inhalation restriction it is the superior most rib that does not move that is the key lesion.

22. *Cervical Spine Segmental Motion*

The next step of the supine exam is screening for cervical segmental mobility or restriction. The examiner stands at the head of the table. First place the patient's head into passive flexion. This can be done by folding the pillow under the head or placing the examiners knee on the table under the pillow. Place a hand on each side of the head, monitor as the patient is asked to look right and turn their head right, then look left and turn to the left. The examiner can apply slight overpressure to confirm the patient has reached end range. Note the degree of rotation and compare side to side. When flexible, 80 degrees is common. The passive cervical flexion is used to limit the contribution of the lower segments and focuses not exclusively but mostly on the rotation of C1 on C2.

Next monitor over the lamina posterior to the transverse processes. The examiner slides their palm posteriorly, extends the second and third fingers to palpate over the lamina, and curls the fourth and fifth fingers to hold the occiput region. Slide the hand and fingers inferiorly until contacting the first rib region. The monitoring second and third fingers are now at the C7 level. Induce passive side to side translation to the cervical segment and feel its relative glide (Figure 16-10). Compare going right to left and left to right. Repeat level by level, moving cephalad looking for asymmetric motion. Remove the pillow and lay the head on the table. Repeat the side-to-side, level-by-level gliding, adding a slight diagonal inferior-to-superior motion to create an *extension movement*. Note whether in *flexion or extension* and record the level and direction of restriction per screening exam worksheet.

To refine this a bit, consistent with the nomenclature used for the thoracic spine, if a restriction is noted in cervical flexion, the vertebrae is most likely (but not always) stuck in an extended position. It is positioned in extension, rotation, and side bending not allowing it to go into the flexed, rotated, and side bent position you are trying to glide it into. Record this as an ERS lesion and note the direction it will not fully glide to. During passive cervical flexion, if C5 cannot fully glide to the patient's right, record it as C5 ERS right. If in extension C3 does not fully glide to the patients left, this would be recorded as C3 FRS left.

The final supine screening technique is to check lower cervical and upper thoracic segmental side bending at the *cervico-thoracic juncture*.

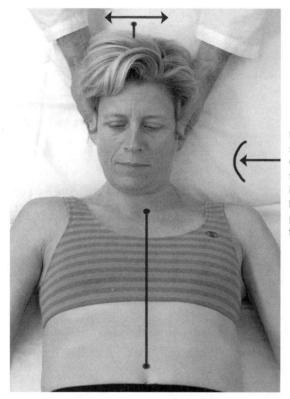

Figure 16-10   Cervical segmental mobility. Cervical segmental translation to patient's right, creating relative left cervical side bending. Head propped on pillow to maintain cervical flexion.

The examiner holds the head in his or her hand, uses the web space between the thumb and index finger to stabilize the cervico-thoracic juncture, and induces side bending. Compare side-to-side and with normals to get a feel for restriction. When flexible, the patient's ear will be within 1-2 inches of their acromium. If severely restricted and not mobilizing in therapy, obtain an x-ray to determine either if arthritic and likely will not move or non arthritic tissue restriction that will need further aggressive mobilization.

D. Prone

23. Ischial Tuberosity Symmetry

The prone exam will look at the symmetry of the ischial tuberosities, sacral base, lumbar spinal segments, and posterior muscle firing. Ask the patient to lay face down. Explain that the alignment of the pelvis, sacrum/"tailbone," and the spine are being examined, and also look at the back muscles. The ischial tuberosity is rounded. The goal is to palpate the same relative spot on each side simultaneously. Prompt the patient to momentarily flex at the knees to hold their feet off the table.

This fires the hamstrings. The examiner palpates the hamstrings bilaterally with thumbs progressing superiorly to the origin on the ischial tuberosities. Have them relax and let their legs onto the table. Now maintain equal pressure at this spot on the ischial tuberosities and scan side-to-side for symmetry or asymmetry in the cephalad-caudal direction. As per earlier exam techniques,·record as being inferior or superior the ipsilateral side at which the standing flexion or one-legged stork was positive.

Unleveling can occur with a pelvic asymmetry, sacral torsion, or ischial shear. In this context, an ischial shear is when the hemi pelvis has slid superiorly or inferiorly on the sacroiliac joint. This is not actually a joint disruption but could be thought of sliding the two structures opposite to each other to the total end range of joint play. If restricted in this position, the prolonged ligamentous and muscle tension can be quite painful. To experience this, pull or twist your little finger to an end stretch and hold it there for awhile. Imagine what it would feel like if stuck that way for days, weeks, or months.

24. *Sacral Base Symmetry*

The sacral base is not the inferior portion of the sacrum but actually the superior portion or "base" that the lumbar spine sets on. To find this location, palpate the underslope of the PSISs as you did for the standing flexion test. Now move medially a thumb width then superiorly two thumb widths. You will find a sulcus that the thumb will drop into. Simultaneously palpate bilaterally with equal pressure in an anterior direction. Observe the depth of your thumbs for symmetry or asymmetry (Figure 16-11). In keeping with prior exam techniques, if asymmetric, record which thumb is posterior on the ipsilateral side at which the standing flexion or stork test was positive. To check this in some degree of lumbar flexion, place a pillow under the lower abdomen/pelvis of thin patients. (Larger patients already have their "pillow.") Evaluate in spinal extension. Have the patient prop prone on elbows, chin supported in their hands to help quiet the paraspinals. As above, check again for symmetry. It is beyond the scope of this chapter to delineate between sacral torsions and unilaterally flexed or extended sacral dysfunctions. For the reader already aware of these, torsion will have asymmetry either in flexion or extension but not both, whereas a unilaterally flexed or extended lesion will maintain its asymmetry relative to the other side in both flexion and extension.

25. *Lumbar Spine Segmental Symmetry*

Lumbar spine segmental mobility and alignment is assessed the same way as the sacrum except the examiner's thumbs palpate over the region of the transverse processes in the gutter between the longissimus and multifidus muscles. The technique is the same as above for the thoracic spine. When asymmetries are present, record whether in flexion or extension, the spinal level, and which thumb is posterior.

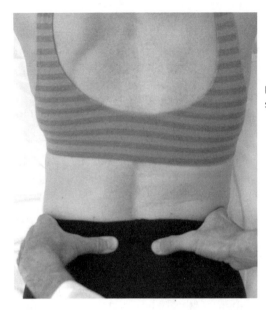

Figure 16-11 Sacral base symmetry.

The propped prone position is excellent for the evaluation in extension. Prone on a pillow is good for major malrotations, but mild to moderate may be missed due to insufficient lumbar flexion. Sensitivity may be increased by screening lumbar flexion while the patient is seated during the thoracic spine evaluation and waiting to screen lumbar extension when the patient is propped prone on elbows. This is also a good position to further screen the thoracic spine in extension.

26. *Prone Leg Extension: Muscle Firing*

Muscle hypertonicity and imbalance can perpetuate biomechanical asymmetries and back pain. A good musculoskeletal physical therapist should do a detailed screen. To be able to follow this and alert the therapist in case they have not done so, a brief in-office screen should look at the firing, mass, and tension generated during activation of the hamstrings, gluteal muscles, lumbar paraspinals, thoracic paraspinals, and deep hip external rotators. This is not comprehensive but is quick and easy to check. If asymmetries or impaired firing are noted, these need to be treated. This tells the clinician that a treatable lesion is present, and suggests that further examination by the clinician or expert therapist will find more specific findings. Monitor muscle firing order, mass, and tension by observation and palpation. Spread your thumb and fingers of one hand across a region of the thoracic paraspinals and a finger or two from the other hand across the lumbar paraspinals. Have the patient perform unilateral prone leg extension, knee held extended/straight, lifting one foot just off the exam table. Note if the monitored muscles fire, when, and compare relative mass and tension developed. Palpate the gluteals and hamstrings. The exact firing order is debated, but in general the ipsilateral hamstrings and gluteals fire, followed by the lumbar paraspinals and then the thoracic paraspinals. Frequently in back pain, one finds the thoracic paraspinals firing first or simultaneously with the hamstrings, the hamstrings with minimal activation not generating much mass, and the gluteal muscles also inhibited with poor firing and limited tension/mass. The compensating muscles may be hypertonic and tender. Stretching to release them is helpful, but the real treatment is to restore the firing and strength of the impaired muscles they are compensating for. The poor firing may be related to tight antagonist muscles such as hip flexors, pain inhibition, deconditioning, or possibly dennervation from nerve impingement.

27. *Iliotibial Band Flexibility*

28. *Deep Hip External Rotator Muscle Firing ("Clam Shell")*

Achiness in the back and hip can be related to tight hip flexors, iliotibial band, and impaired function of the hip external rotator muscles. Ask the patient to lie on their side. Standing behind them, perform Obers position stabilizing the pelvis slightly anterior then bring the superior leg, knee flexed 90 degrees, passively into end range extension followed by allowing the leg to drop into adduction toward the floor. Iliotibial band flexibility is usually sufficient if the knee portion drops halfway or more to the table. If it does not drop, it needs released. Continue the side lying position. Have the patient lie hip and knee flexed about 45 degrees, legs on top of each other. The pelvis should be straight up and down or just slightly rolled anterior. The superior foot remains side lying on the bottom foot. Instruct them to *externally rotate* their top leg so the knee goes up and back as a "clam shell" opens. The femur externally rotates. They should not lift their leg sideways into abduction, just perform rotation. As this occurs, the examiner palpates over the abdominal obliques with one hand while the other monitors the deep hip external rotators just inferior to the the piriformis muscle. Minimal firing and tension should be felt in the abdominal obliques and the iliotibial band muscles. Muscle firing should be felt in the deep hip external rotators If not, notify the therapist to treat this.

29. *Rib Cage Mobility*

The last portion of the manual exam is to obtain a sense of *rib cage mobility* in a side lying position. To limit lumbar spinal rotation, have the patient hip flex to approximately 120 degrees. Allow them to have a pillow under their head, neck slightly flexed, and their upper arm resting out in front of them. Have them reach forward as if to reach for the junction of the wall and floor in front of them. The examiner passively follows the patient's rib cage glide to the end range of motion with overpressure to take the glide to full end stretch. At this point, attempt to continue the motion by adding a posterior-to-anterior nudge to feel the remaining spring of the ribs and connective tissue. Move the examining hand from level to level along the entire rib cage. Note areas of decreased mobility. Have the patient reposition and repeat the process on the other side for comparison.

Conclusion

If the exam reveals neurogenic changes and the manual medicine exam reveals minimal to no significant biomechanical asymmetries, focus on the neurogenic pain evaluation and treatment. If the neurologic and biomechanical exams are essentially normal, further explore the evaluation and treatment per the myofascial algorithm. If workup of all three pathways is negative or inconclusive, consider psychological overlay such as fear of movement or reinjury, hypervigilance, or secondary gain. Especially if work issues are present, refer for specialist intervention as soon as possible in an attempt to minimize the development of chronic pain behaviors.

Once learned, the subacute physical exam can be done in less than 10 minutes. This still may be too long for the busy primary care office, thus an abbreviated version of the manual medicine exam can be useful. The appendix to this chapter is a form that can be used to document the subacute physical examination. An abbreviated examination is indicated with asterisks.

Appendix: Manual Medicine Screening Exam

Items marked with an asterisk (*) are necessary components of an abbreviated exam.

Standing

1. Gait and Posture

Posterior view*
a. Shoulder height
b. Iliac crest height
c. Head tilt
d. T spine paravertebral fullness
e. L spine para vertebral fullness

Lateral view*
a. Cervical lordosis
b. Thoracic kyphosis
c. Lumbar lordosis

d. Head tilt
2. Standing flexion test*
   negative___ positive ___ L___ R___
3. Standing stork test*
   negative___ positive ___ L___ R___
4. Standing side bending test*
   full_ __ restricted ___ L___ R___
5. Standing trunk rotation test: waist stabilized by holding iliac crests or against exam table
   full___ restricted ___ L___ R___
   Can add passive rotation by holding iliac crests/waist and rotating pelvis and trunk (spine) as one unit for a Waddell's sign test.
6. Standing facet loading/foraminal closure; standing extension rotation and side bending of the spine.*
   negative___ positive ___ L___ R___   radiating to:

Seated

If not done, test reflexes, sensation, strength, and seated straight leg raise, then proceed to the following components of the manual exam. Remember to note and compare seated to supine straight leg raise if considering Waddell's signs.
7. Seated flexion test
   negative___ positive ___ L___ R___
8. Upper extremity screen (shoulder abduction and touch dorsum of hands together above head)
   full___ restricted ___ L___ R___
9. Passive trunk rotation seated (can use if questionable effort or relaxation during standing trunk rotation)
   full___ restricted ___ L___ R___
10. Passive trunk side bending seated
    full___ restricted ___ L___ R___
11. Cervical spine range of motion seated (may skip this, wait for no. 20)
    Flexion   full___ restricted___
    Extension   full___ restricted___
    Side bending   full___ restricted: L___ R___
    Rotation   full___ restricted: L___ R___
12. Thoracic spine segmental motion*
    Flexion (ERS lesion) level ___   posterior   L level(s) _____
                                                    R level(s) _____
    Extension (FRS lesion) level ___   posterior   L level(s) _____
                                                    R level(s) _____
13. First rib: r/o superior displacement*
    Can add trunk compression on shoulders or compression on top of head to "load" spine for a Waddell's sign test.

Supine (bridge first)

(Nos. 14,15, and 16: Record according to same side on which flexion tests were positive.)

14. Medial malleolus symmetry*
    level___ superior___ inferior___
15. Anterior superior iliac spine symmetry (ASIS)*
    level___ superior___ inferior___
    (Measure leg length if asymmetric)
16. Pubic symphysis symmetry*
    level___ superior___ inferior___
17. Straight leg raise (monitor ASIS for pelvic rotation)*
    a. Hamstring full___ decreased L _____ R_____ degrees
    b. Nerve root tension negative___ positive @ L_____ R_____ degrees
18. Lower extremity internal-external rotation, passive, 90/90 hip and knee flexion*
    full___ restricted: L_____ R_____ (degrees)
19. Piriformis-gluteal muscle and hip capsule flexibility (consider hip scour and hip capsule exam)*
    full___ restricted: L ___ R___
20. FABERE (flexion, abduction, external rotation, and extension) of the femur*
    full ___ restricted to ___ L degrees _____
                        ___ R degrees _____
21. Rib cage
    a. Alignment (general look for scoliosis, rib cage hump when seated and standing)
    b. Inhalation restriction
    (For a and b: follow along anterior axillary line location of rib up and down during breathing.)
    c. Exhalation restriction
22. Cervical spine segmental motion*
    C1-C2 rotation   full___ restricted to   ___L degrees _____
                                          ___R degrees _____
    Flexion (look for ERS lesions)
                          full___ restricted to   ___L level(s) _____
                                            ___R level(s) _____
    Extension (look for FRS lesions)
                          full___ restricted to   ___L level(s) _____
                                            ___R level(s) _____
    Cervical-thoracic junction
                          full___ restricted to   ___L degrees _____
                                            ___R degrees _____

Prone

23. Ischial tuberosity symmetry (greater than a thumb width asymmetry)
    level___ superior___ inferior___
24. Sacral base symmetry*
    Flexion level   ___ posterior L___ R___
    Extension level   ___ posterior L___ R___
25. Lumbar spine segmental symmetry*
    Flexion (ERS lesion)   level ___ posterior   L level(s) _____
                                                     R level(s) _____
                             (pillow under abdomen if thin person)
    Extension (FRS lesions)   level ___ posterior   L level(s) _____
                                                     R level(s) _____
    (prop prone on elbows, chin supported in hands to quiet paraspinals)
26. Prone leg extension-muscle firing* (exact order is debatable; look for firing and compensation of thoracic paraspinals, for poor firing of lumbar paraspinals or gluteals)
    (Perform passive leg extension stabilizing pelvis to table to assess for hip flexor tightness and to look for femoral nerve stretch dural tension signs).

Side-Lying

27. Iliotibial band flexibility
28. Deep hip external rotator muscle firing ("clam shell")
29. Rib cage*
    Posterior to anterior/inferior gliding motion
    Position patient on side, hips flexed 90-120 degrees, head on pillow, neck slightly flexed. Have patient place upper arm out in front as if to reach for the juncture of the wall and floor. With examiner's hands aligned along the ribs, passively follow the rib cage glide, then add an overpressure challenge to maximize rib cage glide. Identify areas of focal restriction, asymmetry, or global restriction.

■   ■   ■

Key Points

- At weeks 6 to 12, subacute back pain that is not spontaneously resolving warrants a more detailed physical exam to improve the clinician's ability to sort out neurogenic, structural, and myofascial pain.

- The subacute physical exam is basically the same as the acute physical exam with minor modifications and the addition of the manual medicine exam. With practice, it can be accomplished in 10 minutes.
- The abbreviated version of the manual medicine exam can be used by the busy clinician who only needs to answer whether biomechanical lesions are present in order to decide whether to refer to a specialist physician or therapist.
- The sensory examination can be improved by quantifying side-to-side differences, paying attention to hyperesthesia, and looking for neuropathic changes.
- The side of positive standing flexion, seated flexion, or stork test is used to reference an asymmetry noted at the anterior superior iliac spine (ASIS), posterior superior iliac spine (PSIS), medial malleolus, pubic symphysis, or ischial tuberosities.
- Biomechanical dysfunctions (i.e., malalignment with surrounding tissues on prolonged end stretch) can be painful and is treatable.
- Muscle imbalance can create hypertonic tender overused muscle as well as deconditioned poorly firing weak achy muscles. Look for pain inhibition and overactivity of antagonist muscle groups. These imbalances can perpetuate biomechanical structural asymmetries.
- Remember first and second rib dysfunctions in cases of ongoing upper back, shoulder girdle, and arm pain, especially if imaging, EMG, and thoracic outlet studies are negative.

REFERENCE

1. **Greenman PE.** Principles of Manual Medicine, 3rd ed. Philadelphia: Lippincott Williams & Wilkins; 2003.
2. **Greenman PE.** Principles of Manual Medicine, 2nd ed. Baltimore: Williams & Wilkins; 1996.
3. **Greenman PE.** Syndromes of the lumbar spine, pelvis, and sacrum. Phys Med Rehab Clin North Am. 1996;7(4):773-6.
4. **Greenman, PE.** Muscle Energy and High Velocity Thrust Techniques Video tape series. Baltimore: Williams & Wilkins; 1992.

17

■   ■   ■

Imaging of Back Pain

Douglas J. Quint, MD

For the primary care physician, there are two key issues with respect to imaging of patients with back pain: *when* to perform imaging and *which* imaging tests to perform. As is true of any diagnostic test, imaging studies should be performed based on whether the results will determine or alter management decisions. In general, imaging studies are useful for detecting anatomic abnormalities and ruling out serious disease such as infection or neoplasm but should not be used as the sole test to establish a diagnosis and should always be considered in the context of the clinical picture.

The majority of patients with acute back pain either with or without associated focal neurologic symptoms (e.g., sensory changes, motor findings, changes in reflexes) recover in about a month with conservative therapy (e.g., rest, graded exercise, and/or anti-inflammatory medications). Specifically, 50% of patients with new acute "uncomplicated" back pain recover in 2 weeks with 90% of patients recovering in 6 weeks, and the etiology of the pain being determined in less than 15% of patients.

Therefore, as most patients recover in 6 weeks, no imaging should be considered until a patient has failed 6-8 weeks of conservative therapy, except if "red flags" are present (Table 17-1) (see Chapter 9 for a discussion of indications for emergent imaging).

Spinal Imaging Tests

The most common imaging tests for evaluation of the spine include plain radiographs, magnetic resonance imaging (MRI), myelography, computed tomography (CT), and myelography followed by CT scanning (MyCT). Rarely, nuclear scintigraphy and diskography may be considered (Table 17-2).

Table 17-1   Acute Back Pain: Indications for Emergent Spinal Imaging (Red Flags)

- Suspected primary spinal neoplasm
- Suspected metastatic disease in the setting of known malignancy
- Suspected diskitis, osteomyelitis, or abscess (e.g., immunocompromised patient)
- Suspected noninfectious inflammatory process (e.g., spondyloarthropathy)
- Acute spinal trauma (without or with symptoms)

Table 17-2   Spinal Imaging Tests

- Plain radiographs
- Myelography
- Computed tomography (CT)
- Myelography followed by CT (MyCT)
- Magnetic resonance imaging (MRI)
- Nuclear scintigraphy (bone scan)
- Diskography

Radiography

Plain radiographs are relatively inexpensive, universally available, and demonstrate many osseous abnormalities that can cause back pain. In addition, "dynamic" images can be obtained (e.g., flexion and extension x-rays), which can demonstrate abnormal spinal motion. The main disadvantage of plain x-rays is that normal soft tissues such as the spinal cord, nerves, and intervertebral disks cannot be imaged, and most spinal pathologic processes (e.g., herniated disks, non-osseous degenerative changes, tumors, abscesses, hematomas, etc.) cannot be detected (Figures 17-1A, 17-2A, and 17-3A). Plain radiographs may also miss some fractures. Even many intrinsic osseous lesions are difficult to delineate. In fact, until 30% of a bone is replaced by a pathologic process (e.g., tumor, infection), no osseous abnormality will be seen on a plain radiograph.

Plain radiography is indicated for emergency evaluation of possible fracture or red flag, but often subsequent MRI or CT is needed in cases with a high index of suspicion. They are also indicated in the evaluation of potential spondylolisthesis in a young person, but only anterior-posterior and lateral film should be done first, with obliques following only if these films are negative. Special sacroiliac joint views are useful in detecting sacroiliac joint arthritis that occurs in seronegative spondyloarthropathies. Occasionally, flexion-extension x-rays are useful in a patient with indications for surgical fusion when routine MRI or CT do not show the problem.

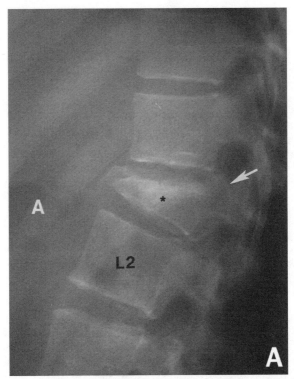

Figure 17-1   Traumatic compression fracture. A 33-year-old status post (s/p) fall from 15 feet. "Unsteady" on feet. Lateral plain radiograph (Figure 17-1A, above) demonstrates L1 compression fracture and possible posterior displacement of a fracture fragment into the spinal canal (*arrow*). Sagittal T₁-weighted MR (Figure 17-1B) redemonstrates the compression fracture and demonstrates encroachment of the fracture fragment (*arrow*) on the distal spinal cord (c). Axial T₁-weighted MR (Figure 17-1C) and axial CT (Figure 17-1D) through the L1 compression fracture confirms that CT is superior to MR for demonstrating fractures whereas MR better demonstrates spinal canal structures. A = anterior; * = L1 compression fracture; c = distal spinal cord; L1 = L1 vertebral body; L2 = L2 vertebral body; arrow = fracture fragment in spinal canal.

Myelography

With myelography, iodinated contrast material is injected into the spinal subarachnoid space via a lumbar puncture (LP), allowing contour abnormalities on or within the contrast column to be observed (Figures 17-4A, 17-4B).

Myelography alone is rarely indicated, primarily for standing flexion-extension views to evaluate dynamic nerve impingement.

Computed Tomography

CT scanning (without administration of intravenous or intrathecal contrast material) can be performed with imaging sections as thin as 1 mm. CT

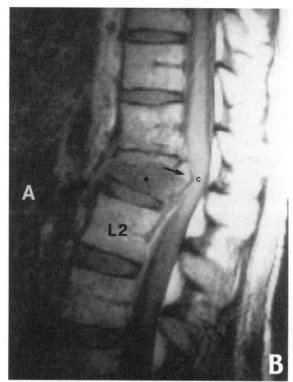

Figure 17-1B. See caption on page 201.

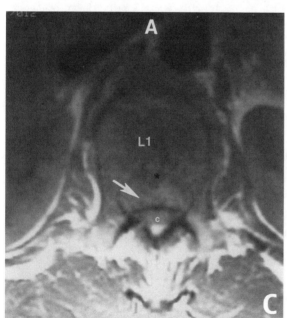

Figure 17-1C. See caption on page 201.

demonstrates acute osseous abnormalities better than any other imaging test (Figure 17-1D). Soft tissue lesions can also be detected with much better sensitivity than plain x-rays or myelography. However, normal soft tissue can still be indistinguishable from pathologic soft tissue on CT scans; this is the reason for performing CT scanning immediately *after* myelography and is also why plain CT and myelography followed by CT are inferior to MRI for the detection of neoplasm and infection (Figure 17-1C vs. Figure 17-1D). CT scanning exposes a patient to the risks of radiation at a dose greater than that for plain radiographs or myelography, which can be of concern when the lumbar spine is being evaluated in females.

Computed tomography is indicated in the evaluation of potential fracture, diagnosis of spondylolysis, and evaluation of fusion. In conjunction with myelography, it may detect some disk lesions or nerve impingement that MRI misses.

Magnetic Resonance Imaging

Magnetic resonance imaging is an imaging technique that does not use ionizing radiation. The rapid application of radiofrequency pulses that temporarily perturb the local magnetic environment of a patient's water molecules can be used to generate an image. MRI best demonstrates soft tissues, can be performed in any plane without the patient having to move

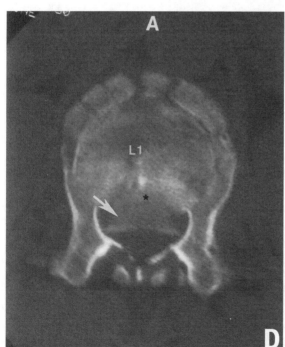

Figure 17-1D. See caption on page 201.

into different positions, and usually does not require administration of any contrast material for the evaluation of back pain (in patients without previous back surgery or suspected spinal neoplasm or infection). MRI is a noninvasive procedure and has no known side effects at the field strengths used for clinical studies. It is the only imaging technique that permits *direct* visualization of the spinal cord (Figures 17-1B, 17-1C, 17-3B, 17-5). Although not ideal for directly visualizing osseous structures (e.g., fractures [Figure 17-1C], cortical erosions reflecting subtle bone abnormalities), it is superb for detecting *intrinsic* osseous abnormalities (e.g., metastatic disease, diskitis/osteomyelitis, etc.; Figs 17-3B, 17-5). MRI is indicated in the evaluation of most red flags, in the diagnosis of radiating low back pain that has lasted more than 6 weeks, in the evaluation of chronic low back pain to rule out treatable lesions, and (usually with contrast injection) in the evaluation of new significant pain in patients with previous surgery.

Nuclear Scintigraphy and Diskography

Other less commonly used imaging tests for the evaluation of back pain include nuclear scintigraphy (i.e., technetium-99 bone scans) and diskography.

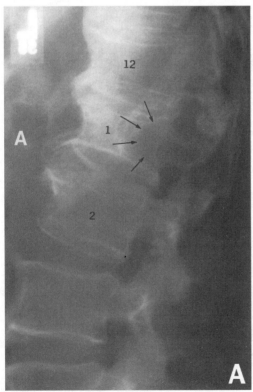

Figure 17-2   Spinal canal neurofibroma. A 73-year-old with 5-year history of back pain; no focal neurologic deficits. Lateral plain radiograph of the lumbar spine (Figure 17-2A, left) demonstrates a mild L1 compression fracture, degenerative changes of the T12/L1 and L1/L2 end plates, and erosion of the posterior aspect of the L1 vertebral body (*arrows*). Whereas spinal canal abnormalities cannot be seen on plain radiographs, sagittal contrast-enhanced T_1-weighted MR (Figure 17-2B) demonstrates a large neurofibroma (N) filling the spinal canal and eroding into the posterior aspect of the L1 vertebral body (*arrows*). N = neurofibroma; 12 = T12 vertebral body; 1 = L1 vertebral body; 2 = L2 vertebral body; A = anterior.

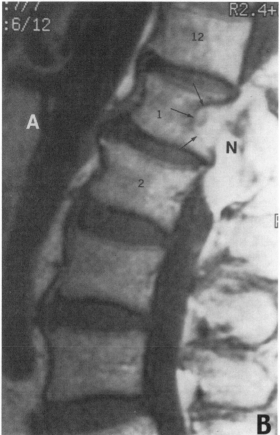

Figure 17-2B.   See caption on page 204.

Bone scans demonstrate turnover of bone as might be seen in degenerative spinal disease, spinal infection, or neoplasm. Although osseous changes will be detected on a bone scan, the cause of the bone changes (e.g., whether the pathologic process is infection, tumor, or degenerative change) and the extent of that inciting process (e.g., whether the process extends into the spinal canal or paraspinal regions) is not delineated. Bone scintigraphy is considered a sensitive but nonspecific test. Essentially, everyone with spinal degenerative changes will have a positive bone scan, but it cannot be determined if there is an associated herniated disk, spinal stenosis, neural foraminal narrowing, or an underlying infection or neoplastic process in most patients. Scintigraphy is considered similar to MRI for the detection of many metastases, but scintigraphy is inferior to MRI for the detection of some neoplasms (e.g., myeloma) and is far inferior for delineating the actual extent of a spinal abnormality. Scintigraphy is useful for detecting osteoid osteomas in children and for the early detection of subtle fractures (e.g., early changes of spondylolysis). Scintigraphy is considered

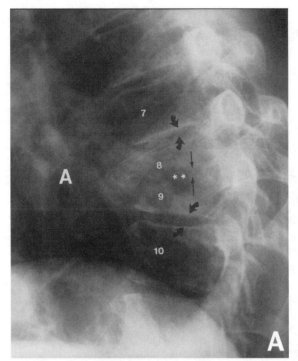

Figure 17-3   *Streptococcus milleri* diskitis with osteomyelitis. A 47-year-old with back pain and fever. Lateral plain radiograph (Figure 17-3A, above) demonstrates loss of the inferior T8 and superior T9 vertebral end plates with apparent "loss" of the T8/T9 intervertebral disk space (*) consistent with diskitis with osteomyelitis. Sagittal contrast-enhanced T_1-weighted MR (Figure 17-3B) redemonstrates the diskitis with osteomyelitis but also shows spinal canal extension by abscess (AB) with spinal cord compression (*large straight arrow*) at this level. A = anterior; 7 = T7 vertebral body; 8 = T8 vertebral body; 9 = T9 vertebral body; 10 = T10 vertebral body; curved arrows = normal end plates; small arrows = absent vertebral end plates; c = spinal cord.

an essentially noninvasive test with radiation exposure less than that of plain radiographs or CT scanning.

Bone scans are indicated in the search for bony metastases, occult fractures, or active spondylolysis in a young person. Focused single photon emission computed tomography (SPECT) imaging can pick up some lesions that a bone scan will miss, and a whole body scan will pick up diffuse arthritis or metastases.

Diskography is a provocative test that attempts to identify an individual intervertebral disk (which may appear entirely normal on other imaging tests) as a cause of a patient's back pain. This test involves placement of a needle into individual intervertebral disks with the injection of contrast material. During the injection, the patient is asked if they are experiencing an exacerbation of their symptoms. If so, surgical fusion of that disk level may result in resolution of patient symptoms. Diskography is a more invasive

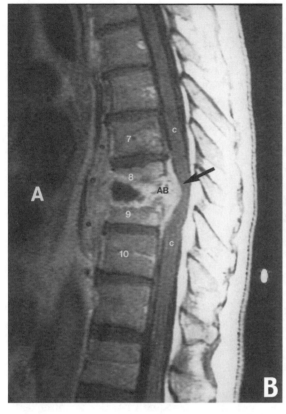

Figure 17-3B. See caption on page 206.

test than myelography and is performed under fluoroscopic guidance, so there are the risks of radiation. The indications for diskography are controversial, but the proponents believe that the test is useful in the evaluation of "diskogenic" axial pain in a patient who is prepared to consider surgery.

Role of Imaging

When performed, imaging of the spine should be used to *confirm* a clinical impression of pathology based on history, physical examination, and basic laboratory tests. When evaluating back pain (or in an asymptomatic patient), imaging tests *cannot* be the sole determining factor for deciding on a treatment regimen. This is because imaging tests are often positive in asymptomatic patients (up to 40% of the time!) (Table 17-3) and, similarly, may also demonstrate abnormalities in portions of the spine that do not correlate with patient symptoms.

Surgery on, or therapeutic injections of, an area of imaging abnormality that does not correlate with patient symptoms will not successfully treat

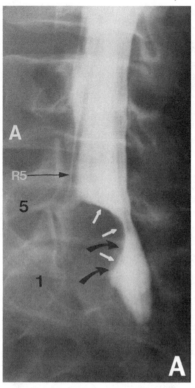

Figure 17-4   Herniated lumbar disk. A-30-year old with right S1 radiculopathy. Right oblique myelogram (Figure 17-4A, left) demonstrates large filling defect (*straight white arrows*) due to herniated L5/S1 disk with compression/displacement of right S1 nerve root sleeve (*closed curved arrows*). Normal right oblique myelogram (Figure 17-4B) for comparison. Note normal right-sided nerve root sleeves (*straight black arrows*). Post-myelogram CT at the L5/S1 intervertebral disk level (Figure 17-4C) directly demonstrates the right dorso-laterally herniated disk (*straight white arrows*) displacing/compressing the right S1 nerve root (*closed curved arrow*). The left S1 nerve root is normal (*open curved arrow*) on the post-myelogram CT (Figure 17-4C). A = anterior; 5 = L5 vertebral body; 1 = S1 vertebral body; R3 = right L3 nerve root; R4 = right L4 nerve root; R5 = right L5 nerve root; S1 = right S1 nerve root; S2 = right S2 nerve root; 5-1 = L5/S1 intervertebral disk.

Table 17-3   Percent of Asymptomatic Patients with Positive Imaging Test

Imaging Test	Asymptomatic Patients with Positive Test
Myelography	24%
CT	34%
MRI	40%

patient pain and may even make the pain worse. For this reason, "clinical correlation" of imaging findings is crucial.

In patients with chronic back pain (more than several months) that is not objectively progressive, psychosocial issues may complicate evaluation and the role of imaging is less clear. This topic is further discussed in Chapters 10 and 25.

Recommendations

• In patients with acute back pain, MRI should be the first test performed, as the widest range of pathology can be evaluated with this test (Figures 17-2B, 17-6). Plain radiographs are of limited value for ruling in or ruling

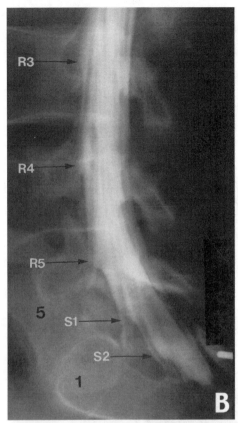

Figure 17-4B.   See caption on page 208.

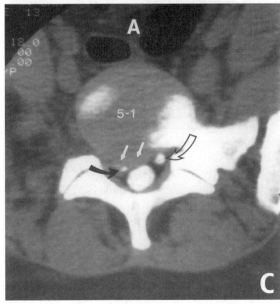

Figure 17-4C.   See caption on page 208.

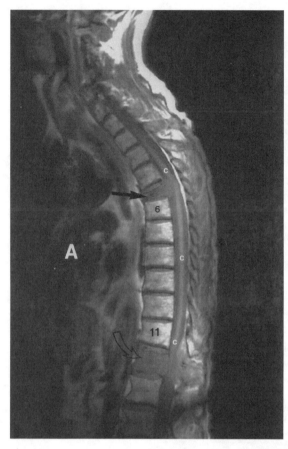

Figure 17-5   Spinal lymphoma. A 58-year-old male with new acute onset lower extremity paraplegia over the past 24 hours. Emergent sagittal noncontrast T_1-weighted MR scan demonstrates two spinal foci of lymphoma invading the spinal canal and compressing the spinal cord-a symptomatic lesion at T12 (*curved arrow*) and an "incidental" lesion at T5 (*straight arrow*). A = anterior; 6 = T6 level; 11 = T11 level; c = spinal cord.

out most pathologic processes. However, occasionally, additional imaging (such as plain radiographs including flexion/extension views to evaluate for spinal instability and/or CT scanning to better characterize osseous lesions) may be necessary.

- If there are contraindications to MRI or the patient is unable to tolerate MRI, myelography followed by CT scanning should be performed. (It should be noted that myelography followed by CT, although more invasive than MRI and associated with greater risks than MRI, is just as sensitive as MRI for the detection of spinal cord compression, central spinal stenosis, and essentially all pathologic spinal processes that require emergent surgical intervention.) Although MRI documents the presence of a herniated nucleus polposus (HNP), the clinical significance of the lesion may range from asymptomatic to severe neuralgic deficit and pain.

Key Points

- Imaging studies should be performed on an urgent basis in the event of trauma or when neoplasm, spinal infection, or a noninfectious inflammatory process is suspected.
- For patients without red flags, imaging studies should not be ordered unless pain has not resolved after 6 to 8 weeks of conservative therapy.
- Plain radiographs are inexpensive and readily available. They are useful for ruling out fractures, but they cannot image soft tissues.
- MRI is the first imaging test of choice, because it is noninvasive, does not use ionizing radiation, and permits direct visualization of the spinal cord, as well as demonstrates soft tissues.
- Myelography, an invasive test, is almost always followed by computed tomography to permit direct visualization of many pathological processes.
- Computed tomography is the best imaging test for the detection of acute osseous abnormalities but is not useful for distinguishing pathologic from normal soft tissue.
- Nuclear scintigraphy and diskography are other, less commonly used, imaging tests.

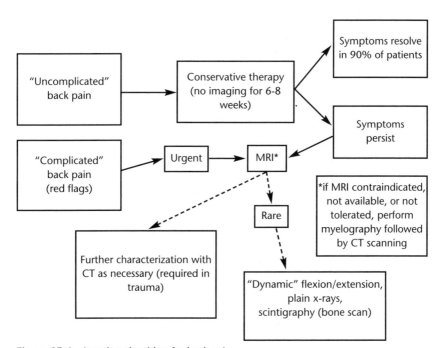

Figure 17-6   Imaging algorithm for back pain.

■   ■   ■

BIBLIOGRAPHY

Boden SD, Swanson AL. An assessment of the early management of spine problems and appropriateness of diagnostic imaging utilization. Phys Med Rehabil Clin North Am. 1998;9:411-7.

Bueff HU, Van der Reis W. Low back pain. Primary Care; Clinics in Office Practice. 1996;23:345-64.

Haldeman S. Diagnostic tests for the evaluation of back and neck pain. Neurologic Clinics. Philadelphia: WB Saunders; 1996;103-117.

Jinkins JR, ed. The lumbosacral spine. Neuroimaging Clin North Am. 1993;3:411-630.

Keim HA, Kiraldy-Willis WH. Low back pain. Rheumatology Rounds. Summit, New Jersey: CIBA-GEIGY Corp.; 1987.

Laredo J-D, ed. Imaging of low back pain I. Radiol Clin North Am. 2000;38:1153-1327.

Laredo J-D, ed. Imaging of low back pain II. Radiol Clin North Am. 2001;39:1-168.

Mooney V, Saal JA, Saal JS. Evaluation and treatment of low back pain. CIBA Clinical Symposia. 1996;48:1-32.

Ross JS, Masaryk TJ, Modic MT. Lumbar spine. In: Stark DD, Bradley WG, eds. Magnetic Resonance Imaging, 3rd ed. St. Louis: Mosby; 1999:1883-906.

18

■　■　■

Electromyography and Low Back Pain

Andrew J. Haig, MD

lectrodiagnostics, also known as electromyography (EMG), is one of the secret weapons in the management of back pain. It is equally sensitive to disk herniation as MRI, provides rare false positives, and is only one third the cost. It is able to diagnose many of the peripheral lesions that mimic radiculopathy but do not show up on scans. It is able to rate the severity and even the timing of the lesion. But this "secret weapon" is poorly understood by many physicians. It is not a test in the same sense as radiography. Rather, it is more accurately a *consultation* with a physician that happens to involve a highly technical tool to extend the physical examination. Only when the primary care physician looks at electrodiagnostics in this light can he or she use it effectively.

With a minimal amount of technical talk, this chapter will briefly outline the process of electrodiagnostic consultation. It will review ways electrodiagnostic consultation can be used for low back pain. Finally, it will review ways the primary care physician can determine whether the consultation has adequately addressed his or her questions.

Goals and Strategy of Electrodiagnostic Testing

The typical referral to an electromyography (EMG) lab reads: "Rule out radiculopathy." However, any good specialist in electrodiagnostic medicine acknowledges the question but then goes on to perform a history and physical examination sufficient to form his or her own differential diagnosis. The real value of the consultation lies not just in confirming or ruling out a radiculopathy but in detecting the frequent other causes of "radiating" back pain. Electrodiagnosis clearly comes up with answers the referring physician does not always expect (1,2). In one study of upper limb neurologic complaints, despite a detailed expert history and physical examination, the electrodiagnostic testing substantially altered or added a diagnosis in about one third of cases (3). A yet-to-be published study of back and lower limb electrodiagnostic consultation shows the same.

The disciplined electrodiagnostic differential diagnosis for radiating pain is shown in Figure 18-1. It begins in the brain and progresses distally. Mechanical low back pain occurs so frequently that it is not at all uncommon for a second cause of the "radiation" to be coincident. The consultant reviews the differential diagnosis as a source for alternative explanations

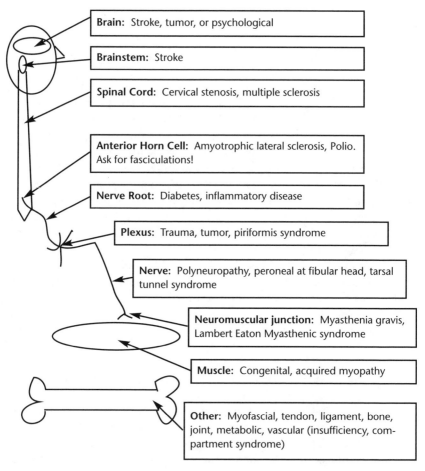

Brain: Stroke, tumor, or psychological

Brainstem: Stroke

Spinal Cord: Cervical stenosis, multiple sclerosis

Anterior Horn Cell: Amyotrophic lateral sclerosis, Polio. Ask for fasciculations!

Nerve Root: Diabetes, inflammatory disease

Plexus: Trauma, tumor, piriformis syndrome

Nerve: Polyneuropathy, peroneal at fibular head, tarsal tunnel syndrome

Neuromuscular junction: Myasthenia gravis, Lambert Eaton Myasthenic syndrome

Muscle: Congenital, acquired myopathy

Other: Myofascial, tendon, ligament, bone, joint, metabolic, vascular (insufficiency, compartment syndrome)

Figure 18-1 Electrodiagnostic differential diagnosis of lumbar disk herniation. More important than the details is acquiring the habit of considering a differential diagnosis in an orderly fashion from the brain down to the muscles.

and also to plan a strategy of testing. For example, in a diabetic, the first test might well be a nerve conduction to rule out a polyneuropathy that would affect the subsequent needle examination.

The physician then picks a strategy to address the differential diagnosis. General test components include needle electromyography and nerve conduction studies. The specific muscles and nerves tested depend on the differential diagnosis, level of suspicion for an abnormal test, the patient's tolerance for the test, and the clinician's training bias. The optimal number of muscles tested to screen for a lumbar radiculopathy has been established at five limb muscles plus the paraspinals (4). If any of the muscles are abnormal, then more muscles may be tested. The goal is to isolate a lesion to a specific nerve or root, to "surround the lesion with normal findings" to be sure that abnormalities are not part of a generalized process such as a polyneuropathy or polyradiculopathy.

Needle Electromyography

Needle electromyography involves "listening" to spontaneous and voluntary electrical activity emitted from muscle cells using a needle electrode. Spontaneous activity, termed *positive waves* or *fibrillations* ("P's and Fibs" on many report forms) suggests that muscle cells are denervated. The doctor inserts the needle into the muscle, then tries to tease out spontaneous activity by quick, very small insertions-maybe six insertions in four different directions. The abnormalities are rated 0 (or negative) to 4+. Even a finding of 1+ suggests pathology.

The next step is to look at voluntary activity in the muscle. A motor unit is a group of muscle cells that are all related to a single anterior horn cell in the spinal cord. *Polyphasic* motor units are jagged looking on the EMG screen and are abnormal. Small polyphasic motor units suggest a myopathy (shrunken muscle cells make it small). Large polyphasic motor units suggest a nerve injury (the anterior horn cell has adopted muscle cells that have lost their innervation). Shorthand notation on some reports, (e.g., "normal" or "polyphasic") is common, but it is hard to tell how much inspection the physician did. A really good electromyographer samples at least 10 motor units to get a sense of what's going on in a muscle and records something like this: "6 of 10 motor units polyphasic, typically 8 turns, duration 10 milliseconds, 4000 microvolt amplitude."

The final step in a given muscle is to look at motor unit *recruitment*, or the order in which motor units help each other out as a person increased effort. If there has been a significant nerve injury-if some motor units have "dropped out" of the picture, then the firing rate of the first recruited motor unit is very fast when another motor unit finally begins to help out. For example, perhaps it is normal for motor unit A to begin firing, then B, C, and D to help out in turn. If B and C are dead, then A fires like crazy trying to move the bone before the spinal cord finally dials up D to help out. Motor unit recruitment is usually recorded simply as "increased," although a real expert will record the actual firing rate of the first motor unit when the second drops in. (e.g., "recruitment less than 20 hertz" is normal)

Nerve Conduction Studies

Nerve conduction studies are helpful adjuncts to the needle examination. The concept is simple. Place an electrode that can pick up small electrical signals over a muscle that a certain nerve attaches to or over the nerve itself. Somewhere else along the course of the nerve, give an electrical stimulation to the skin overlying the nerve. See how long it takes for the nerve to carry the impulse to the recording electrode. This is called *latency*, or if divided by the distance, *conduction velocity*. The size of the signal, *amplitude*, can be compared to norms to determine whether all of the nerve fibers conducted electricity. So anything that kills off nerve axons (an axonal neuropathy, a radiculopathy, or a focal lesion) decreases the amplitude, and anything that damages the myelin cells that surround the nerve and speed its conduction (a demyelinating polyneuropathy or a gradual compression) causes decrease in conduction velocity. Different laboratories have different norms. In planning a consultation, the electrodiagnostician chooses from well over 100 different sensory and motor tests.

A number of nerve conduction studies can test areas where a surface probe cannot go. H-waves are the neurophysiologic equivalent of tapping the Achilles' tendon with a hammer-the impulse goes up the sensory fibers of the nerve, across the spinal cord, synapses with the anterior horn cell, and comes down to a muscle. It is mostly used to assess radiculopathy and neuropathy. In the leg, H-waves can only be obtained from the S-1 nerve root. The H-reflex is generally used to assess S1 radiculopathy. H-waves have overlapping sensitivity with the needle examination. Sometimes the only electrodiagnostic abnormality in a person with radicular pain is the H-wave.

F-waves are a nonphysiologic "trick" in which motor fibers are stimulated and the impulse travels up to the anterior horn cell (and down to the muscle, but that's just another routine motor nerve conduction study). The impulse bounces around the anterior horn cell and about 10% of the time it ricochets down the axon again, causing a motor unit in the muscle to twitch a second time. For spinal disorders, F-waves are almost never abnormal when the needle EMG is normal. But they may be confirmatory, and are useful in evaluation of plexus lesions and polyneuropathy that may enter into the differential diagnosis of low back pain.

Sensory Evoked Potentials

Somatosensory or dermatosensory evoked potentials involve averaging the electroencephalogram brain waves during a large number of stimulations on the skin. Behind all of the noise of brain activity is a consistent brain response linked in time to the stimulus that can be detected after many signals are averaged. Sensory evoked potentials are used to assess sensory neurons in the peripheral and spinal cord pathways, particularly in spinal stenosis and spinal cord myelopathy. Less commonly used are direct nerve root stimulation, in which a needle is introduced near the nerve root to stimulate, and motor evoked potentials in which the brain is stimulated with a strong magnet and the signal is picked up over the muscle. Sensory evoked potentials are not useful in the evaluation of back pain, with one exception: Technically well done dermatomal sensory potentials may add to the diagnosis of spinal stenosis.

Drafting the Conclusion

The final step in the electrodiagnostic consultation is the drafting of the final conclusion. Well done electrodiagnostic conclusions are the result of integration of information from the history, physical examination, and the technical testing-not just the testing alone (3). This final step will be discussed later.

Case Study 18-1

A 47-year-old male had severe low back pain with radiation into the anterior thigh for more than 1 month. The straight leg raise test, reflexes, strength, and sensation were normal. MRI was reported as normal. Because of the severity of pain and suspicion of significant pathology, the physician sent him for an electrodiagnostic consultation.

Sensory and motor nerve conduction testing were normal, suggesting that there was not a polyneuropathy or compressive neuropathy. The needle exam of the limb included at least two muscles that overlapped each nerve root and at least one muscle from each major nerve in the leg: the medial gastrocnemius (S1-S2 roots, tibial nerve), extensor hallucis longus (L5-S1 peroneal nerve), tibialis anterior (L4-L5 peroneal nerve), vastus medialis (L2, L3, and L4, femoral nerve) and tensor fascia lata (L5 and S1, superior gluteal nerve). All were normal except a few subtle polyphasic motor units in the vastis medialis. Paraspinal mapping of the back muscles had a total score of 10 (range of normal, 0-2), with most findings in the L3 distribution. This led to a myelogram with subtle changes at L3-4, and surgery, which demonstrated a moderate to large disk herniation at L3-4. The patient had immediate pain relief and recovered uneventfully.

Discussion

This case illustrates the use of electrodiagnostic testing when the clinical picture does not relate well to the MRI. It also shows the use of quantified paraspinal electromyography, which in this case also localized the lesion to an unusual place. Finally, it demonstrates the problem with high lumbar disk herniations. The pain does not radiate below the knee, and in about half of the cases the clinical exam (hip flexor and adductor weakness, patellar reflex, sensory exam, and reverse straight leg raise test) is not very helpful. About 50% of surgically proven high lumbar disk herniations have negative MRIs (5). On EMG, the limb muscles are often normal or not routinely tested (iliopsoas, adductors), but the paraspinal EMG has high sensitivity (6).

When Is Electrodiagnostic Testing Used in the Management of Back Pain?

Forty years ago, electromyography, along with myelogram, was a gold standard for proving a disk herniation or spinal stenosis existed prior to surgery (7). In the interim, CT scans and MRI scans have fascinated us with their anatomical representation. For a few decades, there was little good research on electrodiagnosis of low back pain. This, combined with the uneven quality of consultation (see below), resulted in a decline in use of electrodiagnosis for low back pain. But in fact, every good quality research paper to date has shown that EMG is equal to myelogram, CT, or MRI in detecting disk herniation. In addition, it can detect the many disorders that can mimic a disk herniation-ranging from tumors in the plexus or nerve, to distal compression, to polyneuropathy. A scan of the spine detects none of these. Furthermore, as we have come to find out in recent years, "pathologic" anatomy on an MRI scan is exceedingly common in asymptomatic people (8).

So why isn't EMG used as a first-line test for radiating low back pain? In the offices of many physiatrists and neurologists, and in many other countries, it is. Because surgeons operate on anatomy, they often prefer the MRI. They will argue that if they order an EMG, they will need to order an MRI anyway if they need to operate. But the percent of primary care patients who go on to surgery is so low that the cost effectiveness is with EMG. In reality, the choice of an MRI is often for "soft" reasons. Doctors and patients like modern stuff, pictures, and painless tests. MRI, by the way, is no better tolerated by patients than EMG and cannot be used in a number of conditions ranging from implanted metal to claustrophobia to obesity.

When an MRI is the first diagnostic test, electrodiagnosis is useful when the MRI does not make sense with the clinical exam-specifically, with apparent false positives and false negatives. EMG will pick up a few of the 10% of disk herniations missed on routine MRI. It will also pick up the other lesions that mimic radiating pain, such as polyneuropathy, and so forth. On the other hand, if an MRI shows a disk herniation, but the physical exam is not classical for herniation, the clinician suspects a false positive MRI. Well done electrodiagnostic testing has rare false positives. Perhaps the most common use of electrodiagnostic testing is the evaluation of equivocal imaging findings. Electrodiagnostic findings tip the scale in the direction of believing or not believing that these findings are clinically significant.

There are less common uses for EMG that are worth keeping in mind. Although mild lesions are not detected in the first few weeks after an injury, severe ones such as an acute onset cauda equina lesion can be detected by analysis of recruitment and H-reflexes (see Case Study 18-2). For clinical and medicolegal reasons, it is sometimes important to determine whether a new back complaint is old or new. EMG can do that, within limits, by evaluation of the size of motor units and fibrillation potentials.

Case Study 18-2

A morbidly obese 50-year-old woman with a significant history of anxiety and frequent health care system use was admitted through the emergency department with a complaint of progressive severe back pain with new incontinence of less than 24 hours duration. Reflexes and strength were intact, though strength was hard to test given her anxiety. Rectal sphincter function was also hard to determine. She was too large for the hospital's MRI scanner. On electrodiagnostic testing, there was no spontaneous activity, and motor units were normal in configuration. Careful analysis of motor unit recruitment showed decreased recruitment (30 hertz) in the medial gastrocnemius (S1-S2, tibial nerve) and the gluteus maximus (S1-S2, gluteal nerves), which could only be reached with a special 75-mm needle.

Rather than discharging the patient, a myelogram was performed. It showed a large L5-S1 disk herniation compressing the thecal sac severely. Given this presentation of acute cauda equina syndrome, emergency surgery was performed. Bladder function returned.

Discussion

The typical and easy to detect findings on EMG-spontaneous activity and motor unit changes-do not occur for at least 2 weeks after a lesion occurs. But immediately after a nerve has moderate to severe damage, there is a dropout of motor units. This emergency surgery was performed only because the referring physician knew of this exception and communicated the special need to the electrodiagnostic consultant.

Ruling Out Radiculopathy

An adequate workup to rule out radiculopathy involves needle electromyography of at least five lower extremity muscles spanning the roots in question and the paraspinal muscles, along with a sensory nerve conduction study to rule out polyneuropathy. The addition of an H-reflex can also pick up rare S-1 lesions that appear normal on needle examination. The F-wave does not appear to add sensitivity to the workup for a radiculopathy. Somatosensory evoked potentials are not typically useful, although Kraft's group has advocated their use in spinal stenosis (9).

Classic proof of a radiculopathy is demonstrated if there are abnormalities in two muscles sharing the same root, but different nerves, and in the paraspinal muscles, assuming the other testing does not detect a more diffuse process (10). Adjacent muscles supplied by different nerve roots should be spared. If the lesion is not "surrounded by normal findings," a polyneuropathy, plexopathy, or polyradiculopathy is considered, and the electrodiagnostic testing continues, maybe involving an arm or the opposite leg.

The paraspinal muscles have substantial importance in the diagnosis of radiculopathy. They cover all nerve roots, so paraspinal EMG serves as an important screening test. Most experts believe that one third of radiculopathies have abnormalities only in the paraspinals. They are also important because a specific newer technique called paraspinal mapping allows quantification of the abnormalities in ways the limb examination cannot (11,12). Quantified paraspinal mapping has led to the first blinded studies in EMG, the first set of norms for this otherwise subjective test, and the first studies of inter-rater reliability. Research has shown that asymptomatic people may have reproducible abnormalities in the paraspinal muscles-more with aging-but that the range of paraspinal mapping scores is low in asymptomatic people (13). This is in great contrast to MRI scans, one third to two thirds of which have significant abnormalities in people without any symptoms. Also, the paraspinal muscles appear to be abnormal in persons with other significant problems-among postoperative patients, paraspinal abnormalities differentiate between ones who have "failed back surgery syndrome" and others, for instance.

Looking for Quality in Electrodiagnostic Consultation

A great electrodiagnostician is easy to spot. He or she provides both an "electrodiagnostic" conclusion based on the technical findings and a clinical conclusion in which the technical findings are integrated into the clinical picture. If the referring physician knows to ask, the electrodiagnostician will provide information about the age of the lesion and its severity. Additional information can be added. Most obviously, electrodiagnosticians are usually expert musculoskeletal physicians, so when the neurophysiologic test is normal, they often pick up previously undetected musculoskeletal conditions (14). For the obsessive patient or the medicolegal case, the consultant may specifically mention the many obscure parts of the differential diagnosis that are "ruled out."

Clearly, electrodiagnostic consultation is a complex process. It should also be clear that much of the process is not transparent. The referring physician cannot tell how much the consultant explored a muscle, whether he or she carefully measured distances for the nerve conduction studies, controlled for temperature variation, and so forth. Although most referring physicians have some sense of neuroanatomy, the subject is complex. The referring physician can get a clue about consultant competency and attention to detail by simply looking at the report format (Table 18-1). Table 18-2 is a good checklist of "soft" evidence of a quality consultation done by a well trained specialist.

Training has a lot to do with competency. At the top end is the American Board of Electrodiagnostic Medicine board certified physiatrist or neurologist. Non-ABEM trained physiatrists still get at least 3, and typically 6 months of training in electrodiagnostic medicine, and are typically quite good. Neurology residencies are highly varied, but the requirement is for surprisingly little EMG training-the assumption is that a neurologist who wants to do EMG will do a fellowship. In many states, allied health professionals such as physical therapists or electrodiagnostic technicians are allowed to do the testing, either independently or under the supervision of a physician who is not trained. Obviously, this kind of background does not prepare one for the complex medical decision making involved in electrodiagnostic testing (15). Finally, more common than one would like to admit, there are frauds. Some clinicians without licenses to use needles have used surface electrodes to test for nerve damage. When the patient says the test was quick and painless and the report indicates that eight muscles were tested in each leg, the primary physician might get a bit suspicious.

Even the primary care physician who has minimal knowledge of the consultation process will soon spot an expert who cares about his or her work. By partnering with this consultant, the physician can take advantage of this great "secret weapon" in the diagnosis of back pain (16).

▦   ▦   ▦

Recommendations

- Find out about the quality of local electrodiagnostic medicine consultants by reviewing a few reports and asking about their training.

Table 18-1   Typical Information Recorded by an Electrodiagnostician

Parameter	Units	Normal Findings
	Needle Examination	
Insertional activity	Normal, increased or decreased	Normal
Spontaneous activity	0-4+ positive waves, fibrillations, complex repetitive discharges, or other rare findings	0
Paraspinal spontaneous activity	MiniPM score	0-2
Motor unit amplitude	Microvolts	800-4000 uV, depending on the muscle
Motor unit duration	Milliseconds	Between 5 and 10 ms
Motor unit configuration	Phases, turns, baseline crossings	80% of motor units sampled have fewer than 4 phases
Motor unit recruitment [decreased]	Firing rate of the first motor unit when a second unit begins to fire (Hz)	0-20 Hz
Motor unit recruitment [increased]	Subjective sense that too many motor units are firing for the force generated	"Increased"
	Nerve Conduction	
Amplitude	Microvolts (μV) or millivolts (mv) (=1000 μV)	Highly dependent on the specific nerve and technique used. Typically: Motor NCS 2-10 mv, Sensory NCS 5-50 uV
Latency	Milliseconds. Sensory measured to onset or peak of the response. Motor measured to onset	Dependent on the nerve and technique used
Conduction velocity	Meters/second	Lower extremity < 40 m/s, upper extremity 50 m/s
Temperature	Degrees centigrade	Skin temperature less than 32°C requires warming or correction
Repetitive stimulation	Percent decrease in motor amplitude between the first and fourth stimulation when stimulated at 2 Hz	< 3% ****check

- Be sure your consultant is aware that you are open to comments beyond the simple diagnosis on electrodiagnostic reports.
- Ask sophisticated questions about severity, timing, and location of the lesion on electrodiagnostic consultations, where appropriate.
- Consider electrodiagnostic consultation as a first- or second-line diagnostic test for subacute radiating back pain.

Table 18-2   Assessing the Quality of the Electrodiagnostic Consultation

From the electrodiagnostic medicine consultant:

- ABEM board certified?
- Technicians (if used) ABET certified?
- What is the physician's testing schedule? (A typical consultation requires an hour or more per patient.)
- Does the laboratory have a quality assurance program (physician peer review or outcome based quality check)?

From the patient:

- Were nerve conduction studies performed by the physician or performed by an ABET certified technician after the physician's history and physical exam?
- Did the physician's needle examination include exploration of each muscle in different directions (adequate inspection for spontaneous activity)?
- Did the physician have the patient gradually tense each muscle with the needle still in it (adequate inspection for motor unit configuration and recruitment)?

From the report:

- Was an appropriate history and physical examination performed?
- Was an appropriate differential diagnosis listed?
- Was the skin temperature recorded or was it noted that the extremity was warmed prior to nerve conduction studies?
- Did the report format suggest that the physician had a flexible examination strategy, or was the physician tied to a "routine" (e.g., a pretyped form with a few muscles or nerves already listed, room for checkmarks or "wnl," but little room for comments or testing of additional nerves and muscles)?
- Did the report record specific quantified data for each parameter for each muscle tested as listed in Table 18-1? (In contrast, a report that lists muscles and simply indicates "Nl" or "0" after the first muscle with a line through the whole column to indicate that other muscles were also normal.)
- Did the report discuss what test results were judged abnormal, and how those results led to the final conclusion in exclusion of the other differential possibilities?

Republished with permission from Haig AJ, Perez A. Electromyography in Occupational Medicine. In: Mayer TG, Gatchel RJ, Polantin PB. Occupational Musculoskeletal Disorders: Function, Outcome, and Evidence. Philadelphia: Lippincott, Williams, and Wilkins, 1999.

Key Points

- Electrodiagnostic testing is a consultation, not a simple test.
- Electrodiagnostics should be considered when imaging tests are negative despite high suspicion of a root lesion.
- Electrodiagnostics should be considered when imaging is positive despite a low suspicion of a root lesion.

■   ■   ■

REFERENCES

1. **Blakeslee MA, Simmons Z, Logigian EL, Koghari MJ.** Does an electrodiagnostic study change clinical management? Muscle Nerve. 1996;19(9):1225.

2. **Danner R.** Referral diagnosis versus electroneurophysiological findings. Two years electroneuromyographic consultation in a rehabilitation clinic. Clin Neurophysil. 1990;30:153-157.

3. **Haig AJ, Tzeng HM, LeBreck DB.** The value of electrodiagnostic consultations for patients with upper extremity nerve complaints: a prospective comparison with the history and physical examination. Arch Phys Med Rehabil. 1999;80(10):1273-1281.

4. **Lauder TD, Dillingham TR, Huston CW, Chang AS, Belandres PV.** Lumbosacral radiculopathy screen. Optimizing the number of muscles studies. Am J Phys Med Rehabil. 1994;73(6):394-402.

5. **Albert TJ, Balderston RA, Heller JG, Herkowitz HN, Garfin SR, Tomany K, An HS, Simeone FA.** Upper lumbar disk herniations. J Spinal Disorders. 1993;6(4)351-9.

6. **Haig AJ, Yamakawa K, Hudson DM.** Paraspinal electromyography in high lumbar and thoracic Lesions. Am J Phys Med Rehabil. 2000;79(4):336-42.

7. **Knuttson B.** Comparative value of electromyographic, myelography, and clinical neurological examination in the diagnosis of lumbar root compression syndrome. Acta Orthop (Scand) 1961; 49 (Suppl).

8. **Jensen MC, Brant-Zawadzki MN, Obuchowski N, Modic MT, Malkasian D, Ross JS.** Magnetic resonance imaging of the lumbar spine in people without back pain. N Engl J Med. 1994;331:69-73.

9. **Snowden M, Haselkorn JK, Kraft GH, Bronstein AD, Bigos SJ, Slimp JC, Stolov WC.** Dermatomal somatosensory evoked potentials in the diagnosis of lumbosacral spinal stenosis: comparison with imaging studies. Muscle Nerve. 1992;15(9):1036-44.

10. **Wilbourn AJ, Aminoff MJ.** The Electrophysiologic Examination In Patients with Radiculopathies. AAEE Minimonograph No. 32. Rochester, MN: AAEE; 1988.

11. **Haig AJ.** Clinical experience with paraspinal mapping I: Neurophysiology of the paraspinal muscles in various spinal disorders. Arch Phys Med Rehabil. 1997;78:1177-84.

12. **Haig AJ.** Clinical experience with paraspinal mapping. II: A simplified technique that eliminates three fourths of needle insertions. Arch Phys Med Rehabil. 1997;78:1185-90.

13. **Haig AJ, LeBreck DB, Powley SG.** Paraspinal mapping: quantified needle electromyography of the paraspinal muscles in persons without low back pain. Spine. 1995;20(6):715-21.

14. **Dillingham TR, Lauder TD, Kumar S, Andary MT, Shannon SR.** Musculoskeletal disorders in referrals for suspected cervical radiculopathy. American Association of Electrodiagnostic Medicine Annual Meeting, September 1997, San Diego, CA.

15. Who is Qualified to Practice Electrodiagnostic Medicine? Position Statement. Approved by the American Association of Neuromuscular & Electrodiagnostic Medicine (formerly AAEM): May 1999. Rochester, MN: American Association of Electrodiagnostic Medicine.

16. **Roija LN, Schneider LB, Ahmad BK.** EMG referral patterns for cervical radiculopathy: the role of the primary care physician in a large multispecialty healthcare system. American Association of Electrodiagnostic Medicine Annual Meeting, October 5, 1996, Minneapolis, MN.

▓   ▓   ▓

KEY REFERENCES

Dumitru D. Electrodiagnostic medicine. Philadelphia: Hanley and Belfus; 1995.

Haig AJ, Perez A. Electromyography in occupational medicine. In: Mayer TG, Gatchel RJ, Polatin PB; eds. Occupational Musculoskeletal Disorders. Function, Outcome, and Evidence. Philadelphia: Lippincott, Williams & Wilkins; 1999:393-409.

A more general review of the use of electrodiagnostic testing, written for the primary care physician. It includes nonspinal lesions such as carpal tunnel syndrome, and more of the technical aspects of the consultation.

Kimura J. Electrodiagnosis in Diseases of Nerve and Muscle: Principles and Practice, 2nd ed. Philadelphia: F.A. Davis Co.; 1989.

Dumitru and Kimura are the two classic electrodiagnostictext books. Dumitru's is an encyclopedic tome. Kimura's, also fairly complete, is a bit easier to digest.

Wilbourn AJ, Aminoff MJ. The Electrophysiologic Examination in Patients with Radiculopathies. AAEE Minimonograph No. 32. Rochester, MN: AAEE; 1988.

A great basic review of the use of electrodiagnostic testing for radiculopathy.

19

■ ■ ■

Rheumatologic Disorders
of the Spine

Vladimir Ognenovski, MD

The rheumatologic disorders of the spine encompass a heterogenous group of inflammatory conditions sharing common clinical features related to inflammation of the spine (spondylitis), the sacroiliac (SI) joints (sacroiliitis), and the entheses-insertion points of tendons, ligaments and joint capsules (enthesitis) (Table 19-1). Some of these disorders are associated with peripheral arthropathy, and many share extra-articular features (Table 19-2). Many of them share the HLA-B27 allele present in the HLA-B locus of the class I major histocompatibility complex (MHS I). Commonly, they are referred to as spodyloarthropathies.

In the acute phase, the specific diagnosis for nonradiating back pain is seldom crucial and most often impossible to obtain. But in the group who continue to complain of pain into the subacute phase, both the odds of finding a specific cause and the consequences of finding a cause increase. It is at this stage that the physician should at least consider the possibility of a rheumatologic disorder. The prevalence of many spondyloarthropathies is fairly high in the population in general, and many people have trivial symptoms. A story of 4-6 weeks of unremitting pain in the sacroiliac region, however, may lead to a diagnostic evaluation for arthritis. If positive, detection of arthritis at this "early" stage may lead to the use of disease-modifying agents and to physical therapy strategies different from that used for mechanical back pain.

Epidemiology and Pathogenesis

The epidemiologic studies of ankylosing spondylitis (AS) suggest strong familial aggregation and high concordance rate among identical twins.

Table 19-1   Inflammatory Disorders of the Spine*

Spondyloarthropathies (SpA):

- Ankylosing spondylitis (AS)
- Reactive arthritis (ReA)
- Psoriatic arthritis (PsA)
- Enteropathic arthropathy-associated with inflammatory bowel disease (IBD)
- Juvenile spondyloarthropathy
- Undifferentiated spondyloarthropathy

*Other, less common, conditions associated with spondyloarthropathy are
1. Behçet syndrome
2. Whipple disease
3. Familial Mediterranean fever
4. Arthropathy associated with intestinal bypass surgery
5. Celiac disease
6. Relapsing polychondritis
7. SAPHO (spondylitis, acne, pustulosis, hyperostosis, osteomyelitis) syndrome
Republished with permission from Van der Linden S, van der Hejde D. Ankylosing spondylitis. Rheum
Dis Clin North Am. 1998;24:663–93.

Table 19-2   Extra-Articular Features

- Ocular inflammation (anterior uveitis, iritis, conjunctivitis)
- Mucocutaneous involvement (psoriasis, erythema nodosum, nail involvement)
- Gastrointestinal (colitis)
- Urogenital (urethritis/balanitis)
- Cardiovascular (aortitis)

Table 19-3   HLA-B27 Associations Among the Spondyloarthropathies

Disorder	HLA-B27 Frequency
Ankylosing spondylitis	90%
with uvetis or aortitis	Nearly 100%
Reactive arthritis	50-80%
with sacroiliitis or uvetis	90%
Juvenile spondyloarthropathy	80%
Inflammatory bowel disease	Not increased
with peripheral arthritis	Not increased
with spondylitis	50%
Psoriasis vulgaris	Not increased
with peripheral arthritis	Not increased
with spondylitis	50%
Unaffected whites	6-8%

Adapted with permission from Taurog JD. Seronegative sponyloarthropathies: epidemiology, pathology,
pathogenesis. In: Primer on the Rheumatic Diseases. Arthritis Foundation. Atlanta. 1997.

Genetic studies show that 94% of patients with AS are HLA-B27 positive. In families with ankylosing spondylitis, 10-20% of those inheriting the HLA-B27 gene developed the disease (1,2,3). High prevalence of HLA-B27 has been found in other conditions associated with spondyloarththropathy (Table 19-3). The observation of chlamydial infections of the urogenital tract and enteric infections triggering reactive arthritis, as well as the presence of bacterial antigens in the synovial fluid observed in rheumatoid arthritis, suggests possible bacterial interaction with the immune system in the perpetuation of the inflammatory process. Taken together, these observations point to genetic and environmental factors in the pathogenesis of the spondyloarthropathies.

Case Study 19-1

A 30-year-old mechanic presented to the rheumatology clinic with a 4-year history of progressive neck pain and stiffness. He recalled neck spasm since age 18. He has been seeing a chiropractor regularly. His examination revealed severe loss of mobility in the thoracic and lumbar spine and mild loss of mobility of the neck. Schober test was 2.5 cm. Radiographs showed syndesmophytes from T-10 to L-1 and complete fusion of the sacroiliac joints. He was diagnosed with ankylosing spondylitis.

History and Clinical Features

The onset of symptoms is characteristically insidious, often lasting for months to years before presentation. Nevertheless, in patients with back pain being followed by a physician, these diseases should be considered and diagnosed in the subacute stage. Typically, the symptoms are prolonged morning stiffness, often several hours, and pain referred to the lower back, the sacrum, and buttocks. The stiffness of the back lasts for several hours and improves with activity, so that patients are less stiff in the latter part of the day. As the inflammation ascends the spine, stiffness, pain, and loss of mobility affect the upper back and neck. Increasing stiffness in the thoracic cage and ribs can lead to severe restrictive lung disease, and the deformity can profoundly affect balance, ambulation, and performance of activities of daily living. Peripheral arthritis may be a presenting symptom. It usually affects a large joint in the lower extremities such as hips or knees. In reactive arthritis and psoriatic arthritis, the presenting symptom may be an acute inflammation of a small joint or a digit, referred to as dactylitis or sausage digit. In reactive arthritis, the onset of articular symptoms typically is preceded by several weeks after the triggering infections, chlamydia in the urogenital tract, and gastrointestinal pathogens in the gastrointestinal tract. In inflammatory bowel disease (IBD)-associated spondyloarthropathy, the peripheral arthritis usually occurs concurrently with the colitis, whereas the spine arthritis is independent of the bowel inflammation. Soft tissue pain due to enthesitis can also be a presenting or accompanying symptom. Occasionally, one may detect one of the extra-articular manifestations, such as urethritis and conjuctivitis in reactive arthritis or uveitis in ankylosing spondylitis, in the early course of the spondyloarthropathies (see Table 19-3). Careful history and examination may reveal subclinical sacroiliitis manifesting with loss of mobility in the sacroiliac/lumbar spine or an abnormal radiograph. The principal features in the history of an inflammatory back pain are summarized in Table 19-4. The presence of any four of these five symptoms raises the probability for an underlying inflammatory back pain to 95-100% (4).

The presence of extra-articular signs and symptoms in a patient with lower back discomfort should be a red flag for the presence of an underlying systemic inflammatory condition (see Table 19-2). The clinical manifestations of spondyloarthropathies are summarized in Table 19-5.

Diagnosis

Physical Examination

The physical examination should include a complete physical exam with a thorough musculoskeletal examination of the spine, the sacroiliac joints (as described in earlier chapters), the peripheral joints, and soft tissues. Attention should be paid to the posture and the range of motion of the entire spine and the sacroiliac joints. In addition, the distance from the occiput to wall (or ear to wall) provides a baseline reference for subsequent assessment of the progression of cervical ankylosis. The thoracic spine ankylosis manifests with decreased mobility of the spine and loss of rib cage expansion. Normal thoracic expansion is at least 5 cm. Ankylosis of

---

Table 19-4   Differentiating Features of Inflammatory Back Pain

- Onset of back discomfort before age of 40
- Insidious onset
- Persistence for at least 3 months
- Prolonged morning stiffness (several hours)
- Improvement with activity or exercise

Table 19-5   Comparison of Ankylosing Spondylitis and Related Disorders

Characteristic	Disorder				
	Ankylosing Spondylitis	Reactive Arthritis (Reiter Syndrome)	Juvenile Spondyloarthropathy	Psoriatic Arthropathy*	Enteropathic Arthropathy‡
Usual age at onset	Young adult <40	Young to middle-age adult	Childhood onset, ages 8 to 18	Young to middle-age adult	Young to middle-age adult
Sex ratio	3 times more common in males	Predominantly males	Predominantly males	Equally distributed	Equally distributed
Usual pattern of onset	Gradual	Acute	Variable	Variable	Gradual
Sacroiliitis or spondylitis	Virtually 100%	<50%	<50%	≈ 20%	<20%
Symmetry of sacroiliitis	Symmetric	Asymmetric	Variable	Asymmetric	Symmetric
Peripheral joint involvement	≈ 25%	≈ 90%	≈ 90%	≈ 95%	Frequent
Eye involvement‡	25-30%	Common	20%	Occasional	Occasional
Cardiac involvement	1-4%	5-10%	Rare	Rare	Rare
Skin or nail involvement	None	Common	Uncommon	Virtually 100%	Uncommon
Role of infectious agents as triggers	Unknown	Yes	Unknown	Unknown	Unknown

* About 5-7% of patients with psoriasis develop arthritis, and psoriatic spondylitis accounts for about 5% of all patients with psoriatic arthritis.
† Associated with chronic inflammatory bowel disease.
‡ Predominantly conjuctivities in reactive arthritis and acute anterior uveitis in the other disorders listed.
Republished with permission from Arnett Jr. FC, Kham MA, Willkens RF. A new look at ankyosing spondylitis. Patient Care. 1989;Nov 30:82–101.

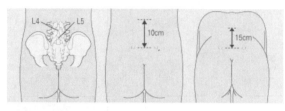

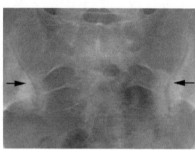

Figure 19-1 Schober test to measure ability to flex the lumbar spine.

Figure 19-2 Sacroiliac joint pseudowidening and joint margin indistinctness due to erosions (Republished with permission from Khan MA. Ankylosing spondylitis: clinical features. In: Kippel JG, Dieppe PA, eds. Rheumatology. Philadelphia: Mosby; 1994;3.25.1-3.25.10.)

the lumbar spine manifests with loss of lumbar lordosis and decreased lumbosacral mobility. Schober's test measures the mobility of the lumbosacral spine (Figure 19-1). Expansion of the lumbosacral spine of less than 5 cm is considered abnormal. Enthesitis manifests with tenderness over the enthesis as a result of inflammation. The tenderness is observed peri-articularly and over the costochondral junctions, spinous processes, iliac crests, greater trochanters, ischial tuberosities, tibial tubercles, Achilles' tendon insertions, and plantar fascia insertion to the calcaneus. Particular attention should be paid to signs of extra-articular manifestations of the underlying systemic inflammatory condition (see Table 19-2).

Radiographs

The physical exam should be complemented with a radiographic evaluation. In early disease, the radiograph may be normal. A bone scan is very sensitive and less specific. It may show an increased isotope uptake in the sacroiliac joints, as well as the spine, entheses, and peripheral joints, suggesting an inflammatory process. Magnetic resonance imaging (MRI) is superior to bone scan and detects early sacroiliac and spine cartilage inflammation. Computed tomography (CT) scan is superior to MRI in detecting bone erosions in the sacroiliac (SI) joints (6). As the disease progresses, the radiographic progression shows initial loss of joint margin indistinctness, erosions with apparent pseudowidening of the joint space (Figure 19-2), and complete ankylosis of the sacroiliac joints in advanced

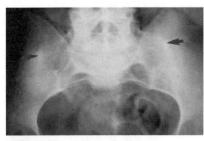

Figure 19-3   Complete ankylosis of the sacroilic joints (Republished with permission from Khan MA. Ankylosing spondylitis: clinical features. In: Kippel JG, Dieppe PA, eds. Rheumatology. Philadelphia: Mosby; 1994;3.25.1-3.25.10.)

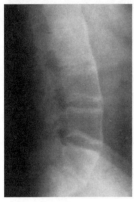

Figure 19-4   Vertebral column ankylosis with "bamboo spine" appearance. (Republished with permission from Khan MA. Ankylosing spondylitis: clinical features. In: Kippel JG, Dieppe PA, eds. Rheumatology. Philadelphia: Mosby; 1994;3.25.1-3.25.10.)

cases (Figure 19-3). In AS and IBD associated spondyloarthropathy, the SI joints are symmetrically affected, whereas in PsA and ReA, one typically sees asymmetric involvement of the SI joints. In the spine, early on one sees signs of osteitis of the vertebral bodies manifesting as shiny (sclerosed) vertebral body corners, progressing to squaring of the vertebral bodies and the appearance of syndesmophytes-calcifying bridges in the intervertebral space. The calcification of the outer layers of the annulus fibrosus, along with calcification of the anterior and posterior ligaments, the syndesmophyte formation leads to ankylosis (fusion) and "bamboo spine" appearance of the vertebral column (Figure 19-4). In PsA and ReA, the syndesmophytes are typically asymmetric and bulky, whereas in AS they are symmetric and linear. Osteopenia of the spine is commonly observed.

Laboratory Evaluation

The laboratory evaluation should be limited to complete blood count (CBC), erythrocyte sedimentation rate (ESR), and C-reactive protein (CRP), which often support presence of a systemic inflammation. Testing for HLA-B27 adds little value to the clinical diagnosis as about 10% of the normal population will be HLA-B27 positive. In certain cases where the clinical picture is incomplete or dominated by one of the extra-articular manifestations of SpA, HLA-B27 testing may be helpful in establishing evidence in favor of SpA. Other serologic markers for immune-mediated arthropathies such as rheumatoid factor (RF) and antinuclear antibody (ANA) are usually negative.

Natural History and Prognosis

The disease course of ankylosing spondylitis is variable and characterized by exacerbation and remissions. More often, the disease outcome is favorable as the disease is self-limited with a mild symptomatology, and patients remain fully functional. The outcome is less favorable in the rare cases of persistent and progressive disease. Those with hip arthritis and akylosis of the cervical spine are more likely to be disabled. Other predictors of poor prognosis include hip arthritis, ESR over 30 mm/h, limitation of lumbar axis, dactylitis, oligo-arthritis, and onset before age 16 (7). Premature mortality is seen after 20 years of diagnosis. In milder cases, the mortality rates are similar to those of the general population.

In IBD-associated spondyloarthropathy, the spinal arthritis occurs in 10% of patients, and the clinical manifestations are identical to ankylosing spondylitis. In contrast to peripheral arthritis, the activity in spinal arthritis is independent of the disease activity in the bowel. Reactive arthritis usually runs a self-limited course lasting 3-12 months. Relapses occur in 15% of patients, and in as many the course is progressive and disabling. About 10% of patients with reactive arthritis will develop ankylosing spondylitis. In PsA, the spinal involvement is often asymtomatic, and the clinical picture is dominated by psoriasis and/or peripheral arthritis. Sacroilliitis has been observed in up to 30% of patients with psoriasis. Spondylitis may affect portions of the spine without concomitant sacroiliitis.

Management

The management of spondyloarthropathies requires a multidisciplinary approach. It involves patient education, pharmacotherapy, physical and occupational therapy, vocational counseling, psychosocial support, genetic counseling, and patient support groups. Patient education about the chronic nature of the illness, possible outcomes and treatment options are essential. Pharmacotherapy is directed toward suppressing inflammation, pain relief, and disease course modification. Nonsteroidal anti-inflammatory drugs (NSAIDs) are the initial choice in suppressing inflammation and relieving pain. Local corticosteroid therapy, delivered intra-articularly or around the inflamed enthesis, is effective. Systemic corticosteroids are generally ineffective in managing the muskulaskeletal symptoms. Disease modifying agents such as sulfasalazine, methotrexate, and imuran have all been used. These agents have been more effective in controlling the peripheral joint inflammation rather than the axial skeletal inflammation. More recently, novel agents targeting cytokines such as tumor necrosis factor (TNF) have shown promising efficacy in retarding the disease progression and joint destruction, both in the peripheral and axial joints (8). Specific doses and the choice of disease modifying agents and specific dosing regimens are complex and changing. They are beyond the scope of this textbook, and often a rheumatologist is consulted at this stage. Iritis and uveitis require prompt ophthalmologic evaluation. Topical steroids and occasionally immunosuppressive agents usually control the inflammation.

Physical therapy is a cornerstone in the management of spondyloarthropathies and complements the pharmacotherapy. It is essential to establish a daily exercise program that would include preservation of good posture, maintenance of spine mobility, prevention/minimization of deformity, and maintenance of good chest expansion. Surgery such as total hip arthroplasty prevents partial or total disability. Vertebral wedge osteotomy offers correction of severe cervical kyphosis, although it carries a relatively high risk of paraplegia.

Recommendations

- In patients younger than 40 years, elicit a history of features of inflammatory back pain (e.g., prolonged morning stiffness) and extra-articular symptoms (e.g., ocular inflammation).
- Physical examination should include occiput-to-wall test to provide baseline to assess subsequent progression of cervical ankylosis.
- Schober test should be done to measure lumbosacral spine mobility.
- Laboratory evaluation should include CBC, ESR, and CRP.
- Plain sacroiliac joint x-ray should be ordered in patients with a suspicion of a seronegative spondyloarthropathy. Bone scan, CT scan, or MRI may be useful in cases where the plain films are not definitive.

Key Points

- The spondyloarthropathies are systemic inflammatory disorders that share the clinical features of inflammation of the spine and sacroiliac joints, as well as extra-articular features.

- Genetic and environmental factors are involved in the pathogenesis of spondyloarthropathies.
- The onset of symptoms is characteristically insidious.
- Symptoms include prolonged morning stiffness and pain referred to the lower back, sacrum, and buttocks. The stiffness improves with activity.
- The management of spondyloarthropathies requires a multidisciplinary approach, involving patient education, pharmacotherapy, physical therapy, and occupational therapy.

■   ■   ■

REFERENCES

1. **Van der Linden S, van der Heijde D.** Ankylosing spondylitis. Rheum Dis Clin North Am. 1998;24:663-93.
2. **Wordsworth P.** Genes in the spondyloarthropathies. Rheum Dis Clin North Am. 1998;24:845-63.
3. **Arnett FC Jr, Khan MA, Willkens RF.** A new look at ankylosing spondylitis. Patient Care. 1989; Nov. 30:82-101.
4. **Calin A, Porta J, Fries JF, Schurman DJ.** Clinical history as a screening test for ankylosing spondylitis. JAMA. 1977; 237:2613-14.
5. **Khan MA.** Ankylosing spondylitis: clinical features. In: Klippel JH, Dieppe PA; eds. Rheumatology, 1st ed. Philadelphia: Mosby; 1994:3.25.1-3.25.10.
6. **Braun J, Bollow M, Sieper J.** Radiographic diagnosis and pathology of the spondyloarthropathies. Rheum Dis Clin North Am. 1998;24:697-735.
7. **Amor B, Santos RS, Nahal R, Listrat V, Dougados M.** Predictive factors for the long term outcome of spondyloarthropathies. J Rheumatol. 1994;21:1883.
8. **Braun J, de Keyser F, Brandt J, Mielants H, Sieper J, Veys E.** New treatment options in spondyloarthropathies: increasing evidence for significant efficacy of anti-tumor necrosis factor therapy. Curr Opin Rheumatol. 2001;13:245-9.

■   ■   ■

KEY REFERENCES

Klippel, JH. Seronegative spondyloarthropathies. Primer on the Rheumatic Diseases, 12th ed. Atlanta: Arthritis Foundation; 2000:239–58.
    Concise, up-to-date chapter on spondyloarthropathies.

Yu David, ed. Spondyloarthropathies. Rheum Dis Clin North Am. 1998;24:663–894.
    An in-depth review of the latest literature and pathogenetic and therapeutic concepts.

20

■ ■ ■

Physician Prescription and Monitoring of Physical Therapy

John M. Koch, MD

P hysical rehabilitation when properly applied can significantly improve the functional outcome of patients with low back pain. There are a multitude of techniques and modalities that can be beneficial in the recovery from low back pain. Not all of these techniques and modalities have been definitively validated by controlled research studies; however, a variety of techniques are available and often are successful on a case to case basis. The purpose of this chapter is to describe the physician's role in initiating and monitoring physical therapy for low back pain and will include the topics of patient selection, writing a detailed therapy prescription, physician assessment of therapy progress, and an overview of various physical therapy techniques that are often used to create an individualized physical therapy program. The decision to refer a patient for physical therapy, which can be quite expensive, is not automatic. There are several reasons not to start physical therapy; most patients with acute low back pain recover spontaneously, others respond to simple exercise instruction given by their primary care physician, and some will present with pain or medical concerns too severe for therapy at the onset.

Patient Selection for Physical Therapy

Many patients with low back pain have potential to benefit greatly from a structured and supervised physical therapy program. After an episode of low back pain has lasted about 2 to 4 weeks, or if there are frequent recurrences of low back pain, it is reasonable to consider physical therapy for treatment. If the patient is off from work or the pain is moderately severe, physical therapy can begin sooner than 2 weeks. Mixed motivation to succeed can occur in patients who are financially or personally rewarded for not working, are in litigation, or are suffering from depression or misunderstanding of the diagnosis. Severe deconditioning is not uncommon. These patients may need to increase their activity level before they can participate meaningfully in specific therapies. Transportation, language barriers, childcare issues, and other practicalities may affect therapy. Once these factors have been assessed, then specific and reasonable rehabilitation goals can begin to be formed. Table 20-1 lists some common goals when prescribing physical therapy for low back pain.

A thorough history and physical examination with close observation of movement is valuable in assessing candidates for physical therapy. Observing gait and documenting range of motion of the back and major joints can be very useful to determine the patient's baseline flexibility. This will assist in goal setting. Observing the patient's ability to move about on the exam table can provide additional clues to flexibility and movement patterns.

Sometimes, rehabilitation candidates with low back pain will also have significant comorbid medical conditions that need to be considered before prescribing physical therapy. The primary care physician often assumes that the therapist knows and understands the comorbid condition and understands how to construct restrictions to proceed safely with therapy. In fact, the responsibility for outlining restrictions is the physician's. If a therapy prescription contains no restriction, the conscientious therapist may vastly underestimate the patient's ability to participate in therapy, and the less skilled therapist may injure the patient. Occasionally, the therapist also needs to know of issues that may affect his or her own safety. Sometimes, a severe medical problem will preclude therapy or will make it impossible for therapy to accomplish the required task. For instance, in a patient with severe emphysema, the rate-limiting factor to exercise is the lung. Large muscles will not get fatigued; thus they cannot be trained. Table 20-2 lists some of the comorbid conditions and the therapy precautions that may result from them.

Table 20-1   Typical Therapy Goals for Low Back Pain Patients

- Decrease pain
- Stretch contracted muscles
- Strengthen weak muscles
- Decrease mechanical stress to spinal structures
- Stabilize hypermobile segments
- Improve posture
- Improve mobility
- Improve fitness to prevent injury
- Give patient confidence in resuming normal activity

Table 20-2   Diseases and Restrictions That Should Be Considered Before Therapy

Disease	Possible Restriction
Angina	Keep heart rate < 75% maximum; keep nitroglycerin available at all times for chest pain
Diabetes	Have juice available; modify insulin schedule
Emphysema	Train only one muscle at a time; monitor with oxymeter and provide oxygen for saturation less than 90%.
Seizure disorder	Protect from unexpected falls
Knee arthritis	Maintain good knee mechanics, but okay to fatigue quadriceps with isometrics
Osteoporosis	Avoid trunk flexion exercises
Peripheral vascular disease	No physical modalities to the limbs
Psychosis/dangerous personality disorder	(Phone call to discuss safety issues)
Bleeding disorder	Avoid falls or impacts
Learning disability	Provide pictorial instructions

Getting Started

After determining whether the patient will benefit from physical therapy, the physician writes a physical therapy prescription to initiate the specific therapies that will give the patient the best chance of recovery (see Choosing a Physical Therapy Program for Spine Diagnosis later in this chapter).

Writing the Prescription

A detailed physical therapy prescription enhances communication between physician and physical therapist. The components of a physical therapy prescription include the patient's name, date, diagnosis, duration of requested therapies (either in weeks or number of sessions), frequency of therapies (e.g., 2-3 times/week), goals for therapy, precautions or activities to avoid, possible use of modalities or assistive devices, and approximate date of physician follow-up. The physician should list the pertinent items from the patient's past medical history as precautions on the physical therapy script. For example, the notation "Precaution: seizures, diabetes, hypertension" provides the therapist and any emergency personnel with the conditions to be aware of in the event of an emergency while at physical therapy (2). A case report example showing a detailed physical therapy prescription is described below.

The initial referral to therapy usually includes duration and frequency of therapy. Research has not determined the optimal duration of therapy.

In general, acute back pain only requires 3-4 visits if the therapist has a well-organized protocol for acute back pain. For subacute back pain, it is reasonable to refer for therapy 2-3 times/week for a month. Most experts feel that lack of improvement in that time frame suggests that either the therapist does not have sufficient skills, the patient is noncompliant, or further therapy will not work. But some patients with severe contractures or difficult to treat sacral or rib dysfunctions do require more time. Physiatrists who know the quality of their therapists and have good lines of communication over time with the therapists will often defer to the therapist on a case-by-case basis, as their long-term expectations are known.

Case Study 20-1

Mr. X is a 48-year-old male with low back pain radiating into his anterior calf after a lifting injury at work 2 weeks ago. There is hypertonicity of his paraspinal muscles as well as stiffness and guarding with movement. An MRI was obtained showing an L4/5 paracentral disk herniation. Diagnostic and clinical findings are consistent with an L5 radiculopathy. He has a past medical history of diabetes, hypertension, right hip arthritis, tibial bone fracture 15 years ago, and appendectomy. He is motivated for physical therapy and wishes to start as soon as possible.

Physical Therapy Prescription
Date: 12/1/04   **Patient:** Mr. X
Physical therapy: 3/week, 3-5 weeks.
Diagnosis: L5 radiculopathy
     Please include L-S extension based program, progressive range of motion (ROM), education on proper lifting techniques, stabilization and home exercise program (HEP). Modalities as needed.
Precautions: Right hip DJD, diabetes, hypertension
Goals: Improved flexibility, 50-75% pain reduction, return to work
Physician follow-up: 3 weeks
(Note: The therapist will be careful not to stretch the hamstrings to the point of increasing neural tension/nerve root pain.)

In a busy practice, it is often difficult to have the time to write a highly detailed prescription. Additional ways to improve communication between physical therapist and physician might be to send the physical therapist a copy of the physician's dictated chart note or to discuss the case with the therapist by telephone or in person. This communication will further enhance the therapist's understanding of the patient's condition and will keep physician and therapist goals consistent. It will also allow the therapist to work on specific therapeutic regimens individualized for the patient's condition, which will optimize chances for significant recovery.

Choosing a Physical Therapy Program for Specific Spine Diagnoses

The optimal and most effective exercise regimens for specific spinal conditions and diagnoses continues to be an area of ongoing research. Table 20-3 offers some general established therapy guidelines and suggestions for initiating an appropiate exercise program for various spinal diagnoses (3,4). However, it should be remembered that exercise regimens need to be individualized based not only on diagnosis, but also by factors such as age, co-existing medical and spinal conditions, baseline flexibility, fitness level, pain radiation pattern, and motivation.

Table 20-3   Typical Therapy Approaches to Common Spinal Disorders

Spinal Diagnosis	Therapy/Exercises
Spinal stenosis	Lumbo-sacral flexion program
	Stretch hip flexors
	Posterior pelvic tilts
	Reduce lumbar lordosis
	Hamstring stretching
	Trial of traction
	Abdominal strengthening
	Gluteal strengthening
Facet syndrome	Lumbo-sacral flexion program
	Manual therapy techniques for mobilization of facet joints
	Avoid hyperextension
	Trial of a back support during activity
Radiculopathy/disk herniation	McKenzie extension program
	Gradual transition to lumbo-sacral stabilization program
	Trial of traction
	Limit excessive back flexion
	Education on proper lifting techniques
	Hamstring stretching (not to point of neural tension)

Continued on page 242.

Table 20-3   Typical Therapy Approaches to Common Spinal Disorders
(Cont'd from page 241)

Spinal Diagnosis	Therapy/Exercises
Spondylolisthesis	Lumbo-sacral flexion program
	Decrease lumbar lordosis
	Trial of a back support
	Abdominal strengthening
	Avoid hyperextension of spine
	Proper posture training
Sacroiliac joint dysfunction	Manual therapy techniques to correct asymmetries and restore normal motion
	Mobilization of sacroiliac joint
	Piriformis stretches
	Gluteal strengthening
	Modalities, ultrasound
	Trial of SI belt for hypermobile joints
	Home exercise program with self-correction techniques
Back strain/sprain	Modalities
	Stretch paraspinals
	Stretch hamstrings, hip flexors
	Abdominal strengthening
	Education on proper lifting techniques
	Soft tissue mobilization
	Aerobic conditioning
Spondyloarthropathy	Lumbo-sacral extension-based program
	Proper posture training
	Prevent forward stooping
	Prevent loss of chest motion
	Deep breathing exercises
Compression fracture	Lumbo-sacral extension-based program
	Avoid excessive flexion
	Trial of back support

Exercise Programs

Exercises can increase strength, elasticity, range of motion, and endurance (5) and are categorized as either passive or active. *Passive* exercise is completed externally (e.g., from a therapist) without any voluntary contraction of muscles by the patient. These exercises are most useful in the initial phases of improving flexibility and joint range of motion. *Active* exercises require muscular contraction from the patient. This may include isometric, isotonic, or isokinetic forms of exercise.

Ultimately, the goal is to restore flexibility, mobility, and alignment of the musculoskeletal system, symmetric muscle firing, strength, good balance/coordination, and a home exercise program is a necessary part of the overall exercise regimen.

(Therapeutic exercises and modalities are defined in Chapter 24.)

Flexion-Based Exercises

Flexion exercises are used for posterior spinal pain that may be reduced or centralized in a flexed spine position. The goal is to open intervertebral foramina and facet joints. The Williams flexion-based program is commonly used and has been modified over the years (1). Flexion exercises are used to decrease facet joint compressive forces and stretch the lumbar extensors, including the posterior ligamentous and myofascial tissues. Stretching of hip flexors, strengthening gluteal muscles, and abdominal strengthening are also usual components of the flexion-based program. It has been reported that strong abdominal muscles can protect the spine from supporting excessive loads.

Flexion exercises are contraindicated in patients with acute disk herniation, as flexion induced on the lumbar spine will increase intradiskal pressure. Additional contraindications include segmental hypermobility, spinal instability, or peripheralization of pain into the lower extremity. An increase in low back pain is a relative contraindication.

Extension-Based Exercises

Extension-based exercises such as the McKenzie program are based on the theory that repeated posterior compression of the disk causes anterior migration of the disk material and subsequent relaxation of neuromeningeal tension on the nerve root (6). These exercises may be useful with patients who have a radiculopathy due to disk herniation. The McKenzie program uses exercises that facilitate "centralization" of pain away from the feet, legs, and buttocks, while pain may sometimes persist at the back. Normal lumbar lordosis is encouraged and paraspinal muscles are strengthened.

It should be noted that extension-based exercises may likely exacerbate symptoms in patients with facet joint dysfunction, lateral recess stenosis, or central spinal stenosis. Contraindications to extension exercises include segmental hypermobility, instability, uncontained disk extrusion, bilateral sensory or motor symptoms, or an increase in radicular pain.

Stabilization Exercises

Stabilization exercises work to maintain a neutral spine, improve muscular proprioception and posture, and to strengthen the paraspinal musculature. In theory, this position provides the greatest functional stability, decreases tension on associated ligaments and neural elements, and balances forces between the disk and facet joints. The neutral spine posture is taught to the patient to incorporate in their daily posture and lifting techniques. It is hoped with this program of exercises that the stabilized neutral spine will allow for improved patient comfort and prevention of re-injury.

Manual Therapy

Manual therapy has the goal of normalizing alignment and mobility throughout the spine, sacrum, pelvis, and associated musculoskeletal system using specific mobilization techniques. The mechanism by which manual therapy relieves pain remains unclear. Theories include releasing abnormally tight "spasming" muscles, stretch of contracted soft tissues, improvement in microcirculation, and desensititization. Regardless of the mechanism, it is clear that mechanical joint dysfunctions such as sacroiliac joint dysfunction or segmental restrictions at facet joints can often be successfully treated with manual therapy techniques (7). Specialized training for the therapist or physician is necessary to practice manual therapy successfully.

Physical modalities are not emphasized in the treatment of subacute back pain. Heat, cold, surface electrical stimulation, ultrasound, iontophoresis, phonophoresis, and other physical treatments have been studied and do not appear to change the course of the disease. Although therapists may teach patients how to use physical modalities at home for temporary relief, the prohibitive cost of physical therapy makes therapist-applied modalities inefficient. Further discussion of manual therapy techniques and its applications can be found in Chapter 24.

Corsets and Braces

Back supports such as corsets and braces are occasionally beneficial in the treatment of some types of low back pain. The rationale for use is that increased pressure applied to the abdomen and lumbar spine from use of a back support can distribute the pressure more diffusely around the back and abdomen, thereby decreasing the total load that would be placed on the lumbar spine. There are a variety of types of back supports available. The simplest type of back support device is the lumbo-sacral belt, which is a four to six inch wide band of elastic material that fits around the waist. These simple orthoses do not prevent lumbo-sacral flexion or extension but do serve as reminders to patients to limit their back activities and to use proper posture during lifting. A taller version called a lumbo-sacral corset may have the addition of posterior stays to the corset to offer additional resistance to movement of the lumbar spine. The restriction of back motion can be further improved by the addition of a formed plastic insert such as the "Warm-n-Form" back support. Rigid back braces covering the trunk and low back called thoracic lumbo sacral orthoses (TLSO) provide the greatest amount of restriction of back motion. They are used when there is potential instability or severe pain with movement from bony lesions in patients with spondylolisthesis, spondylolysis, compression fractures, advanced multilevel degenerative disease, and scoliosis (1,8). A significant limitation of back supports is that chronic use can potentially lead to disuse atrophy of muscles of the lumbo-sacral spine and abdomen. Assuming a stable spine, in general patients should be reminded to continue to work on strengthening exercises, remove the back support daily to minimize disuse atrophy, and wean from their use as quickly as possible.

Monitoring Physical Therapy

Physical therapy needs to be monitored and reassessed at periodic intervals. Therapist progress notes, patient verbal reports, and serial physical examinations are the tools that allow the physician to determine if the course of physical therapy is improving the patient's function, or if progress has reached a plateau. (Chapter 33 discusses in greater detail what factors are to be considered when stopping physical therapy.)

After physical therapy has been initiated, especially for the acute injury, physician follow-up should occur within 2 to 3 weeks to assess progress in therapies and to determine if any therapy adjustments need to be made. It is expected that the primary physical therapist working with the patient will send a therapy progress note to the physician for use at the follow-up visit. Progress notes and requests for continued treatment should document gains of function, future goals, type of treatment, and anticipated duration.

During the follow-up, these questions should be answered:

- Has the patient been conscientious in attending therapies?
- How many sessions have been completed?
- What are the documented therapy goals?
- Have the therapy goals been reached? Or partially reached?
- Has there been no progress?
- Are the goals appropriate and individualized? (For example, an elderly patient with back pain living at home with supervision may have the goal of simply improving flexibility and reducing pain to move around the house easier, whereas another person may have goals of returning to a strenuous job or high-level sport.)
- Is pain level improving?
- Is flexibility or strength improving?

Goals should be continually reevaluated between physician, patient, and therapist. Continued physical therapy without improvement should be discouraged especially if it consists only of passive modalities (see Chapter 33).

One of the most important goals of therapy is to have the patient learn a home exercise program. To find out if the patient is doing the home exercises, the physician may ask the patient to demonstrate some of the exercises in the clinic room. If the patient cannot recall or demonstrate the exercises, then they are likely not doing them at home.

It is also useful to ask the patient what happens in physical therapy. Does the patient report receiving primarily passive modalities such as heat and ultrasound, or does the patient participate in active exercises under supervision and assistance as needed? Inquire whether the patient is receiving primarily one-on-one care with a trained physical therapist; is the patient on their own during therapy or working in a group with distant supervision. Depending on progress, adjustments in level of therapist supervision may need to be made.

Occasionally, the patient may report new symptoms since the onset of physical therapy. It needs to be determined if the new symptoms are related to the physical therapy itself or another factor. Re-examine the patient to determine if progression of existing symptoms or a new injury may be present. Close attention to gait, reflexes, strength, and range of motion will be especially helpful. Adjustments in the types of exercises may need to be recommended. For example, a patient with new clinical findings consistent with lumbo-sacral facet syndrome may experience exacerbation of symptoms with hyperextension maneuvers. It may be necessary to write a therapy addendum recommending avoidance of hyperextension exercises.

Sometimes, the patient will demonstrate improved flexibility and less muscle hypertonicity but report no improvement in pain symptoms. At follow-up, review the history and reexamine the patient to determine if this is due to a persistent inflammatory etiology, muscle guarding, repetitive trauma, ongoing problem that is now more evident, or a new problem. Sometimes, the addition of a TENS unit to act as a counter-irritant can help to control the pain symptoms (9). Also, "secondary gain" or other psychosocial variables may be factors of continued pain. When these are suspected, consider referral for a multidisciplinary evaluation to sort out the most significant factors contributing to persistent pain and disability. An example of this is a Spine Team Assessment, discussed in Chapter 27.

■   ■   ■

Recommendations

- Clear goals and time frames should be established.
- Close communication should be maintained between the patient, therapist, and physician.
- The first follow-up visit should occur within the first 2 to 3 weeks after the patient has begun physical therapy.
- Progress should be reassessed at regular intervals.

■   ■   ■

Key Points

- Writing a detailed prescription with specific rehabilitation goals in mind will maximize the efficiency of physical therapy and the patient's functional outcomes. Remember to add medical precautions.
- Specific therapy programs, such as flexion-based programs, extension-based programs, and manual therapy techniques, have a role in the treatment of various types of low back pain syndromes.
- Back supports may have a limited beneficial role in conditions such as spondylolisthesis, spondylolysis, compression fractures, and scoliosis.

■   ■   ■

REFERENCES

1. **Borenstein DG, Wiesel SW Boden SD.** Low Back Pain: Medical Diagnosis and Comprehensive Management, 2nd ed. Philadelphia: W.B. Sauders; 1995:595-601.

2. **Schramm-Bloodworth DM.** Physical therapy in the pain clinic setting. In: Abram SE, Haddox JD, eds. The Pain Clinic Manual. Philadelphia: Lippincott Williams & Wilkins; 2000:85-101.

3. **Sinaki, M, Mokra B.** Low back pain and disorders of the lumbar spine. In: Braddom RL, ed. Physical Medicine and Rehabilitation. Philadelphia: W.B. Saunders; 1996:813-51.

4. **Saal JA, Saal JS.** Physical rehabilitation of low back pain. In: Frymoyer JW, ed. The Adult Spine: Principles and Practice. Philadelphia: Lippincott-Raven; 1997:1805-19.

5. **Wilkinson HA.** The Failed Back Syndrome, 2nd ed. New York: Harper & Row; 1992:111-27.

6. **Welsh T, Wolfe RM. In: Wolfe RM, Borenstein DG, Wiesel SW; eds.** Low Back Pain, 3rd ed. Charlottesville: Matthew Bender & Company; 2000:587-627.

7. **Greenman, P.** The osteopathic approach to rehabilitation. In: Kirkaldy-Willis WH, Bernard TN, eds. Managing Low Back Pain, 4th ed. New York: Churchill Livingstone; 1999:341-350.

8. **Steiner ME, Micheli IJ.** Treatment of symptomatic spondylolysis and spondylolisthesis with the modified Boston brace. Spine. 1985;10:937-43.

9. **Conti A.** Back, spine, and chest. In: Buschbacher RM, ed. Musculoskeletal Disorders: A Practical Guide for Diagnosis and Rehabilitation. Stoneham, MA: Andover Medical Publishers; 1994:113-31.

■   ■   ■

KEY REFERENCES

Greenman P, Boers T. The osteopathic approach to rehabilitation (Ch. 19) and Manual therapy (Ch. 17). In: Kirkaldy-Willis WH, Bernard TN, eds. Managing Low Back Pain, 4th ed. New York: Churchill Livingstone; 1999:341-50.
An excellent review of the manual examination for low back pain.

Snook SH, Webster BS, McGorry RW, Fogleman MT, McCann KB. The reduction of chronic nonspecific low back pain through the control of early morning lumbar flexion. Spine. 1998;23:2601-7.
Very interesting article describing a simple self-care measure for patients to reduce the severity of back pain.

21

■   ■   ■

Interventional Therapy in Disorders of the Spine

Anthony Chiodo, MD

S pine injection therapy is a developing technology in the treatment of patients with spine pain and disease. Treatment success depends on patient selection, interventionalist technique, and result interpretation. Spine injection therapy is usually combined with medication and physical therapy and is rarely a stand-alone intervention. The order, timing, and type of strategies chosen will have an impact on patient pain control and function. In combination, these will often maximize efficiency or minimize unproductive therapy treatment, undue discomfort, time delay, or overzealous interventional treatment. This chapter will review important tenets of spine interventional techniques, their utility in the treatment of spine disorders, and describe some of the more common interventions. Detailed technical discussion of the procedures can be found in the references listed at the end of this chapter.

Goals of Treatment

Interventional spine techniques have three main purposes:

1. Treat the spine disorder
2. Clarify the underlying diagnosis
3. Direct further treatment.

The injection of a local anesthetic and corticosteroid at the site of a pain generator will result in immediate symptom relief secondary to the anesthetic. If the pain is inflammatory mediated, sustained benefit will occur from the anti-inflammatory properties of the corticosteroid, allowing for progression of rehabilitation and function. Interventional spine techniques thus can help clarify the diagnosis: If pain is not immediately relieved after

Table 21-1   Types of Injection for Spinal Pain Generators

- Invertebral disk: diskography
- Annulus: epidural
- Posterior longitudinal ligament: epidural
- Nerve root: epidural
- Facet joint: intra-articular facet or medial branch block
- Muscle or tendon: local injection
- Vertebral body: epidural
- Posterior bony structures: medial branch block

injection at the site of the presumed pain generator, an alternate diagnosis must be considered. With fluoroscopic control, there is no doubt about the location of the injection. Table 21-1 lists the type of injection used to anesthetize spine pain generators.

With the response to injection data in hand, one is in a better position to direct further therapy. Questions that these data can answer include:

1. Is the pain generator identified?
2. If identified, what is the degree of relief sustained?
   a. What impact does this have on the rest of the treatment plan?
   b. Can activity restrictions change?
   c. What is the best course of action at this point?
3. If the pain generator is not identified, what are the likely pain generators?
   a. How can I clarify the diagnosis?
   b. If no other potential pain generators are likely, are there psychosocial issues that confound this evaluation?
   c. How can they be addressed?

Indications

In making the initial and succeeding decisions about whether interventional therapy is needed, the optimal location of the injection, and what type of spine injection to use, focused patient evaluation and selection is needed. It is also important that the injectionist/interventionalist be someone that the primary care physician can communicate well with, in order that all necessary information about the patient is taken into account at the time of making a choice about a spine intervention. Factors to be considered in making a diagnosis and in determining whether to use injection therapy are shown in Table 21-2.

Different spinal injections require different levels of diagnostic certainty. For epidural injections, most clinicians want magnetic resonance imaging (MRI) or computed tomography (CT) scan to confirm that a lesion exists and to rule out lesions that may be harmed by injection, such as

Table 21-2   Factors to Be Considered in Determining the Usefulness of Spinal Injections

- Presence of axial vs. radiating pain
- Pain with activity vs. at rest
- Pain with extension vs. flexion
- Pain with compression vs. stretch
- Psychosocial factors
- Severity of pain
- Risk of permanent neurological impairment
- Presence of trauma
- Unusual history or physical signs
- Litigation and workers' compensation issues

tumor. In cases where the imaging study has multiple findings, electrodiagnostic testing is often used to localize the most traumatized nerve roots. Facet injections also typically require MRI or CT. Sacroiliac joint injections are often done after plain x-ray, or the injector takes advantage of the fluoroscopic image to assure himself or herself that there is no surprising pathology. The diagnostic needs of physicians performing diskograms are not clear, while intramuscular injections typically are done without previous diagnostics in patients with clear history and physical examination.

The presence of litigation or workers' compensation claim requires attempts to determine whether issues such as secondary gain, worker satisfaction, or compensation satisfaction are playing a role in the patient's presentation. The presence or absence of Waddell's signs during physical exam will give the practitioner further information as to the likelihood of a specific anatomical structure as the pain generator versus the possibility of superimposed somatosization and generalized pain. Consideration of this and degree of clinical confidence in the diagnosis based on the physical examination and history need to be balanced in making the decision whether to proceed with injection treatment or to proceed with diagnostic testing. If spinal injection will be an early part of treatment, appropriate anatomic diagnostic testing will be needed. Concern about a relative high risk of neurological injury, presence of trauma, low confidence of the diagnosis, presence of unusual history or physical danger signs, and the presence of litigation and secondary gain issues would make early diagnostic testing more likely.

Interventionalist Training and Qualifications

Interventionalists should be board certified in pain management. An American Board of Medical Specialties practitioner wishing to be designated as a specialist in pain medicine must pass an exam given by the ABMS. *Qualified* practitioners who pass the ABPM exam will then be board certified in pain medicine by the primary board to which they have already been credentialed. There are other organizations such as the American Academy of Pain Management, the American Academy of Pain Medicine, the American Society of Regional Anesthesia and Pain Medicine that are dedicated to research and education in the field of comprehensive pain management, of which injection therapy is an important facet. The quality of the spine intervention is highly dependent on the skill of the interventionalist.

Mechanisms of Action

Therapeutic injections of anesthetic agents and glucocorticoids have been studied for the treatment of radiculopathy, foraminal stenosis, central stenosis, and facet joint syndrome. Investigators have reported that local anesthetics may have an anti-inflammatory effect by inhibiting phagocytosis, reducing leukocyte enzyme release, and diminishing superoxide anion release. Animal experiments have shown improved intraradicular blood flow after nerve root block. It is well-known that glucocorticoids stabilize neural membranes, have anti-inflammatory properties, and may suppress discharges of sensitized nerve fibers (1).

Risks

Potential risks secondary to injection are bleeding, infection, vasovagal response, intravascular injection, hematoma, nerve infiltration, and allergic reaction. The risk of bleeding is minimal and is minimized by avoiding injection in a patient with a blood coagulation abnormality or using an anticoagulant. It is not necessary to hold nonsteroidal anti-inflammatory therapy. It is advised that Coumadin be held for 3 days and heparin for 24 hours prior to the injection. The risk of infection is minimal with good sterile technique. However, the intervertebral disk has a difficult time fighting potential infection due to minimal vascularity and perfusion. If intradiskal therapy is being done, consideration of intradiskal Kefzol or Ancef, 30-50 mg, further lessens the risk of infection. (It should be made certain that the patient has no known allergy to cephalosporin.) It is imperative to avoid injection therapy in a patient with a systemic infection (fever, chills, etc.) to avoid contaminating deep structures in the spine at the time of injection. Although the risk of a vasovagal response is present for all injections, IV line placement before the procedure is necessary only when doing procedures in the cervical spine. The risk of vascular injection into the venous plexus needs to be considered with transforaminal lumbar epidural injection. During transforaminal cervical epidural injection, care is taken to minimize the risk of injecting the vertebral artery. Thorough knowledge of anatomy, experience, and technique should avoid these vascular complications.

Contraindications

Contraindications are anticoagulant therapy (Coumadin, heparin, Lovenox), bleeding disorder or active infection. Relative contraindications include pregnancy, allergy to injectants, and glucose intolerance.

Patient Tolerance

Most interventional spine techniques are well tolerated. The use of local anesthetic agents and verbal encouragement lessen discomfort. The actual procedure takes just a few minutes to complete in most cases. The need for intravenous sedation is usually only necessary for radiofrequency nerve ablation techniques and sympathetic ganglion blocks. Intravenous sedation may limit the ability of a patient to give simultaneous feedback during a procedure, making it difficult for them to confirm the location of a pain generator. However, in the presence of high patient anxiety, low pain tolerance, and difficulty remaining still in the treatment position, the practitioner would likely elect to use intravenous sedation to ensure a successful injection experience.

Procedures

Fluoroscopic guidance is strongly recommended to insure proper anatomic localization and delivery of medication to the intended target tissue. Studies have revealed that epidural injections performed blind, without fluoroscopic guidance, fail to reach the epidural space in 25-30% of cases.

Epidural Injection (Transforaminal, Translaminar, Caudal)

Epidural injections are useful for the treatment of radiating pain due to nerve root inflammation in disk disorders, lumbar stenosis, fibrosis, as well as axial pain mediated by the annulus fibrosis and posterior longitudinal ligament. They can be used for the subacute and chronic situation. Acute use is recommended for radicular pain that is severe or not responsive to a brief course (2-4 weeks) of medication and physical therapy techniques. Except in the patient with progressive neurological loss, epidural steroid injections are likely to be successful and a step to consider prior to surgical treatment. This is supported by the fact that the natural history of disk herniation is highly favorable in the vast majority of patients (2,3).

Several techniques have been used historically. In a *transforaminal approach*, the needle enters the epidural space between the disk space anteriorly and the facet joint posteriorly, lateral to the mid-facet line. Figure 21-1 illustrates a transforaminal injection. A similar block can be done at the Sl nerve root at the neuroforamina of that nerve in the sacrum. Anterior-posterior (AP) and lateral fluoroscopic views are used to confirm needle placement in the thoracic and lumbar spine while a 45 degree oblique view is used as well in the cervical spine. Avoiding the lumbar venous plexus just posterior to the vertebral body is important, as is avoiding the vertebral artery posterior and lateral to the vertebral body in the cervical spine.

This injection allows isolation of a single nerve root, which is excellent for diagnostic purposes. It also allows concentration of a small volume of medication at the presumed pain generator site. Administration of a contrast agent is recommended to insure proper needle placement and prevent intravascular injection. Additionally, injection of contrast along the nerve root can allow an epidurogram to assess for evidence of stenosis or fibrosis. This technique avoids the risk of dural puncture or spinal headache.

Another common epidural approach is the *translaminar approach*. This is done initially with an AP view and then lateral to evaluate needle

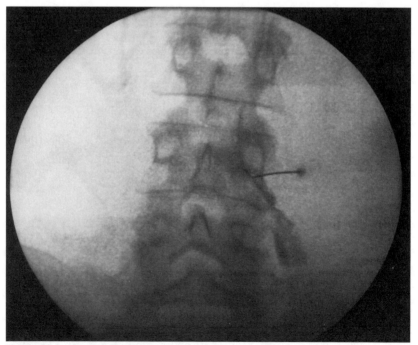

Figure 21-1   Dye injection for a transforaminal epidural steroid injection. The needle on the right is causing a black cloud of dye in the nerve root sleeve.

depth. The use of a loss of resistance technique minimizes the risk of dural puncture, which can be as high as 15% with its risk of spinal headache that sometimes requires a dural blood patch. If done without fluoroscopic control, the miss rate in the skilled practitioner may be as high as 30%. Injection of a contrast agent can evaluate the presence of stenosis or fibrosis. This injection type is less selective and yields less helpful diagnostic information than the transforaminal approach. However, this approach may be helpful in the patient with prior posterior fusion where transforaminal approach may be very difficult.

Caudal epidural injections are also commonly used. These injections require injection at the sacral hiatus, through the sacrococcygeal ligament at the base of the sacrum. It is the least selective procedure and only delivers medication to the L4-5 level. The presence of stenosis or fibrosis may also further limit the flow of medication. This approach is now also being used for more advanced techniques such as lysis of adhesions with the use of a flexible epidural wire or with epiduroscopy, which remains an experimental technique in the fiberoptic evaluation and treatment of spine disorders.

Site of Injection

The site for epidural injection is selected based on patient symptoms, electromyography (EMG) data, and MRI. A more midline disk herniation with impingement of a descending nerve root may be best treated by epidural injection at the level of the affected nerve root rather than the level of disk herniation. If facet hypertrophy contributes to narrowing at the affected nerve root, combined epidural injection and intra-articular facet block should be considered. Sciatica due to facet synovial cyst may be relieved with intra-articular facet injection alone. Radiating pain in the thorax may be treated with epidural injection or intercostal nerve block depending on the site of nerve irritation or damage.

The patient with epidural fibrosis is a special case for whom more advanced injection therapy may be effective. As epidural scar formation is unlikely to be amenable to surgical treatment due to the likelihood of further scar formation except in the case where the patient has progressive neurological signs, more aggressive injection therapy should be considered. Corticosteroids and mechanical pressure from injection have an effect on scar formation. Lysis of adhesions with hyaluronidase, a proteolytic enzyme, or 10% hypertonic saline should be considered. Use of other mechanical means to treat scar formation can be done with a caudal or transforaminal approach with a flexible guide wire under fluoroscopic control. In these circumstances, the use of intravenous sedation and higher doses of epidural anesthetics should be considered.

Intra-Articular Injection (Facet Block, Sacroiliac, Costovertebral, Hip)

Facet-mediated pain can be addressed with two different techniques. If intra-articular pathology is noted on plain film, CT or MRI, intra-articular injection should be considered. *Intra-articular injection* can also be effective in treating patients with segmental hypomobility and pain. *Facet injections* could be considered after a brief trial of medication and physical therapy (2-4 weeks) to improve pain control and correct faulty joint dynamics. If this is not effective or if anatomic tests are normal, *medial branch block* is preferred. The facet joint is innervated by the medial branch of the posterior division of the nerve roots that exit the spinal canal at the same neuroforamina level and the level above the facet joint to be treated. The S1 medial branch also provides innervation to the L5-S1 facet joint. If medial branch blockade yields temporary relief that can be reproduced, radiofrequency ablation can be considered.

Other joints can be injected if they are sites of pain or pain with decreased motion. Clarification of the diagnosis is the same as other areas of the spine. Consideration for injection should occur after appropriate diagnostic testing and after failing a conservative treatment course with physical therapy and medication. Fluoroscopic injection of the hip joint, SI joint, and costovertebral joints are easily accomplished with high likelihood of success. Injection of omnipaque to create an arthrogram is done prior to injection of corticosteroid and anaesthetic.

Diskography

Intradiskal pain is axial pain that increases with lumbar flexion. As radiating pain is possible, this cause should be considered in the patient with radiating pain without nerve root tension signs that does not decrease with transforaminal epidural injection. If physical therapy intervention is not helpful and diagnostic testing does not reveal another pain source, the diagnosis can be clarified with diskography. Figure 21-2 illustrates a discogram. A positive response is one where there is concordant pain on injection of dye that is relieved with bupivacaine injection. Fluoroscopic evaluation for full or complete annular tear(with epidural extravasation) should be done. Further anatomical clarification can be accomplished with post-diskogram CT scanning. If a positive response is noted, intradiskal radiofrequency ablation or intradiskal electrotherapy can be done. Neuroplasty can be considered in patients where chronic radiating pain in the presence of a positive diskogram that has a well-maintained architecture except for the inciting annular tear/lesion. Surgical options should also be entertained.

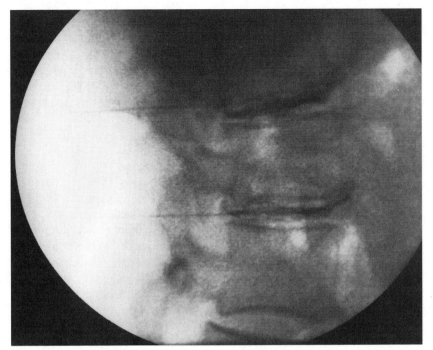

Figure 21-2   Dye injection for a lumbar discogram. The pain reproduction, not the shape of the dye mass, is important.

Case Study 21-1

A 54-year-old welder is injured while doing some work on an automobile restoration. In spite of activity restriction, medication, and physical therapy, he continued to have pain that was worse with prolonged sitting, prolonged standing, and bending activities. Lying down significantly eased his pain. He had some pain radiating into his right hip, but 80% of his pain was in his back. Neurological examination was normal with no dural tension signs. Physical examination showed mild paraspinal spasm in the right lumbosacral spine. No focal spinal malrotations or restrictions were noted to account for his pain. Forward bending reproduced his pain, which was not reproducible on palpation of the spine and paraspinal muscles. He continued to work in spite of his complaints. MRI evaluation revealed right eccentric disk bulges at L4-5 and L5-S1. Serial transforaminal injections at the right side of these two levels done 2 weeks apart resulted in no transient or sustained pain improvement. They ruled out nerve root irritation or compression at the foramen were thus were diagnostic. Diskography at these two levels identified the L5-S1 level as the level with condordant pain production. Right-sided L5-S1 intradiskal radiofrequency ablation resulted in improved pain control.

Myofascial Injections

Axial pain due to soft tissue structures can be addressed with injection therapy when physical therapy intervention is not effective in relieving the symptoms. Pain may localize to tendons, muscles, or ligament structures. Connective tissue structures can be injected with corticosteroids and local anesthetic. Muscle tender or trigger points can be injected with local anesthetic and/or botulinum toxin. Pain in these areas may also be controlled with medial branch block or ablation.

Cervical Whiplash

Special consideration should be given to the patient with cervical whiplash injury or cervicogenic headaches. They are taken together here, as the approach to intervention is similar. Clarifying the diagnosis with careful history, physical examination, and radiological testing is important to detect the pain generator(s). Evaluation for spine stability may be warranted if the mechanism and severity of trauma indicate. Headaches may be from soft tissue, facet, or nerve root (commonly C2) causes. An injection therapy strategy is then devised from these findings and the results of physical therapy intervention. Unusual interventions may include CO-l and Cl-2 facet blocks, greater and lesser occipital nerve blocks, C2 nerve root block, cervical plexus block, or accessory nerve (cranial nerve XI) block. As with other spine therapy, the presence or absence of immediate and sustained benefit from injection will dictate the ensuing treatment recommendations.

Conclusion

Spine injection therapy is a powerful tool used in the evaluation and treatment of patients with spine disorders. Injection therapy should never be used in isolation but as part of an overall management plan that includes patient education and may include medications, physical therapy, and other modes of treatment. For spinal injections, with the diagnosis hypothesized by the pattern of consistency between the history, physical examination, and diagnosis tests, the physician can apply interventional therapy techniques to clarify the diagnosis, improve patient pain control, and improve patient function. If done expediently, improved patient outcome at less cost can be accomplished. Future research will undoubtably identify other effective injection medications as well as identify the most favorable situations for their use.

Key Points

- The quality of the spine intervention is highly dependent on the skill of the interventionalist and the ability of the examiner to put together the clinical information in a manner to identify the pain generator.
- Each intervention completed provides important diagnostic information to assist the clinician in the further care of the patient.
- Contraindications and complications are few and minimized by careful evaluation and technique.
- Spine interventions are another tool in the management of patients with spine pain. Comprehensive management strategies incorporate these techniques with other treatments including medications, therapies, and exercise. Spine interventions can improve the efficacy and efficiency of these other treatments.

▨   ▨   ▨

REFERENCES

1. **Slipman WC, Chow DW.** Therapeutic spinal corticosteroid injections for the management of radiculopathies. Phys Med Rehabil Clin N Am. 2002;13:697-711.
2. **Bush K, Cowan N, Katz D, Gishen P.** The natural history of sciatica associated with disc pathology: a prospective study with clinical and independent radiologic follow-up. Spine. 1992;17:1205-12.
3   **Saal JA, Saal JS, Herzog R.** The natural history of lumbar intervertebral disk extrusions treated nonoperatively. Spine. 1990;15:683-686.

▨   ▨   ▨

KEY REFERENCES

Cannon D, Aprill C. Lumosacral epidural steroid injections. Arch PMR. 2000;81(3):S87-98.

Waldman SD, Winnie AP. Interventional Pain Management. Philadelphia: WB Saunders; 1996.

22

■ ■ ■

Surgical Treatment for Back Pain

Paul Park, MD

Julian Hoff, MD

Even with significant advances in radiographic and electrophysiologic testing, the cause of low back pain is often unclear. In fact, radiographic imaging of the lumbosacral spine can be misleading: A small disk herniation or mild slippage of the vertebral bodies known as spondylolisthesis is a common finding and frequently asymptomatic. Nevertheless, these findings are often thought to be the primary cause of low back pain and have resulted in unnecessary operations. The history-taking and physical examination are therefore of prime importance. Although today we have sophisticated diagnostic tools such as computed tomography (CT), magnetic resonance imaging (MRI), and electromyography (EMG) to help confirm the diagnosis and define structural anatomy, in many cases all that is necessary to determine the cause of back pain is an accurate history and careful physical examination. Establishing the correct diagnosis is essential in determining whether surgical treatment is indicated for low back pain. Unfortunately, there are many patients with low back pain of unclear etiology in which the history, physical examination, radiographic and electrophysiologic studies do not support a specific diagnosis and, as a result, are poor surgical candidates.

Indications for Surgical Treatment

Once the diagnosis of a potentially surgically treatable problem is made, indications for intervention include pain refractory to conservative measures, motor weakness, severe sensory deficit, or cauda equina syndrome. Surgery is usually not the first option for pain without neurologic deficit, as most patients suffering from back pain will improve with medication, rest, and time (1). Those individuals with associated neurological deficits, however, may be less responsive to conservative measures. The presence of a tumor in the lumbar spine, either extradural or intradural, may be an indication for surgical treatment, depending on the type of tumor. Metastatic tumors that cause neurological deficits may be treated with surgery in conjunction with other modalities appropriate for the primary cancer. Intradural tumors, on the other hand, are relatively benign and can potentially be treated conservatively. However, if there is growth in the tumor and/or presence of neurological deficit, surgery is indicated. Timing of surgery is usually dependent on the type and severity of symptoms. Progressive weakness or cauda equina syndrome is an urgent indication for surgery. On the other hand, surgery for the presence of pain alone, even if severe and chronic, is considered an elective operation.

Sometimes a significant abnormality such as a large slippage of the vertebral bodies is identified by diagnostic studies. Symptoms, however, may be mild or absent. In this situation, a reasonable option is to defer surgery until symptoms develop or become more severe. Of course, there are circumstances in which an operation to prevent onset of neurological deficit may be considered; for example, the patient with a large L4-5 ruptured disk and moderate low back pain but no neurologic deficit anticipating a rigorous backpack trip.

Common diagnoses that respond to surgical treament are herniated disk, foraminal stenosis, lumbar stenosis, spondylolisthesis, some tumors, and potentially unstable compression fractures. For a detailed description of these conditions, see Chapter 5.

Surgical Options

Surgical procedures for back pain and their potential indications are summarized in Table 22-1.

Diskectomy

Diskectomy may be indicated for a herniated disk. A typical lumbar diskectomy consists of a small incision in the midline of the lower back that is followed by unilateral retraction of the paraspinal muscles away from the laminae of the lumbar spine. The ligamentum flavum, located between

Table 22-1   Surgical Procedures for Back Pain and Potential Indications

Procedure	Indication
Laminectomy with diskectomy	Disk herniation
Multilevel laminectomy	Spinal stenosis
Foraminotomy	Lateral recess or foraminal stenosis
Fusion (various hardware)	Spondylolythesis, segmental hypermobility

adjacent lamina, is then identified. A small portion of the laminae is removed superiorly to provide adequate exposure. The ligamentum is incised and removed until the dural sac and nerve root are found. A ruptured disk is often seen compressing the nerve root. The herniated fragment is then resected. In the case of a symptomatic bulging disk, the annulus is first incised and then the protruding disk material is removed. A microdiskectomy is essentially the same procedure but involves the use of a microscope for better visualization of the lesion. A smaller incision is usually possible with a microdiskectomy.

Recovery

A lumbar diskectomy usually takes about an hour to perform under general anesthesia. The patient is often allowed home the same day or the following morning. Wounds are now closed with absorbable suture and Steri-Strips, eliminating the need for suture removal. Activity is progressive so that the patient can drive within 1 week and often return to work within a couple of weeks. For those involved in physical labor, recovery may take 2-3 months including physical therapy and work hardening.

Outcomes

There is little comparative literature on the outcomes of spinal surgery. Two randomized controlled trials of diskectomy versus conservative treatment show that the surgical group had better short-term outcomes, but the long-term outcomes were not significantly different (2). Subjects with "severe" and "mild" pain were not included in the trials, however. One randomized controlled trial of fusion compared with unsupervised "conservative" management showed fusion to be superior, but two subsequent trials in which the rehabilitation was actively managed showed no difference in outcome (3-5). Surgical outcomes are often judged with a global scale of excellent to poor, which may be defined in terms of pain, satisfaction, medication use, work status, and other parameters. Here we discuss surgical outcomes in terms of our observations, knowing that outcomes vary considerably based on patient selection and surgical skill.

In our experience, patients who have undergone lumbar diskectomy can expect good to excellent results 85% of the time. Those who do not recover continue to have back and, at times, radicular pain symptoms. Five percent of failures can be attributed to a recurrent disk herniation. The remainder fail to improve because of technical difficulties, scar formation at the site of surgery, or other ill-defined factors including nerve injury from prolonged compression prior to diskectomy.

Case Study 22-1

A 33-year-old engineer complains of back and left leg pain. There is no history of trauma or excessive physical activity. He reports waking up the previous week with severe low back pain. Two days after the development of back pain, he experiences a shooting pain radiating into his left buttock and down the posterior aspect of his leg. Interestingly, his back pain has improved, but his leg pain is much worse. He now notes difficulty walking, particularly on uneven surfaces. Upon examination, he has a profound weakness of dorsiflexion of his left foot. Straight leg raising is positive and he has decreased sensation along the dorsum of his foot. An MRI is ordered and shows a large ruptured disk (Figure 22-1). Given his significant weakness, a diskectomy is recommended.

Foraminotomy

Foraminal stenosis may be treated by foraminotomy. Similar to a diskectomy, a foraminotomy involves exposure of the lamina followed by removal of bone and ligamentum flavum until the symptomatic nerve root is identified. The exiting neural foramen for that nerve root is then found. Visualization of the foramen is difficult, so palpation is used to assess the degree of stenosis. As noted previously, the foramen is bounded by the pedicles, disk, and superior and inferior facets. Curettes and rongeurs are used to remove a small portion of the superior facet and thereby enlarge the foramen.

Recovery and Outcomes

The recovery after foraminotomy is the same as that after diskectomy. In the appropriate patient, the outcome of a foraminotomy is very similar to that of a diskectomy. Persistent symptoms are attributed to technical difficulties, scar formation, or prolonged compression prior to surgical decompression.

Laminectomy

Laminectomy is typically a part of the diskectomy surgical procedure used to remove a herniated disk. It is also used to decompress a small spinal canal or to expose the spinal canal so that tumors,cysts, or other lesions can be removed. A laminectomy also consists of a midline incision, but with bilateral retraction of the paraspinal muscles to expose the spinous process, both laminae, and the joint facets of the vertebral body. In general, the spinous process is removed along with the laminae. The often hypertrophic ligamentum flavum present between adjacent lamina is removed as well. Care is taken not to disturb the facet joints laterally. The dura is exposed, but the nerve roots are not typically visualized. The neural foramen are evaluated by palpation and are opened if thought to be stenotic. A laminectomy usually does not disturb the stability of the lumbar spine unless there is some underlying defect such as spondylolisthesis.

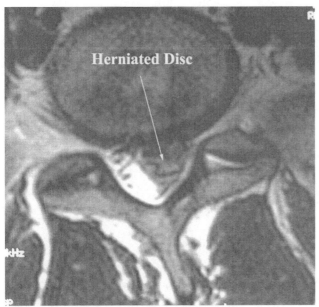

Herniated Disc

A

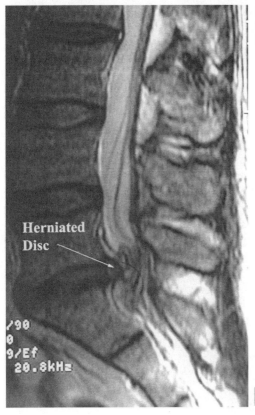

Herniated
Disc

B

Figure 22-1   MRI showing a left-sided herniated disk. (A) Axial image. (B) sagittal image.

Recovery

A single level laminectomy requires approximately 1 to 1.5 hours to perform under general anesthesia. The hospital stay after a lumbar laminectomy is approximately 1-2 days. Patients undergoing this procedure are typically older and, as a result, the hospital stay tends to be a bit longer. Total recovery from a laminectomy may require as little as 1 month or as long as 3 months, depending on the motivation and physical fitness of the patient.

Outcomes

Patients undergoing lumbar laminectomy for stenosis have about a 75% chance of resolution of their leg symptoms. Improvement of back pain is less predictable. Success rates are lower due to the often diffuse problems found in the arthritic back of the aging patient.

Case Study 22-2

A 60-year-old woman presents with complaint of low back and bilateral lower extremity pain. Previously active, she finds that walking and even standing is now difficult due to leg pain (neurogenic claudication). Sitting, however, tends to relieve her pain. Neurologic exam is normal, although MRI reveals significant spinal canal stenosis (Figure 22-2). Conservative management is attempted but her pain persists. Decompressive laminectomy is recommended.

Spinal Fusion

The goal of any spinal fusion is to eliminate motion between adjacent vertebral bodies. To accomplish this objective, there are now a multitude of techniques available. Posterolateral fusion is a common procedure that begins by exposing the vertebral bodies to be fused. Adjacent bony surfaces including the transverse processes are then decorticated and autologous bone is placed to bridge the segments. Decortication or "roughing up" the bony surfaces and placement of the patient's own medullary bone serve to promote new bone formation. Similar to an arm cast for a broken bone, external immobilization in the form of a rigid brace is then used to limit motion while the vertebral segments fuse. More recently wires, hooks, pedicle screws, and rods have been used to provide additional internal immobilization between vertebral segments and, as a result, the fusion success rate has increased significantly (6). Other fusion techniques involve interbody constructs in which the lumbar disk between adjacent vertebrae is replaced with metallic cages or bone dowels. Interbody fusions can be performed from an anterior or posterior approach and can be combined with an instrumented posterolateral fusion. Candidates for interbody fusions are typically patients that are believed to suffer from diskogenic pain,

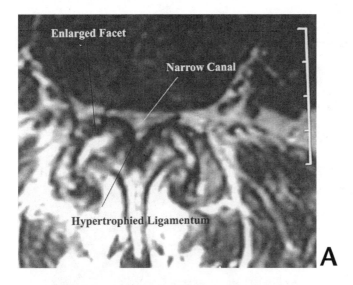

Enlarged Facet

Narrow Canal

Hypertrophied Ligamentum

A

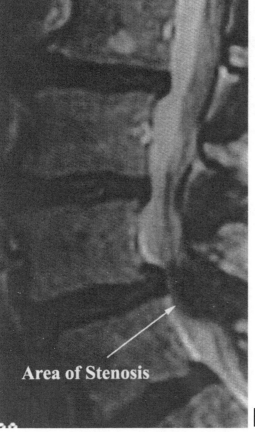

Area of Stenosis

B

Figure 22-2   MRI showing lumbar stenosis. (A) Axial view showing compromise of the spinal canal by facet hypertrophy, posterior ligamentous hypertrophy, and anterior disk bulge. (B) Sagittal view showing canal stenosis from a disk bulge anteriorly and ligamentous hypertrophy posteriorly. (C) Axial view of a normal spinal canal.

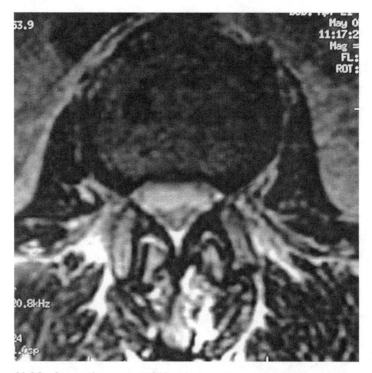

Figure 22-2C   See caption on page 267.

as the disk is removed in the procedure. The technique used, as well as either anterior or posterior approach, is determined by numerous factors including the disease being treated, body habitus, and surgeon preference.

Recovery
The length of operative time required for a spinal fusion will vary depending on the route and number of vertebrae involved. Blood loss can be substantial. Patients typically will have wound drains for a day or two after the procedure. Three to five days in the hospital after an fusion is common. As with a diskectomy or laminectomy, activity is progressive. A rigid brace is commonly worn for at least 3 months when out of bed. Serial x-rays are also obtained to follow the extent of fusion and check the integrity of the instrumentation.

Outcomes
Depending on the technique used, spinal fusion rates can exceed 90%, particularly with the addition of instrumentation. The success of fusion, however, does not necessarily equate with pain relief. One extensive review suggested that although some improvement was found in 75% of patients, 50% or less had significant or complete pain relief after spinal

fusion for back pain (6). Of course, in certain patients such as those with spinal instability, outcomes are often better. The often multifactorial nature of back pain likely accounts for at least part of the relatively poor outcomes associated with spinal fusion.

Case Study 22-3

A 45-year-old male presents with a long history of lower back pain. He feels that his back pain is worsening. Neurologic exam is normal. An x-ray is obtained, showing significant slippage of the L4 vertebral body forward (Figure 22-3). On flexion/extension films, there is approximately 3 mm of movement between the L4 and L5 vertebral bodies. The patient undergoes aggressive conservative management but feels his pain is no better and is severely limiting his normal activities. Given his persistent pain and failure of maximal conservative management, a L4-L5 fusion is considered.

Surgical Treatment of Tumors

As in the case of spinal fusions, the surgical treatment of spinal canal tumors will depend on many factors including the specific disease, its location, and prognosis. For most lumbar intradural tumors, a laminectomy is performed for exposure of the dural sac. The dura is then opened and the tumor is removed using a microscope for better visualization. Most extradural tumors

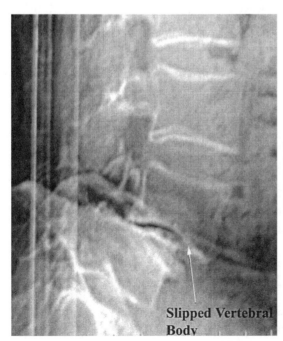

Figure 22-3   X-ray of a patient with L4-5 spondylolisthesis. Note the slippage of the L4 vertebral body relative to the L5 body.

are metastatic and have bony involvement. Surgical resection of the tumor often results in spinal instability necessitating fusion with instrumentation to maintain stability.

Recovery

With intradural tumors, patients are kept flat in bed for 1-2 days after the surgery to prevent spinal fluid leaks. They are then encouraged to be active. Typically, patients without significant neurologic deficit stay in the hospital 3-5 days. Those with deficits are seen by physical therapists and the rehabilitation service for disposition. With metastatic tumors, recovery depends on many factors including the type of primary tumor and its systemic involvement. In a relatively healthy individual, recovery is similar to that of a spinal fusion.

Outcomes

Outcomes for spinal canal tumors depend on the type of tumor as well as the degree of neurologic deficit prior to surgery. Many intradural tumors are benign and can potentially be cured with surgery. In certain circumstances, tumor tissue is purposely left attached to a nerve root because its sacrifice is potentially disabling. The residual tumor must then be followed serially with imaging to detect recurrence.

Case Study 22-4

A 43-year-old male presents for evaluation of back and left leg pain. He reports the rather sudden onset of back pain. Interestingly, he notes that his back pain is much worse in the recumbent position, particularly at night. He feels that his pain is better with standing and walking. Neurologic exam is normal. An MRI shows an intradural, ring-enhancing lesion (Figure 22-4). A laminectomy was performed to remove the tumor.

Vertebroplasty

Compression fractures commonly occur in older individuals due to osteoporosis. Traditional treatments for this problem involve bracing and pain medications. Recently, however, percutaneous transpedicular vertebroplasty has been shown to improve pain in those individuals unresponsive to conservative management. This procedure is designed to deliver acrylic cement into the compressed vertebral body. Pain relief is believed to occur from either the heat generated by the cement mixture with subsequent destruction of nociceptive nerve fibers or from the improvement in mechanical stability produced by the cement (7).

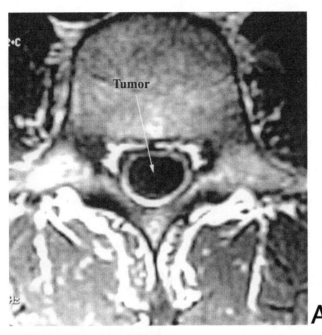

A

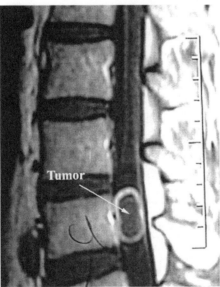

B

Figure 22-4   MRI of a lumbar schwannoma. (A) Axial view showing the tumor (ring-enhancing) filling the spinal canal. (B) Sagittal image.

Recovery

A percutaneous vertebroplasty is commonly performed under monitored anesthesia. Patients are observed for several hours after the procedure while the cement hardens and then are discharged to home.

Outcomes

Most patients appear to benefit from percutaneous vertebroplasty. In a large study by Amar et al., approximately 75% of patients had some improvement in their quality of life (7).

■　■　■

Recommendations

- In patients without neurologic deficits, conservative management, rather than surgery, should be considered the first option for back pain.
- Progressive weakness or cauda equina syndrome is an urgent indication for surgery.
- Metastatic tumors that cause neurologic deficits or intradural tumors that grow or are accompanied by neurologic deficits should be treated with surgery.
- If significant abnormality is identified by imaging studies but the pain is mild or absent, surgery may be deferred until pain develops or becomes severe.
- Patients without a specific diagnosis for back pain are poor surgical candidates.

■　■　■

Key Points

- Establishing the correct diagnosis is essential to determine if surgery is indicated for low back pain.
- Radiographic studies alone are insufficient to determine the cause of back pain. Although diagnostic tools such as CT, MRI, and EMG may help confirm the diagnosis, in many cases all that is necessary to determine the cause of back pain are an accurate history and careful physical examination.
- Patients without a specific diagnosis for back pain are poor surgical candidates.
- Common conditions that respond to surgical treatment are herniated disk, foraminal stenosis, lumbar stenosis, spondylolisthesis, some tumors, and potentially unstable compression fractures.
- Pain refractory to conservative measures, motor weakness, severe sensory deficit, and cauda equina syndrome are indications for surgery.
- Surgical options include diskectomy, foraminotomy, laminectomy, spinal fusion, and vertebroplasty.

■　■　■

REFERENCES

1. **Deyo RA, Weinstein JN.** Primary care: low back pain. N Engl J Med. 2001;344:363-370.

2. **Weber H.** Lumbar disc herniation. A controlled, prospective study with ten years of observation. Spine. 1983;8(2):131-40.

3. **Brox JI, Sørensen R, Friss A, et al.** Randomized clinical trial of lumbar instrumented fusion and cognitive intervention and exercises in patients with chronic low back pain and disc degeneration. Spine. 2003;28(17):1913-1921.

4. **Fairbank J, Frost J, Wilson-MacDonald JS, Yu L-M, Barker K, Collins R, for the Spine Stabilisation Trial Group.** The MRC Spine Stabilisation Trial: A randomised controlled trial to compare surgical stabilisation of the lumbar spine versus an intensive rehabilitation programme on outcome in patients with chronic low back pain. International Society for the Study of the Lumbar Spine Annual Meeting 2004, Porto, Portugal.

5. **Fritzell P, Hagg O, Wessberg P, Nordwall A, Swedish Lumbar Spine Study Group.** 2001 Volvo Award Winner in Clinical Studies. Lumbar fusion nonsurgical treatment for chronic low back pain: a multicenter randomized controlled trial from the Swedish Lumbar Spine Study Group. Spine. 2001;26(23):2521-2532.

6. **Hanley EN, David SM.** Lumbar arthrodesis for the treatment of back pain. J Bone Joint Surg Am. 1999;81:716-730.

7. **Amar AP, Larsen DW, Esnaashari N, Albuquerque FC, Lavine SD, Teitelbaum GP.** Percutaneous transpedicular polymethylmethacrylate vertebroplasty for the treatment of spinal compression fractures. Neurosurgery. 2001;49:1265-1115.

23

Subacute Rehabilitation: The Injured Worker

Deborah S. Heaney, MD, MPH

I n the subacute phase of back pain (6-12 weeks), having the patient return to work and restoring function is crucial. It is during this period that the practitioner has the opportunity to prevent a back pain case from becoming chronic, where full recovery and return-to-work and function become progressively less likely. In addition to medical treatment of these patients, providers should focus on rehabilitation, reconditioning, and return to normal daily function.

This chapter will address issues of return-to-work and return to premorbid functioning in daily life. It will give direction regarding work restrictions and job modification, areas where many primary care physicians lack training and experience. The importance of working with employers and insurers in order to keep the case moving and to achieve the goal of providing the patient with a safe and healthful return to the workplace is also discussed. Congenial and cooperative relationships among all parties involved in this process provide for a smoother and less stressful transition for patients and providers.

Work Restrictions

Impairment versus Disability

Impairment refers to the physical inability to perform a task, whereas the definition of disability takes into account the impact that inability has on the person's life at home or at work (13). Providers are experts in prognosis and treatment, whereas disability determination is a social and political construct (2). It is the provider's responsibility to determine capability, or functional impairment, not disability. It is the employer's administrative responsibility to determine whether workplace accommodation can be made and thus whether the impairment makes the employee "disabled." Although physicians generally cannot be sued for their opinions concerning a workers' ability to work, physicians can be sued for interference with employment administrative issues. For example, it is not the physician's responsibility to determine the essential functions of the job, to arrange accommodations, or to make ultimate job placement decisions. These limitations of the physician's responsibilities actually make things simpler for the physician. Keeping in mind that many companies have modified work available, after determining impairment the physician only needs to issue appropriate work restrictions (10). This is further discussed later in this chapter in the context of the Americans with Disabilities Act in the section "Job Modification."

Job Description

A detailed knowledge of the patient's job demands is helpful to the treating physician when considering work restrictions. Many employers have an occupational medicine clinic or human resources department that may be able to provide a written job-to-work decision. Details regarding an employee's position are important, as considerable variability exists in the tasks and level of activity engaged in by workers with the same job title. For example, a custodian in an office setting may do relatively light work compared to a custodian in a heavy industrial setting. Similarly, the term *production worker* gives little insight into job specifics (1,3,4).

The patient should be asked to describe his or her job tasks in detail. These include physical and mental demands, hazardous exposures, and the use of personal protective equipment. For example, the patient may be required to do heavy lifting and stand for prolonged periods of time while wearing a supplied-air respirator. The physician should encourage the patient to be specific about job tasks, such as weight of objects moved, bending, twisting, pulling, pushing, body positions, work at heights, duration of tasks, and the use of assistive devices such as lift tables and hoists. The provider should also inquire about ergonomic worksite configuration, such as the height of a worktable or the reach required to pick up a part (1,3,4).

Writing the Restrictions

Work restrictions may be necessary or prudent to facilitate healing or protect the worker from further tissue damage. A subacute back pain patient who has a sedentary job or has recovered completely may be able to be returned to full duty. However, it is not necessary to wait until a patient is capable of doing his or her full job to return him or her to work safely.

Regardless of whether a patient says that his employer requires a full release for him to return to work, it is good practice to issue restrictions. It is important to remember that the decision to accommodate an employee in the workplace or whether the impairment should constitute disability is the employers, not the physician's. An employee who insists there is no light duty available may be told, "I will write down what it is safe for you to do, and then it is up to your employer to determine if they can accommodate your restriction or if they will chose to send you home."

Although functional capacity evaluations can be a valuable tool in issuing restrictions in the return-to-work process, they are costly and should be reserved for refractory or chronic cases and are not typically needed when caring for a patient in the subacute phase (1). The treating provider should evaluate a patient, identify the impairment, and write restrictions that would keep him from worsening his condition or harming himself. In order for an employer to find appropriate modified work, functional restrictions must be clearly outlined. In other words, you should state what the worker should or should not do in terms of motions, repetitions, force or load, use of tools or machinery, or restricted hours of work. "Light duty" is meaningless to most employers and supervisors and does not help in job placement (2). There should always be an expiration date for restrictions, and work limitations should be reconsidered at each clinical follow-up, progressing as appropriate for the patient's progress (1). Physicians tend to dislike calls requesting clarification of restrictions, yet it is usually vague restrictions or lack of an expiration date that prompt those calls.

Some of the occupational risk factors that contribute to low back pain include lifting and forceful movements (pushing and pulling), frequent bending and twisting of the trunk, and whole body vibration. Although restrictions are addressed on a case-by-case basis specific to the impairment, these issues will likely be addressed (3,4). Providers must take care to express work capabilities in specific terms useful to the employer and to individual supervisors (5). A restriction for lifting should address poundage. "No repetitive work with hands" should probably more appropriately be written to address forceful grasping or pinching or whatever is specific to the particular impairment. "No repetitive work" makes it virtually impossible to accommodate an employee in an industrial setting. "No repetitive wrist extension and supination" would be a great restriction for someone with lateral epicondylitis, except that it is incomprehensible to a supervisor who does not have medical training. The challenge of writing restrictions is translating that into layspeak. "No forceful grasping" may be what ends up being written. Limiting work hours is an option, but it may make more sense for the employee to work a full shift in a safe job than half of a shift in an unsafe one. If an employee with back pain is doing a desk job where he can change positions and work at his own pace, how would 8 or 9 hours a day be more harmful to him than four?

Case Study 23-1

A 51-year-old assembly-line worker was lifting a tray of parts when he felt a sudden pull in his left low back. He had had several bouts of back pain in the past 3 years, and x-rays showed degenerative joint disease in the lumbar spine. He was seen and diagnosed with a lumbar strain previously at another institution. He was placed on Motrin and Flexeril.

The patient reports that his typical job requires heavy lifting and frequent bending, so the physician he is now seeing decides that he should ot return to work for 6 weeks. After 6 weeks, the employee is feeling better but still has discomfort with prolonged standing and walking and with bending. He has not tried to lift anything heavy and feels like he is generally weak. He does not feel that he is ready to return to work. The physician extends his disability another 2 weeks and prescribes physical therapy. The insurance company's nurse case manager has called requesting medical documentation regarding why this employee is totally disabled from work.

The case manager indicates that though the patient's regular job is physically demanding, his company has a modified work program that could accommodate a back-injured patient. With appropriate restrictions, he could return to work. Therefore, this man was impaired but not "disabled" by the employer. The physician is mildly aggravated by the extra work but issues a restriction of no lifting, bending, or twisting. Later that day, the employer calls for clarification. The physician is busy dictating records and starts to think it was easier to just keep him off of work. The employer says the job they have in mind requires him to inspect 5-pound parts. He would also have to bend to adjust the conveyor if it gets stuck, which can happen several times a day. They want to know if lifting 5 pounds is okay and if it is okay if he bends over briefly up to 10 times a day. The physician responds that she meant "heavy lifting" and that it is okay if the patient bends once in a while. The physician clarifies that she just meant no repetitive bending. If the restriction had stated "no lifting over 10 pounds" and "limited bending and twisting" or "no repetitive bending and twisting" the physician may have been spared the phone call. In fact, the employer had this job, and even lighter ones, available all along, and the worker probably could have been returned to work several weeks ago.

Job Modification

Title I of The Americans with Disabilities Act of 1990 (ADA) states that employers are obligated to provide reasonable workplace accommodation to employees with disabilities. However, even if an employee has a "disability" in the workers' compensation arena (i.e., unable to work), he or she may not have a disability for ADA purposes. Impairments resulting from occupational or personal injury may not be severe enough to substantially limit a major life activity or they may be only temporary (the ADA applies to permanent disability), thus not qualifying for protection under the ADA. It follows that the employer is not required to provide reasonable accommodation for an employee with an injury, occupational or otherwise, who does not have a disability as defined by the ADA (6).

Though there is no legal mandate for providing modified work in most subacute back pain cases, employers are increasingly amenable to providing transitional work. Many employers who have chosen to offer modified work have come to realize that to prevent deconditioning and to help maintain mental and physical well-being, a patient should be kept as active as possible, which means remaining in the workplace. When the condition is work-related, the employer has additional motivation to find modified work, such as decreasing workers' compensation costs and manpower issues. Employers with more than 10 employees are required to keep a log of work-related injuries and illnesses and count workdays lost. This is a significant motivator for many employers who are judged by corporate offices based on these records. Employers in small companies, however, may have less of an ability to modify work content during a period of impairment from back pain (2).

Employers in small companies, however, may have less of an ability to modify work content during a period of impairment from back pain (2). Employers may also be less likely to make the extra effort to find modified work for employees when their condition is not work-related. Some employers preserve what may be limited modified work for workers' compensation cases. Others are concerned that a personal back injury aggravated in the workplace will become an occupational back injury, according to workman's compensation law in many states.

Though most subacute back pain patients may have only temporary impairment and thus their conditions may not be covered under the ADA, The Equal Employment Opportunity Commission's Enforcement Guidance on the ADA neatly summarizes the employer's responsibility regarding modified work assignment, which is applicable regardless of ADA status. They state that the employer should gather information from the provider and other parties regarding the employee's specific functional limitations and abilities. The employer may solicit suggestions for reasonable accommodation. The employer then bears the ultimate responsibility for deciding whether an employee with a disability (or in the generic case, impairment) is ready to return to work. The employer, rather than the provider, must determine whether the employee can perform the essential functions of the job, with or without reasonable accommodation (6). The employer is not required to accommodate the worker if the accommodation would cause undue hardship or if the worker would not qualify for the accommodated job. The goal of transitional work is to match physical capacity to ergonomic job demand (5).

Employer Relations

Health care providers should be encouraged to gain more knowledge about the job requirements of their patients by communication with employers, or in the ideal situation through personal visits to job sites. Better communication between the employer and the provider on issues such as the importance of early return to work, work restrictions, and possible transitional or modified work is helpful for all parties involved. An occupational physician or case manager may be a facilitator in this interaction of the various parties involved (5).

In a multistate injured worker self-report survey that was done at 6 and 18 months postinjury, it was found that whether or not modified duty leads to better outcomes was a result of physician-employer cooperation. Employees who reported that their employer worked with their doctor to find appropriate modified duty and return to work had significantly higher levels of physical and mental functioning than those whose employers and physicians did not cooperate. They also had significantly shorter median time away from work (7).

One cohort study suggested that physician proactivity alone (discussing work issues with the employee) did not influence the duration of disability in the subacute or chronic back pain patient once workplace issues were considered. These authors emphasized the necessity of having the provider work with the employer to encourage ergonomic and other changes, which the physician cannot bring about on his own. The impact of workplace factors (physical and psychosocial, such as time spent binding and lifting and job strain) on duration of disability suggested that the employers' contribution to the return to work problem is not insignificant and is a necessary factor in the equation (8).

Several other studies have noted that essential elements of the success in returning patients with subacute back pain to work have been to involve the workplace explicitly in the management process and to clearly communicate a return-to-work management plan to all parties: the provider, the worker, the employer, the insurer. This is not surprising, given that failure to return to work within a few weeks is often the result of no workplace accommodation (9). When communicating with the employer, the provider should be aware that medical information must be kept confidential at the worksite and should be limited only to what is necessary for appropriate job assignment. Supervisors are only entitled to the restrictions (10).

Insurer Relations

Many providers have little knowledge or interest in the legal, administrative, and insurance parts of the work injury process. Dialogue often occurs only in adversarial situations. It has been suggested that meaningful, non-adversarial communication between provider and insurer can facilitate problem solution and a better perception by each party of the position of the other (5). Physicians may do the most good for their patients by working with insurers early on to assist their return to work (2). Keeping open communication with insurers and case managers is important. Haig et al. have outlined the complex relations between case managers and physicians (12). The case manager needs information from the provider to do his or her job effectively. Similarly, the case manager often has information helpful to the provider, such as relevant company personnel records, investigator reports, history of previous injuries and absenteeism, and so forth (11). Though many providers may think that only medical information is relevant to their treatment of the patient, in the setting of return-to-work (for a work-related or personal medical condition) or workers' compensation, this additional information is often helpful and in many cases necessary for successful case management and claim progression. For example, a worker with an exemplary attendance and performance record is less likely to be challenged about his or her motivation to return to work.

The insurer expects that the treating provider will return the worker to restricted duty if appropriate work is available. Complete and quality medical records are crucial, providing detailed information to the insurer on a clinical rationale for the presence (or absence) of work impairment (13,2). Providers are often required to fill out a plethora of forms from employers, government officials, and insurers. Filling forms out fully and clearly and providing detailed chart notes may limit the additional forms being sent (10). For example, the treating provider should inform insurance carriers, case managers, and the employers about the patient's work ability in every issued report (5).

Patient Relations

The physician should place some responsibility on the patient as to what the patient expects the recovery rate to be. It is helpful to share with the patient information regarding work capability and restrictions that have been given to the insurance company. Workers must be reassured that the provider is their advocate, and the patient should be included in all decisions (2).

The patient should be advised that staying active and continuing activities as normally as possible may lead to a faster recovery, a faster return to work, and less chronic disability. It is important to give the patient reassurance intended to reduce fear of movement. Providers sometimes respond to patients' anxieties and fears about return to work by keeping them off work, thereby feeding their fear. Fear and avoidance regarding work and activity are strongly related to work loss due to low back pain. In one study, 2 months after seeking care for back pain in a primary care setting, a large proportion of patients reported being worried that a wrong movement might injure their back. Patients reported concern about being unable to do things and continued activity limitations because of the fear of risk for injury and because of concern that their pain indicated that there was something serious wrong with them. Twenty-four percent to thirty-five percent of patients reported that they had decreased or ceased housework, sexual activity, walking, and standing. Though these limitations were not indicative of total disability, they suggest that many patients have sustained decreased quality of life because of their pain. The study showed that a large proportion of primary care patients with back pain still had significant activity limitations that continued at 1 year, further suggesting the need for interventions that support resumption of normal activities, including work (14,15).

In a survey of injured workers 6 and 18 months postinjury, physical function scores were significantly better when the physician and the worker discussed activities that could be safely performed, prevention of reinjury, and a return-to-work plan. Time off work was 2-4 weeks shorter when the physician and the worker discussed these as well as other topics (7). In one cohort study, 37% of workers recalled that their initial primary treating physician talked to them only a little or not at all about their preinjury job, and 27% felt their physician did not understand their job. Only 64% of patients were told by their provider that they were ready to go back to work. A positive return-to-work recommendation during the subacute phase was associated with shorter disability durations (8). Another study of chronic pain patients found that significantly more patients who were directed to return to work did so (60%) than did patients in another group who were similarly treated but for whom return-to-work was not directed (25%). Patients in the group who were given a return-to-work directive also needed less additional treatment for their pain (16).

Case Study 23-2

The patient of Case Study 23-1 is very reluctant to return to work. For 8 weeks he has being doing nothing but sitting around the house watching television, and he feels that his work is too strenuous for him. He experiences pain when he walks for short distances, and he is afraid he is going to do "permanent damage" to himself. His physician encourages him to return to work and, after discussing the work situation with the patient, writes a note giving permission to for him to return to work with a 10-pound lifting restriction. Two days later, he comes back to see her, unscheduled. He says that he is having increased pain in his back. He says that despite his restriction not to lift over 10 pounds, he has to lift racks of parts that weigh 30 pounds apiece. He says the employer is not honoring the restrictions. The physician issues a note that entitles the patient to another medical leave.

The employer calls to ask why the physician's opinion has changed. Her first instinct is to not take the call, as she does not want to be in the middle of this. She reluctantly agrees to talk with the supervisor and tells him that the patient has informed her that the work restrictions were not being honored, and that his continuing to lift heavy items will delay his recovery. The employer, however, replies that the patient has been instructed not to lift the trays of parts and that there is another employee who has been assigned to do that lifting. The physician then calls the patient at home. He tells her that he finishes all of his parts assembly before the assigned coworker arrives to give him new stock, so he just does the lifting himself. She tells him that it is his responsibility to protect himself and to advocate for his well-being and that if he feels his restrictions are not being honored he needs to speak with his supervisor or case manager if available. In this case, the worker needs to wait for the other employee to arrive to give him new stock. If this slows down his production, that is not his concern. The physician reassures her patient that some increased pain is expected when returning to work, but if he follows the work restrictions, he will not be harming himself and will in fact be improving his strength and endurance, which will lead to a quicker recovery.

Conclusion

Prolonging work incapacity in patients with subacute low back pain can lead to angry patients, employers, and insurers. In fact, prolonging work incapacity contributes to chronicity of back pain and disability, which in turn results in increased societal costs. It is important to realize that the system can work well, and patients' best interests are served if all parties involved-employers, employees, insurers, and providers-have clear and open communication. The provider needs to communicate to the patient's employer work restrictions that are detailed, specific, and easy to understand. With the patient, the provider needs to discuss a return-to-work plan early in the course of treatment and to give reassurance that resuming activities will not be harmful to the patient. Early communication facilitates return to work, particularly when this involves job modification. This sends a clear message to the employer and insurer that both the provider and patient are trying to work together to help the patient resume employment.

Recommendations

- As the first step in writing work restrictions, ask the patient to describe his or her job in detail. Ask for specific information about job tasks, such as what bodily movements are involved, what is the weight of objects being lifted or moved, and what is the height of the worktable.

- Write specific restrictions that are useful to the employer. For example, rather than simply writing "no lifting, bending, or twisting," specify "no lifting objects over 10 lbs" and "no repetitive bending (no bending more than 10 times per day)."
- Functional capacity evaluations should be reserved for refractory or chronic cases; they are not usually needed for patients with subacute pain.
- Include the patient in all decisions. The patient should feel assured that the physician is his or her advocate.
- Encourage the patient to remain active, and advise him or her that inactivity and avoidance of returning to work may actually prolong the pain condition. Reassure the patient that the pain may increase upon return to work, but that this pain does not mean that the condition is worsening. Remind him or her that resuming work will improve strength and endurance.

Key Points

- It is the provider's responsibility to determine impairment, not disability.
- Many employers offer modified work programs that can prevent disability in patients with low back pain, with appropriate restrictions from providers.
- Work restrictions should be detailed and able to be interpreted by a non-medical person.
- Open communication among employers, insurers, and providers leads to a smooth progression of the case. It can help prevent animosity between parties and in the long run serves the best interest of the patients.
- Enlisting the patient in the return-to-work plan and assuaging fear about resuming activity is crucial to success in the subacute rehabilitation process.

REFERENCES

1. **Wyman D.** Evaluating patients for return to work. Am Fam Physician. 1999;59(4):844-8.
2. **Carey TS.** Disability: how successful are we in determining disability? Neurol Clin. 1999;17(1):168-176.

3. **Dasinger LK, Krause N, Deegan LJ, Brand RJ, Rudolph L.** Physical workplace factors and return to work after compensated low back injury: a disability phase-specific analysis. J Occup Environ Med. 2000;42(3):323-33.

4. **Gerr F, Mani L.** Work-related low back pain. Primary Care; Clinics in Office Practice. 2000;27(4):865-76.

5. **Wyman E, Cats-Baril W.** Working it out: recommendations from a multidisciplinary national consensus panel on medical problems in workers' compensation. J Occup Med. 1994;36(2):144-54.

6. **U.S. Equal Employment Opportunity Commission.** EEOC Enforcement Guidance: Workers' Compensation and the ADA. EEOC Notice. 915.002. Available at www.eeoc.gov/policy/guidance.html.

7. **Harris J, Lee A.** Effective practices in workers' compensation medical care and care management. OEM Report. 2002;16(3):17-23.

8. **Dasinger LK, Krause N, Thompson PJ, Brand RJ, Rudolph L.** Doctor proactive communication, return-to-work recommendation, and duration of disability after a workers' compensation low back injury. J Occup Environ Med. 2001;43(6):515-25.

9. **Frank J, Sinclair S, Hogg-Johnson S, Shannon H, Bombardier C, Beaton D, et al.** Preventing disability from work-related low-back pain: new evidence gives new hope—if we can just get all the players onside. Can Med Assoc J. 1998;158(12):1625-31.

10. **Colledge AL, Johns R Jr, Thomas MH.** Functional ability assessment: guidelines for the workplace. J Occup Environ Med. 1999;41(3):172-9.

11. **Haig AJ, Hadwin K, Palma-Davis L, Rich D.** Insurance case managers' perception of quality in back pain programs: a focus study group. Am J Phys Med Rehabil. 2001;80(7):520-5.

12. **Haig AJ.** Commentary: the influence of insurance case managers. Am J Phys Med Rehabil. 2001;80(7):526-7.

13. **Pye H, Orris P.** Workers' compensation in the United States and the role of the primary care physician. Primary Care; Clinics in Office Practice. 2000;27(4):831-44.

14. **Von Korff M, Moore J.** Stepped care for back pain: activating approaches for primary care. Ann Intern Med. 2001;134(9 Part 2):911-17.

15. **Waddell G.** A fear-avoidance beliefs questionnaire (FABQ) and the role of fear-avoidance beliefs in chronic low back pain and disability. Pain. 1993;52(2):157-68.

16. **Catchlove R.** Effects of a directive return to work approach in the treatment of workmans' compensation patients with chronic pain. Pain. 1982;14(2):181-91.

24

Therapies for Subacute Back
Pain: A Glossary Approach

i. Physical Therapy
Elizabeth A. Wiggert, PT

ii. Rehabilitation Therapies
Quaintance L. Miller, MS, OTR
Sandra Dodge, COTA

iii. Surgery and Injection Treatments
Andrew J. Haig, MD
Matthew W. Smuck, MD

i. Physical Therapy

Elizabeth A. Wiggert, PT

Physical therapy is one of the most frequently prescribed treatments for back pain. The purpose of this chapter is to provide a quick reference to many types of physical therapy that may be used in the treatment of back pain. It is not intended to be all-inclusive or individually detailed, rather a listing with a brief description of therapy types, indications, contraindications, goals, and expectations. *Physical therapy* was the term originally given to the practice of using physical modalities such as heat, light, and sound to treat pain and disability. That rather archaic definition has been broadened, and even replaced, by the current practice that often focuses more on exercise, patient education, and manual therapy than modalities.

Therapist Education

A licensed physical therapist in the United States has graduated from an accredited 2- to 3-year program. There are practicing physical therapists that graduated with a bachelor's degree; however, those programs now offer at least a master's degree. For the current programs, a college degree is a prerequisite for admission. Most physical therapy programs are graduating students with an entry-level master of physical therapy degree, or MPT. This is in the process of being replaced by the DPT, or doctor of physical therapy degree. The American Physical Therapy Association has stated that by the year 2020, all physical therapy (PT) schools will offer the DPT as the entry level physical therapy education. This means that in the year 2005 there are physical therapists currently in practice that may have a bachelor's, master's, or doctorate degree. It is important to keep in mind that these are all entry level degrees, and in fact at this time, the therapists with the doctorate degree will most likely have less clinical experience than the therapist with the older bachelor's degree. The differences in the bachelor versus doctorate degree curricula are slight with the latter including more administrative courses. Subspecialty advanced degrees are available. For example, a therapist may elect to have further training to obtain an advanced master's in orthopedic physical therapy, cardiopulmonary physical therapy, pediatric physical therapy, geriatric physical therapy, to name only a few. Their credentials will usually be written as Jane Doe, MS, PT. The same holds true for advanced PhD degrees.

Regardless of the degree, physical therapy education is very broad. The techniques of how to treat the outpatient with back pain are only a portion of what is taught while in school. Detailed education and clinical experience in treating back pain is done, for the most part, on a continuing education basis.

Each state does require minimum qualifications for licensure of physical therapists. However, not all states require evidence of continuing education to maintain the license. There are some subspecialty programs that offer advanced training and certification (for example, the MacKenzie approach and the Orthopedic Manual Physical Therapist). These programs provide systematic education and testing for minimal qualifications, as well as specialization certification for the particular focused treatment approach. The American Physical Therapy Association offers a clinical subspecialty in orthopedics (OCS, or orthopedic clinical specialist) via testing. Unlike the others, it does not include formal didactics. Knowledge of the orthopedic treatment for the entire body is tested rather than being limited to the spine. There is no current advanced specialty certification in a broad-based multimodality treatment approach for the patient with back pain.

One reasonable approach to determining the skill of a physical therapist is to ask for a list of courses attended and the top three most common diagnoses of the patients they treat. Just because a therapist has attended a course by no means assures his or her mastery of the techniques taught. Work is in progress to develop clinical skills testing, but at present there is no national broad-based certification of skill in the field. Ultimately, referring patients and monitoring the efficacy of treatment by an individual therapist remains the best way to determine that individual's skill.

Treatment Goals

The primary goal of physical therapy is to return a person to the highest level of independent functioning possible. The code of ethics of the American Physical Therapy Association states that the therapist must identify realistic long-term and short-term goals, anticipated duration of treatment to reach goals, expected outcome of treatment, and timely discharge. The patient must be discharged when either the goals have been met or there has been a plateau of functional progress.

The treatment plan should be designed for the advancement of function. Formal physical therapy is not a palliative approach and is not intended for maintenance. (The home exercise program, on the other hand, is meant to focus on those aspects of therapy.) During physician evaluation of a patient, if considering referral to physical therapy, it is important to remember the following: if the patient has no further gains to be made, is not functionally limited, or has plateaued, physical therapy is not the treatment of choice. Not surprisingly, third-party payers have embraced this component of the practice act and usually will not reimburse for what could be considered palliative or maintenance care. Retrospective reviews are occurring more frequently with payment being denied for those sessions provided for inappropriate referral, nonacute exacerbation of a chronic condition, or continued therapy after progress has plateaued. Each progress note written by the physical therapist and requests for continued treatment should document objective gains of function, future goals, type of treatment to be delivered, and anticipated duration to warrant continuation of care. Of course, interval physician patient interview and follow-up exam is also a key component in making this decision.

Treatment Descriptions

Physical Modalities

Therapeutic Ultrasound

CONTINUOUS

Definition: The use of a continuous high-frequency sound wave to generate heat in the underlying tissue. Ultrasound (US) may increase temperature in structures up to 5 cm. deep (1). Temperature increases of 4 to 5 degrees centigrade may be found at depths of 8 cm (2).

Uses

- Decrease muscle spasm, tone
- Decrease pain
- Facilitate soft tissue or joint extensibility

Contraindications

- Should not be used over metal implants
- Should not be used near pacemaker or active implantable cardiac defibrillator
- Presence of malignancy

Comments

- Should not be considered a treatment in and of itself. It should be used as an adjunct to increase extensibility or decrease pain to facilitate stretching and or mobilization.

PULSED

Definition: As above, except that waveform is pulsed rather than continuous (1).

Uses

- Decrease pain
- Decrease inflammation
- May increase extensibility

Contraindications

- Should not be used near pacemaker or active implantable cardiac defibrillator
- Presence of malignancy

Comments

- Very useful in presence of active inflammation
- For very acute injury or pathology, may be used in isolation
- For chronic conditions, should not be viewed as independent treatment

Phonophoresis
Definition: The use of ultrasound to drive a steroid cream carried in a water-soluble base into soft tissue.
Uses

- Decrease pain
- Decrease inflammation

Contraindications

- Allergy to steroids
- Should not be used over metal implants
- Should not be used near pacemaker or active implantable cardiac defibrillator
- Presence of malignancy

Comments

- Great debate exists whether any medication crosses the skin with this procedure. It has been shown with pigskin that the carrier for the medication blocks the transmission of sound waves entirely. Many feel that continuous wave form should be used, as it is more likely to drive the medication in. However, because this modality is often used for its anti-inflammatory effect and continuous use increases heat in the underlying tissues, this seems counterproductive. Certainly, this procedure is waning in popularity.

Iontophoresis
Definition: The use of a direct electrical current to drive a medication into a soft tissue (frequently dexamethasone 4 mg/cc).
Uses

- Decrease pain
- Decrease inflammation

Contraindications

- Allergy to steroids
- Pain intolerance to direct current
- Presence of pace maker or active implantable cardiac defibrillator

Comments

- Clinically, this is a very useful technique. It almost always affords the patient immediate pain relief. Experimentally, iontophoresis has been shown to be superior to phonophoresis in the delivery of medication. If the patient cannot tolerate the electrical current, however, and the amplitude is subsequently lowered, the medication may dissipate from the tissue before enough is delivered to provide a therapeutic dose.

Biofeedback

Definition: The use of surface electromyography (EMG) to measure the electrical activity of muscle and display in a visual and/or auditory manner.

Uses

- Increasing active contraction of intact, but inhibited muscle
- Decreasing contraction of painful, shortened muscle

Contraindications

- None

Comments

- This is especially useful in patients with pain-related fear of movement, co-contraction of antagonistic muscles groups limiting passive motion, or patients with poor postural habits.
- For multidisciplinary teams, psychology and physical therapy often work together with the patient using biofeedback.

TENS (Transcutaneous Electrical Nerve Stimulation)

Definition: The use of electrical waves transmitted through surface electrodes to preferentially stimulate the A delta fibers and thus "close" the gate to inhibit ascending nociceptive information.

Uses

- Chronic, unretractable pain
- Neurogenic pain

Contraindications

- Mental status/cognitive limitations of patient
- Skin sensitivities

Comments

- Use needs to be limited/restricted to a few hours a day. Clinically, it has been noted that when overused, the nervous system seems to quickly habituate to the waveform, requiring increased amplitude to get same pain-relieving benefit. Eventually, the unit is no longer useful. Newer models have many choices of waveform parameters, thus decreasing the risk of habituation. Using two channels and thus "crossing" the involved nerve can be very effective in the management of radiculopathy, post-herpetic neuralgia, and so forth.

Hot Pack
Definition: The use of a warm moist compress directly on the skin.
Uses

- Decrease pain
- Increase soft tissue extensibility
- Facilitate relaxation

Contraindications

- Insensate skin

Comments

- Hot packs should be viewed as a modality to facilitate the patient's relaxation to better tolerate therapy. The heating is only superficial, probably has no direct effect on subcutaneous structures.

Cold Pack/Ice Massage
Definition: The use of a cold compress (crushed ice, gel) or ice cube applied directly to the skin.
Uses

- Decrease pain
- Decrease muscle spasm
- Decrease inflammation

Contraindications

- Insensate skin
- Raynaud or other circulatory impairment (relative precaution)

Comments

- Clinically, ice can be very useful in acute pain problems such as muscle tears, ligamentous sprains, bone contusion, or any local inflammation. Ice is also useful for pain after joint mobilization or stretching.

Mechanical Traction
Definition: The use of a mechanical device to provide a longitudinal force in the axial plane of the spine.
Uses

- Radicular type pain
- Pain that is alleviated by such a force

Contraindications

- Spinal instability

Comments

- The reasons why traction can be successful continue to be a subject of debate. Some clinicians believe that enough force is provided to actually separate the intervertebral region, allowing more room for the nerve root. Others believe the stress of the joint distraction reduces inflammation, and thus nerve root irritation. Still others believe it stretches the deep spinal musculature more adequately than any other means. Regardless of the mechanism, traction should be viewed as an adjunct to a more comprehensive program and not a stand-alone treatment.

Manual Therapy

Definition: Therapeutic approaches in which the practitioner uses his or her hands to restore normal joint mechanics and stretch contractile and noncontractile soft tissue. "The goal of the [manual therapies] is to restore maximal, pain-free movement of the musculoskeletal system in postural balance" (3). There are a great number and variety of manual therapy approaches. Below is a noninclusive list of several popular types.

Types

BIOMECHANICAL MODEL (OSTEOPATHIC APPROACH)

- Muscle Energy: "a manual medicine treatment procedure that involves the voluntary contraction of patient muscle in a precisely controlled direction . . . against a distinctly executed counterforce applied by the operator" (3).
- Cranial Manipulation: application of the principles of biomechanics to the minimal movement of the skull sutures.
- Strain Counterstrain: "Relieving spinal pain . . . by passively putting the joint into its position of greatest comfort. . . . Relieving pain by reduction of and arrest of the continuing inappropriate proproiceptor activity" (4).

NORWEGIAN APPROACH (KALTENBORN, OMPT)

- "In the Nordic System, range (hypomobility, hypermobility or normal mobility) and quality of movement [of a joint] is evaluated using translatoric movement in addition to rotational movements. In treatment, translatoric traction and gliding movements rather than rotational movements are preferred to avoid compressing a joint that is already strained by pathology" (5).

MACKENZIE APPROACH

- A system in which pain alleviating positions are used to diagnosis and treat spinal pathology.

CRANIOSACRAL THERAPY

- A type of therapy in which the practitioner is believed to feel the pulse of the motion of the cerebrospinal fluid within the dura. By palpating this motion indirectly via the skull and spine and gently manipulating it, the restrictions of the spine and skull are treated (6).

MASSAGE

- A generic term applying to many traditions of rubbing the soft tissues (primarily muscle and fascia).

MYOFASCIAL RELEASE

- A more specific type of soft tissue treatment that stretches the fascial structures of the body along its inherent planes.

Exercise

Types

STRETCHING

Definition: Exercises in which the patient holds a position to lengthen shortened soft tissue structures.

STRENGTHENING

Definition: Exercises in which the patient moves against a force (including gravity) to increase muscle torque production.

REEDUCATION

Definition: Exercises in which the patient practices movements to affect the quality of the muscle recruitment; that is, rather than performing hip abduction as a gross movement, specific movements that incorporate gluteus medius firing are performed.

AEROBIC CONDITIONING

Definition: Exercises that increase the cardiovascular endurance of the patient.

FUNCTIONAL RESTORATION

Definition: Activities or exercises that use the patient's vocational or avocational movement requirements to restore performance of these activities.

TREATMENT PARADIGM APPROACHES

Definition: Traditional physical therapeutic approaches that incorporate exercise as both part of the evaluation and treatment of spinal dysfunction. These include:

- MacKenzie
- Williams

MOVEMENT THERAPIES

Definition: Systems that are not traditionally physical therapy, but sometimes are incorporated by physical therapists, that use specific movements
to retrain the body in normal movement patterns, and to reduce pain.
These include, but are not limited to,

- Alexander technique
- Chi Kung (Qigong)
- Feldenkrais
- Pilates
- Tai Chi Chuan (Taijiquan)
- Trager
- Yoga

The efficacy of all the different physical therapeutic approaches and
types has not been substantially validated to date. There have been some
studies looking at specific therapeutic approaches, but these have been
small, poorly controlled, and highly inconclusive.

Treatment Paradigm

In general, the following approach seems to be successful in the majority
of low back pain cases:

1. Educate and instruct the patient about what they do themselves; this is
   the real key to success.
2. Restore optimal range of motion and alignment. Address any joint tightness. This may present as joint capsule tightness, muscle imbalance, or
   malalignment referred to as "somatic dysfunction" or "manipulative
   lesion." The extremity joints such as the hips need to be evaluated and
   treated, as they influence the spine.
3. Address any muscle shortness.
4. Evaluate for agonist/antagonist inhibition of muscle firing, postural
   muscle imbalance, and correct patterns of dysfunction.
5. Address muscle weakness.
6. Introduce aerobic conditioning or work reconditioning.

In general, modalities should be used as an adjunct to the above, not as
treatment alone. Modalities can be very useful to either increase elasticity
or to decrease pain so the patient may better tolerate stretching and so
forth, but should rarely, if ever, be used in isolation.

There are many techniques to be used to accomplish efficient and good
treatment of the patient with back pain. The skilled, experienced therapist
will cover all of the issues above by picking and choosing treatments to
create the most useful program for the individual patient. One therapist
may have better skill and success with one technique, whereas another
uses a different regimen. As long as efficient objective progress is being
made, then the reviewing physician does not need to focus on specific

techniques. If the same old routine is used time and time again and the patient does not progress as well as hoped, a review is in order.

Most physical therapists who are skilled and experienced in this field do agree that the home program prescribed is the most important intervention. The approach outlined above can be, in some cases, accomplished with a home program in conjunction with periodic physical therapy sessions to ensure compliance and proper performance, upgrade of the program, when necessary, and reinforcement of goals.

The home program is only as effective as the patient is compliant; thus it cannot be emphasized enough that both the physical therapist and the physician need to consistently reinforce the importance of the home program and to regularly check that the patient is following it. The patient should be asked regularly to demonstrate his or her performance of the program; remember that, except at the early stages of treatment, if the patient has to think too long or requires handouts to perform his or her home program, it is likely not being done at home.

A basic home program takes each joint through its range of motion once a day (see Table 24-1 for a representative home program). That takes the spine, sacrum, and bony pelvis through all of the normal physiologic range of motion and therefore can be good as both preventative as well as self-treatment for recurrence.

■   ■   ■

Recommendations

Physicians should expect communication from the physical therapist after the initial evaluation is performed. This may be via electronic, written, or verbal means. The significant findings, subsequent functional disabilities, goals, and treatment plan should be included in this communication. The physician should also receive information from the physical therapist when:

- The goals have been met, and the patient has been discharged.
- The patient has plateaued, and no further physical therapy is warranted.
- There is change in the patient's status that requires medical attention.
- The patient is to be seen by the physician for follow-up.

■   ■   ■

Table 24-1   General Low Back Pain Home Program

Name	Purpose	Comments
Pubic self-correction (Fig. 24-1)	Aligns the base of the pelvis.	Needs to be done first.
Segmental sit-backs (Fig. 24-2)	Eccentrically strengthens abdominals, restores spinal segmental flexion, stretches hamstrings and heel cords.	Should be used with caution in any patient with adverse neural tension (i.e., positive straight leg raise).
Anterior innominate self-correction (Fig. 24-3)	Posteriorly rotates an anteriorly rotated hemi-pelvis.	Can be done bilaterally without harm.
Diagonal hip sinks (Fig. 24-4)	Restores segmental flexion, and posterior nutation of sacral base, Stretches quadratus lumborum, posterolateral hip joint capsule, piriformis, and lumbar paraspinals. Eccentrically strengthens gluteus medius.	Can be done bilaterally without harm.
Unilateral prone press-up (Fig. 24-5)	Restores segmental extension and anterior nutation of sacral base. Anteriorly rotates a posteriorly rotated hemi-pelvis. Stretches anteriorhip capsule and uniarticular hip flexors.	Should be used with caution with patient with spinal instability (e.g., spondylolisthesis) or spinal stenosis. Can be done bilaterally.
Pelvic clock (Fig. 24-6)	Affords lumbar spine and sacrum all available motion. Initiates abdominal strengthening and proprioception.	Should be done by all patients. Should be performed last.

Adapted with permission from Bookhout MAR. Exercise as an adjunct to manual medicine. Handout and lecture presented in Ann Arbor, Michigan; February 1997.

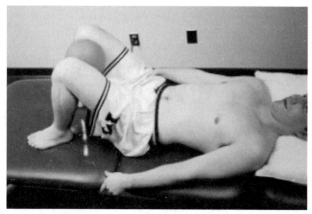

Figure 24-1 Pubis self-correction. Lie on your back with your hips and knees bent so your feet are flat on the table and together. Put a firm object (soccer ball, video-tape) between your knees. Use your knees to squeeze the object. Try to push the same with both knees.

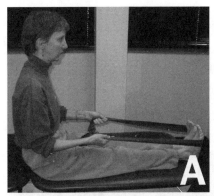

Figure 24-2 Abdominal sit-backs. Sit on the floor with your legs extended out in front of you. Place a long strap around the balls of your feet, holding an end in each hand. Using your arms (via the belt) to assist you as much as you need , start lowering your back down to the floor. Work from the bottom up: the sacrum touches the floor first, then the lowest lumbar vertebra up to the top. Make sure the low back remains rounded. Return to a seated position, trying to curl up in reverse order (or using your arms as needed). Repeat 10 times.

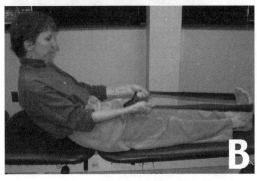

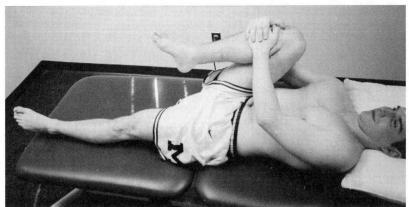

Figure 24-3 Anterior innominate self-correction (right leg). Lie on your back with the left leg straight. Bend your right hip and knee and bring your right knee to your right shoulder. Hold your right leg with both hands below your knee. Push your right leg into your hands, resisting the movement with your hands so your leg does not move. Hold for 4-5 seconds. Relax and bring your right knee closer toward your right shoulder.

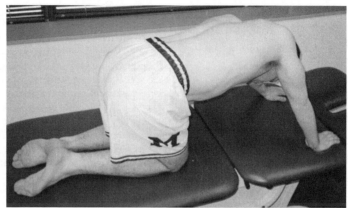

Figure 24-4   Hip sinks. Start on your hands and knees. Sit back to the right, letting your spine curve so the right side of your spine elongates. Allow your elbows to straighten and your pelvis to drop.

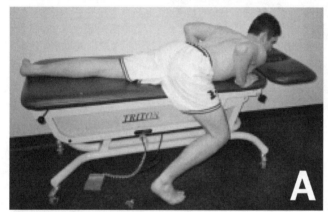

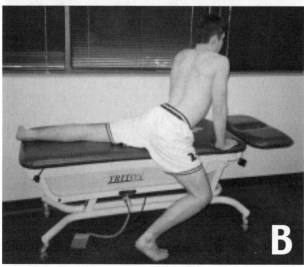

Figure 24-5
Unilateral prone press-up. Lie on your stomach on a table with your left foot planted on the floor. Keep your right leg on the table, knee straight with the hip slightly to the side and your toes pointing toward the right. Put your hands under your shoulders with your palms flat on the table. Use your arms to push your chest up. Keep your lower back relaxed. Try to completely straighten your elbows, but do not allow the belt line to come up.

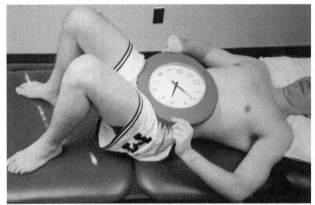

Figure 24-6   Pelvic clock. Lie on your back with your hips and knees bent so your feet are flat on the floor. Put your feet about your hips' width apart. Pretend there is a clock on your stomach. Your navel is 12:00, the bottom of your pelvis is 6:00, your left hip is 3:00, and your right hip is 9:00. Move your lower back and your pelvis to touch 12:00 to the floor, then 6:00 to the floor. Then practice rotating your pelvis so you can touch 3:00 to the floor, then 9:00 to the floor. Then practice rotating your pelvis to move clockwise, touching each number; then counter-clockwise touching each number on the clock. Try to have full and smooth movement in each direction.

REFERENCES

1. **Michlovitz SL.** Thermal Agents in Rehabilitation. Philadelphia: F.A. Davis Company; 1986.

2. **Lehmann JF, DeLateur BJ, Stonebridge JB, Warren CG.** Therapeutic temperature distribution produced by ultrasound as modified by dosage and volume of tissue exposed. Arch Phys Med Rehabil. 48:662-666, 1967.

3. **Greenman PE.** Principles of Manual Medicine, 2nd ed. Baltimore: Williams & Wilkins; 1996.

4. **Jones, LH.** Strain and Counterstrain. Indianapolis: American Academy of Osteopathy; 1981.

5. **Kaltenborn FM.** The Spine: Basic Evaluation and Mobilization Techniques, 2nd ed. Minneapolis: OMPT; 1992.

6. **Upledger JE, Vredevoogd JD.** Craniosacral Therapy. Seattle: Eastland Press; 1983.

KEY REFERENCES

Bookhout MR. Exercise and somatic dysfunction. Phys Med Rehabil Clin North Am. 1996;7:845-62.
This reference provides the theory and techniques of exercise as an adjunct to manual therapy in a very thorough and clinically applicable way.

Greenman PE. Principles of Manual Medicine, 2nd ed. Baltimore: Williams & Wilkins; 1996.
This text is considered by many to be the "master text" of the osteopathic approach. Provides theory, treatment techniques, and exercise prescription.

Janda V. Muscle Function Testing. London: Butterworths; 1983.
This text is the basis for much of Bookhout's work.

ii. Rehabilitation Therapies

Quaintance L. Miller, MS, OTR

Sandra Dodge, COTA

I t is fairly well established that, for patients with spinal disorders, pain and function are not strongly related. Rehabilitation therapies are designed to restore function, not necessarily to relieve pain. Although the separation between physical medicine and rehabilitation is somewhat arbitrary, certain interventions, more clearly designed to improve function at home and at work, are especially indicated in the subacute phase of back pain. They may include occupational therapy, some aspects of physical therapy, exercise training, counseling, vocational rehabilitation, case management, and worksite modification. Sophisticated multidisciplinary approaches are often the most useful, especially in complex patients who appear headed toward chronic disability.

Occupational Therapy

Occupational therapists specialize in improving function in activities of daily living, work, and avocational activities. According to the American Occupational Therapy Association, with acute onset, postsurgery, or with chronic pain conditions, occupational therapy (OT) may be indicated where education in activities of daily living is necessary to maintain or avoid certain postures and positions in patients with these pain conditions. Interventions focus on the individual's ability to function in a variety of performance areas (i.e., self-care, home management, dependent care, leisure, functional mobility, work, etc.). Additionally, as some patients have unresolved pain, OT may address psychosocial factors including self-concept, role performance, coping skills, time management and self-control (1).

Physical Therapy

The many tools of physical therapists have been described in Part I of this chapter. Only some are intended primarily to rehabilitate. For a patient who is deconditioned or has physical restrictions in relationship to his or her work or life activity, stretching, strengthening, and endurance training are oriented to rehabilitation. This work is typically coordinated by a physical therapist, as the physical therapist is most skilled at assessing specific deficits. Alternatively, an exercise physiologist is often very effective and inexpensive, although often not reimbursed. Sometimes, occupational therapists take on parts of this role. At a most basic level, the patient can do this work at a health club, in an aerobics, yoga, or Tai Chi type class, depending on the complexity and severity of deficits and the patient's ability to exercise independently.

Psychological Therapy

Psychologists may instruct in pain coping strategies and use cognitive-behavioral approaches to impact a patient's pain and mood control. Biofeedback, stress management, and relaxation training are frequently included as part of treatment. Interventions addressing comorbid psychological problems such as depression and anxiety, and posttraumatic stress disorder are not uncommon in patients with back pain.

Vocational Rehabilitation

Vocational rehabilitation counselors assist persons with disabilities in finding and maintaining meaningful work in their communities. Services include vocational counseling and guidance, as well as assistance with job placement. Plans are developed that take into consideration the clients' aptitudes, education, physical abilities, and career goals. Vocational rehabilitation counselors can be contracted directly by the physician. They are typically available through larger rehabilitation clinics, state agencies, or workers' compensation insurance companies.

Case Management

Confusion about treatment choices, conscious or subconscious delay on the part of the patient or providers, insurance, social, and financial issues may all delay effective treatment and decision making. Case managers, coming from a variety of social or health care backgrounds, are paid to facilitate treatment and decision making for the patient with complex problems. As a patient's problem drags into the subacute phase, the risk of chronic disability makes case management more cost effective. Occasionally, case managers work for sophisticated multidisciplinary rehabilitation or surgical programs. Sometimes, they work for state vocational rehabilitation agencies. Most commonly, their employer is an insurance company or the patient's employer. They are assigned to patients when the risk of long-term cost has increased sufficiently. In this circumstance, their primary goal is to save their employer money. The needs of case managers, rights of patients, and appropriate use by physicians are complex issues, but undeniably case managers are important and influential members of the rehab team (1). Although they are ethically and often legally prohibited from influencing the patient's choices of treatment or practitioners, they are not prohibited from trying to convince the primary physician of a course of action. It is suggested that primary care physicians cooperate with case managers by meeting with them and the patient only after the physician and patient have completed their clinical visit in private. This time is reimbursable, and a good case manager can greatly facilitate treatment.

Jobsite Analysis

Often, the workplace is poorly designed for the worker, especially the worker with back pain disability. Changes in the worksite are often effective in facilitating return to work for the patient and typically involve very low cost modifications that benefit overall productivity. A jobsite analysis involves the objective observation, evaluation, and recording of a client's job as it relates to use of machines, equipment, and tools within a specific environment; task sequencing; and cognitive and physical demands that are required to complete the essential job tasks. Assessment of risk factors and suggestions for modification are made. Occupational therapists, ergonomists, vocational rehabilitators, and physical therapists may offer these services.

Multidisciplinary Approaches

Functional Restoration Program

A functional restoration program is a comprehensive multidisciplinary treatment approach for chronic back pain disability aimed at restoring functional movement and capacities, minimizing self-limiting behaviors, and reducing deconditioning syndrome. Individuals who successfully complete the program are discharged with a home program. The program is minimum of 3 weeks in length, with interventions provided by any/all of the following disciplines: psychology, occupational therapy, physical therapy, and exercise physiology.

Pain Management Program

This label encompasses a wide variety of rehabilitation programs. At the University of Michigan, the Pain Management Program is a multidisciplinary rehabilitation program for chronic spine pain conditions including physical and occupational therapies, psychology, and the referring physician. Treatment focus is exercise based, with the primary objective to remediate musculoskeletal dysfunctions through the application of therapeutic exercise. Treatment goals are to reduce pain and enhance functional activity. These are facilitated by the use of proper body mechanics, activity pacing, and the use of psychological strategies for enhanced physical functioning and pain control. In other places, pain management may forego any manual physical therapy in favor of more teaching and counseling.

Geriatric Spine Rehabilitation Programs

Older persons are under less pressure to perform and often have preconceived notions that they must simply resign themselves to increasing disability with age. Geriatric spine rehabilitation programs are designed to impact this perception. This kind of program is new; just beginning to evolve. The prototype, the Senior Restoration Program at the University of Michigan, is an 8-week program designed to increase function and quality of life for seniors who are experiencing spine pain greater than 3 months in duration and for whom other medical and surgical interventions have been unsuccessful. Occupational therapy, physical therapy, exercise physiology, and psychological interventions include cardiovascular, balance, strength and flexibility training, activity tolerance enhancement, education, and counseling.

Work Hardening and Work Conditioning

"Work conditioning and work hardening programs are intensive, highly structured, job oriented, individualized treatment plans based on an assessment of the patient's work setting or job demands, and designed to maximize the patient's return to work. These programs must include real or simulated work activities" and may also include physical conditioning and other functional activities designed to restore strength, endurance, movement, flexibility, motor control, and cardiopulmonary function (1). Physical therapy, occupational therapy, and exercise physiology may be involved in these services.

Work conditioning usually refers to a general exercise program, often in a group setting. It may or may not take into account the specific work requirements of the individual. Work hardening may be much more extensive, perhaps involving a few different types of therapist. The program typically mimics actual work activity of the worker, in an attempt to provide physical conditioning that is relevant to the specific work tasks and to build worker confidence in his or her return to actual work. A more recent trend is to return the worker to the actual workplace, with graded increased activity. But this depends on a cooperative employer, work tasks that are relatively safe for the worker, and good worker understanding and compliance.

■   ■   ■

Recommendations

Physicians are advised to study these different types of rehabilitation treatments and to understand their differences.

■   ■   ■

Key Points

• Physicians dealing with back pain will interact with individual and team rehabilitation treatments.
• Knowledge of the language and types of program will help physicians to treat back pain with more sophistication.

■   ■   ■

REFERENCES

1. **Larson B.** Occupational Therapy Practice Guidelines for Adults with Low Back Pain. Bethesda, MD: American Occupational Therapy Association, Inc.; 1996:7-9.

iii. Surgery and Injection Treatments

Andrew J. Haig, MD

Matthew W. Smuck, MD

P hysicians are frequently asked about invasive treatments for back pain. Is IDET better than a PLIF? How about kyphoplasty and vertebroplasty? As in other areas of surgery, the trend in spine surgery is toward the less invasive. Newer procedures hit the 10 o'clock news before they hit the medical journals. The terminology for older procedures alone is substantial. So, a chapter that briefly defines the common invasive procedures is useful.

Many new procedures are called minimally invasive. Sometimes this refers to a new open surgical technique and sometimes to an intervention performed through a needle. When a procedure is done through a needle, it is called *percutaneous*. All procedures can be classified as either surgical or percutaneous. To avoid confusion, we will stick to that general organization. We will also describe the implantable devices currently used to treat chronic pain.

Percutaneous Procedures

Caudal epidural: Injection from the sacral hiatus, a small opening on the sacrum near the coccyx, through the sacral canal into the distal epidural space. Accuracy is better with fluoroscopy but can be done without.

Diskogram or **Diskography:** A purely diagnostic test used to identify which disks are true pain generators. Its only purpose is to direct more invasive spine procedures when a patient has failed all available conservative treatments. Needles are inserted into the center of several adjacent intervertebral disks. One at a time, radioopaque dye is injected into each disk to increase the pressure inside the disk. Abnormal leakage of dye from the disk will locate tears. More importantly, the patient is constantly monitored for reproduction of pain. A positive diskogram requires reproduction of the patient's usual pain at one or more disks, along with at least one painless control disk. Some have advocated use of pressure control monitors to provide more objective results. However, usefulness of pressure controlled diskography on clinical outcome of subsequent interventions has been limited.

Epidural injection: Injection of a medication into the epidural space (not the deeper intrathecal space, which is filled with cerebrospinal fluid). In the spine, the epidural space is a potential space filled mostly by fat. Steroid medication is most often used in injections for back pain and radicular pain. Often, a local anesthetic is included for immediate pain control, and sometimes as a diagnostic aid. Other medications such as morphine have been tried, but with less proven efficacy. Epidurals are done with or without flouroscopy. Accuracy is improved significantly when fluoroscopy is used. Radioopaque dye is injected to confirm proper epidural placement of the drugs. Along with increasing use of fluoroscopy, there is a trend to use selective transforaminal injections. Epidurals have been around for decades. The newer specific injections combined with the inclusion of epidurals as a presurgical treatment option in practice guidelines has made them much more popular recently. In the lumbosacral spine, there are three possible epidural techniques: transforaminal, interlaminar, and caudal.

Facet joint injection, Zygoaphophyseal injection, or **Z-joint injection:** Injection into the facet joint, a true synovial joint. This procedure is performed with fluoroscopy; accuracy without fluoroscopy has not been demonstrated. For therapeutic purposes, corticosteroids are used. Diagnostically, the injection may include sham injections into neighboring joints or use of anesthetics of different half-life to identify which are true pain generators.

Interlaminar epidural: Injection from a posterior approach. The same approach as with lumbar puncture, but stopping in the epidural space. Accuracy is better with fluoroscopy but can be done without.

Intradiskal electrotherapy, Intradiskal electrothermal annuloplasty, or **IDET:** The first invasive alternative to fusion surgery for chronic disk pain that has failed all conservative treatments. Only considered if diskogram (see above) is positive. A radiofrequency heating wire is inserted along the internal portion of the posterior annulus of the intervertebral disk. The heating treatment was initially thought to modify abnormal disk collagen. This occurs only in very close proximity to the heating wire. Heat is sufficient to denervate nearby nerve fibers, another proposed mechanism for improvement of pain. Initial clinical studies have produced varied results, much like the data on fusion surgery for low back pain. Long-term outcome is unknown.

Kyphoplasty: A treatment for vertebral body compression fractures. Different from vertebroplasty by use of a balloon to partially reduce the compression deformity and create a potential space for the plastic cement. The balloon is inserted into the vertebral body through a needle, then expanded in place. After the balloon is removed, the potential space it created is filled with plastic cement (e.g., polymethylmethacrylate). It can reduce a kyphotic deformity shortly after a compression fracture.

Theoretically safer than vertebroplasty, as lower pressure is required to inject the plastic cement, reducing the risk of further displacement of bone fragments into the spinal canal.

Medial branch block: A purely diagnostic test. Injection of anesthetic onto the medial branch nerve of the posterior primary ramus, done with flouroscopy. The medial branch is the sensory nerve to the facet joint and its synovial capsule. To assist with diagnostic interpretation, the injection may include sham injections of neighboring joint medial branch nerves or use of anesthetics of different half-life to identify which facets are true pain generators.

Percutaneous microdiskectomy: A treatment for back and radicular pain due to specific types of disk herniations. Over the years, this has come in many forms: chymopapain (an enzyme), nucleotome (a cutting and suctioning probe), laser, and nucleoplasty (radiofrequency). Each of these treatments is through a needle into the center of the intervertebral disk. Each, by a different method, removes disk material. Percutaneous microdiskectomy has been validated in randomized trials. Only the nucleoplasty and laser techniques still find wide use in the United States. The other techniques are still in use in Europe and elsewhere.

Prolotherapy: Injection of sclerosing, or scar-forming materials. Proposed benefits are from scarring down lax ligaments, denervation of the tissue, or irritation of reflex arcs. Around for years, research on clinical efficacy is limited.

Radiofrequency medial branch ablation, Radiofrequency facet ablation, or **Selective dorsal rhizotomy:** A treatment used after diagnostic facet joint injections or diagnostic medial branch blocks have provided temporary relief of pain. A radiofrequency probe is inserted to the medial branch nerve of the posterior primary ramus. The medial branch is the sensory nerve to the facet joint and its synovial capsule. Radiofrequency heat is used to traumatize the nerve, denervating the facet joint. Only recently subjected to research scrutiny.

Sacroiliac joint injection (SI injection): Injection of steroid medication into the sacroiliac joint. The procedure is performed with fluoroscopy; accuracy without fluoroscopy has not been demonstrated. Like injections of the facet joints, it is done for both diagnostic and therapeutic purposes. An old intervention with ambiguous proof of efficacy, but still considered the gold standard for diagnosis of intra-articular sacroiliac joint pain.

Transforaminal epidural or **Selective nerve root block:** Injection of medication into the epidural space and nerve root sleeve at the neuroforamen. This procedure is performed with fluoroscopy; accuracy without fluoroscopy has not been demonstrated.

Trigger point injections: Use of local anesthetic, or sometimes a dry needle, to destroy or "reset" trigger points. This has been around for decades and has demonstrated short-term but not long-term benefit.

Vertebroplasty: A treatment for vertebral body compression fractures. Injection of plastic cement (e.g., polymethylmethacrylate) into the body of a recently collapsed vertebra. Used for both osteoporotic and malignant compression fractures. A relatively new procedure not yet subjected to critical or long-term research.

Surgical Procedures

Artificial disk: A metal or plastic device inserted in the place of an injured disk. A new procedure not yet validated by sufficient research. Patients desire this on an intuitive basis, and theoretically the idea of maintaining a disk space makes sense. Indications are unclear, the procedure is substantial, and long-term outcomes and complications are not yet well understood.

Cage: A small cylindrical device placed into the disk space during fusion. The cage may hold bone matrix along with chemicals that stimulate bone ingrowth.

Diskectomy: A treatment for back and leg pain due to disk herniations. Removal of herniated disk material, typically with removal of some intact nucleus pulposis. Typically done with a laminectomy or partial laminectomy. Less invasive forms have been developed and are described below.

Laproscopic diskectomy: A treatment for back and leg pain due to disk herniations. Diskectomy using laproscopy. Recovery times are thought to be faster than routine diskectomy.

Microdiskectomy: A treatment for back and leg pain due to disk herniations. Diskectomy using a dissecting microscope. Fairly routine now, it causes less damage to paraspinal soft tissue than the routine diskectomy.

Foraminotomy: Enlarging the neuroforamen, usually by removing a portion of the adjacent superior articular process. This provides more room for the exiting nerve root.

Fusion or **Arthrodesis:** Joining of two adjacent vertebrae. Done to prevent abnormal or painful motion. Various procedures are listed below. Most recent research shows no clear advantage of one over another for simple fusion procedures.

Anterior lumbar interbody fusion (ALIF): Fusion via an anterior approach through the abdominal wall, joining the anterior portions of the adjacent vertebrae.

Anterior posterior fusion (AP fusion) (also called *Circumferential fusion):* Fusion through an anterior and posterior approach, joining both the anterior and posterior portions of the adjacent vertebrae.

Instrumented fusion: Any fusion involving screws, rods, or plates. Noninstrumented fusion implies use of bone grafts and wire alone.

Laproscopic fusion: A new laproscopic technique for anterior fusion.

Posteriolateral gutter fusion: Fusion using a muscle splitting technique to arrive at the transverse processes. The transverse processes are fused.

Posterior lumbar interbody fusion (PLIF): Fusion from a posterior mid-line approach, joining the posterior portions of the adjacent vertebrae.

Laminectomy: Removal of the lamina. Partial laminectomies are done to provide visualization of the epidural space for diskectomy. Full laminectomies may be used for the same purpose, or for decompression of spinal stenosis. *Hemilaminectomy* implies removal of the lamina on one side (right or left).

Pedicle screws: Screws placed through the pedicles into the vertebral body. They are attached to various rod systems to support the spine.

Rods: Any of a group of different devices used to hold vertebrae together during a fusion. They may attach by wires and hooks (e.g., Harrington rods) or by pedicle screws.

Implantables

Dorsal column stimulator, Spinal cord stimulator, or **Epidural electrical stimulator:** An implanted stimulator with electrodes on the thecal sac. For chronic pain only. The electrical stimulation may cause less noxious signals to override pain signals in the dorsal column of the spinal cord and brain.

Intrathecal morphine pump: An implantible pump used to deliver morphine directly to the thecal sac. For chronic pain recalcitrant to oral narcotic treatment. Morphine side effects are thought to be less with the pump.

■   ■   ■

BIBLIOGRAPHY

Brodke DS, Dick JC, Kunz DN, McCabe R, Zdeblick TA. Posterior lumbar interbody fusion. A biomechanical comparison, including a new threaded cage. Spine 1997;22(1):26.

Carette S, Marcoux S, Truchon R, Grondin C, Gagnon J, Allard Y, et al. A controlled trial of corticosteroid injections into facet joints for chronic low back pain. N Engl J Med. 1991;325:1002-7.

Derby R, Howard MW, Grant JM, Lettice JJ, Van Peteghem PK, Ryan DP. The ability of pressure-controlled discography to predict surgical and nonsurgical outcomes. Spine. 1999;24(4):364-71.

Garvey TA, Marks MR, Wiesel SW. A prospective, randomized, double-blind evaluation of trigger-point injection therapy for low-back pain. Spine. 1989;14:962-64.

Nelson DA. Landau WM. Intraspinal steroids: history, efficacy, accidentality, and controversy with review of United States Food and Drug Administration reports. J Neurol Neurosurg Psychiatry. 2001;70(4):433-43.

Ongley MJ, Klein RG, Dorman TA, Eek BC, Hubert LJ. A new approach to the treatment of chronic low back pain. Lancet. 1987;2:143-6 [about prolotherapy].

Slipman CW, Lipetz JS, Plastaras CT, Jackson HB, Vresilovic EJ, Lenrow DA, Braverman DL. Fluoroscopically guided therapeutic sacroiliac joint injections for sacroiliac joint syndrome. Am J Phys Med Rehabil. 2001;80(6):425-32.

Stitz MY, Sommer HM. Accuracy of blind versus fluoroscopically guided caudal epidural injection. Spine. 1999;24(13):1371-6.

Watts NB, Harris ST, Genant HK. Treatment of painful osteoporotic vertebral fractures with percutaneous vertebroplasty or kyphoplasty. Osteoporosis Int. 2001;12(6):429-37.

Zuniga RE, Schlicht CR, Abram SE. Intrathecal baclofen is analgesic in patients with chronic pain. Anesthesiology. 2000;92(3):876-80.

SECTION IV

CHRONIC BACK PAIN

25

■ ■ ■

Chronic Low Back Pain

Andrew J. Haig, MD

Sean Kesterson, MD

C hronic back pain has about as much to do with acute back pain as
the common cold does with metastatic lung cancer. True, the
common cold and lung cancer both involve the same organ. They
both can present with similar features. But one is self-limiting; the other is
seldom cured. One is a trivial inconvenience that most people work
through without medical help. The other is the complex purview of tertiary
care subspecialists. Physicians seldom order tests for the first; they use up
the HMO's bank with the other.

The analogy stops here, though. Today, metastatic lung cancer left untreated is usually fatal. Back pain, on the other hand, is not. The primary
care physician will have to deal with it forever unless the patient moves
away. For back pain, though, appropriate management has a high chance
of improving quality of life and alleviating pain. In this chapter, we will
provide an overview of chronic back pain. The rest of Section IV of this
book discusses management in great detail.

The Evolution of the Chronic Pain Patient

Earlier, we discussed some important issues in relation to chronic pain. The
natural history of acute pain is quite favorable, but the few who become
chronically disabled have a very poor prognosis for return to work. Factors
that predict onset of chronic disability are primarily psychosocial.

What happens that makes a person become chronic? Some patients just
"are" chronic. They are the overusers of clinics for sore throats, carpal
tunnel syndrome, and irritable bowel syndrome. Why? Primary care physicians may suspect depression, anxiety and other psychiatric diseases

(Table 25-1). Personality traits such as dependency and a need for validation, and so forth, bring people to doctors. Social factors are important. At
the extreme are abuse and neglect. More common are frustration with work
or home situations.

Other patients find themselves in a position where chronic pain is an
adaptation. Their family may give them social support for the disability
role. They may get time off from boring or stressful work. They may be
nearing retirement, in the midst of all the psychosocial adaptations people
make before starting life without a punch clock. Or they may just be starting at a new job, physically and emotionally stressed without social support. Most researchers believe that only a very small minority of patients
with chronic pain complaints are purely "in it for the money." But the
promise of money-both the financial support and the validation of symptoms caused by cold cash-is a strong force in industrialized society.

Table 25-1   Psychopathology and Chronic Pain

- Premorbid psychopathology is common in persons with chronic pain.
- Social rewards such as financial secondary gain are often in play (e.g., spouse sup-
  port, staff attention, or avoidance of military service).
- Specific psychosocial correlates of chronic pain
    ◊ Premorbid personality disorders
    ◊ Dysthymia or depression
    ◊ Anxiety disorder
    ◊ Thought disorders
    ◊ Alcohol and drug abuse
    ◊ Hysteria
    ◊ Malingering
    ◊ Fictitious disorders
    ◊ Tendency to avoid pain
    ◊ Mistrust or excessive faith in health care providers
    ◊ Physical, sexual, or emotional abuse
    ◊ Impending major social change-layoff, divorce, etc.
    ◊ Resultant fear
    ◊ Posttraumatic stress disorder
    ◊ Financial or legal secondary gain
    ◊ Sleep disorders
    ◊ Medication-related delirium
    ◊ Unrealistic medical goals
    ◊ Abandonment
    ◊ Financial crisis
    ◊ Social handicap

As we discussed in Chapter 4, chronic pain is often out of proportion to tissue damage. It can be confusing but appears less so when one takes into account the behavioral adaptations that must occur for many patients to cope with the pain. Patients learn to avoid the pain by avoiding movements-they become profoundly deconditioned in terms of strength, endurance, flexibility, and coordination. This in itself becomes disabling and causes pain under circumstances that would not cause others to hurt.

Patients become vigilant-searching for ways to avoid pain. When pain is truly unavoidable, the vigilance is frustrated-almost a laboratory experiment in anxiety. Anxiety, along with life stresses and sleep deprivation, results in depression.

Most texts do not list hints about suicide as "red flags," and the risk of suicide in persons with acute low back pain may not be much greater than that in the general population. But in dealing with chronic back pain, there is a high incidence of depression and anxiety, and certain personality types are more prone to get into distress as a result of chronic back pain disability. When dealing with chronic back pain patients, it is important to judge the patient's mood and to ask questions such as "do you sometimes feel like you wish you just weren't around?" which can lead to the diagnosis of major depression and suicidal risk (1).

Successful treatment looks beyond the severe or obvious DSM-IV diagnoses to personality traits and coping styles. These factors may be assets or barriers in planning successful treatment.

Chronic Back Pain Algorithms

Management of chronic back pain is very complex. The role of the primary care physician is equally complex, interwoven with those of subspecialists and allied health professionals. Occasionally, primary care physicians fall into the role of rehabilitation team leaders. For example, the author owes a great debt of gratitude to Rowland Hazzard, MD, an internist, an influential colleague at The University of Vermont's Spine Center of New England. But in the vast majority of cases, the primary care physician is advising the patient as he or she seeks out different forms of subspecialized care, whether that be surgery or rehabilitation. Of course, after all the subspecialized work is done, it is often the primary care physician who has the important role of health maintenance.

It is important for the primary care physician to understand something of the specialists' roles if he or she is to act as a player in this interwoven web. Therefore, this chapter introduces two algorithms. The first outlines the roles of typical primary care physicians. The second reaches into the workings of specialized teams.

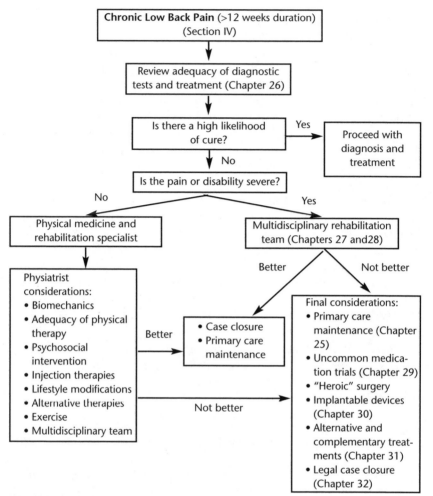

Figure 25-1   Chronic low back pain algorithm for primary care.

Primary Care Management

Figure 25-1 presents a primary care algorithm for managing chronic low back pain. Chronic back pain patients present to the primary care physician two different ways. The new patient who presents with longstanding pain or disability is obvious. Tougher is recognition of the date and time when a patient already being managed by the primary physician for subacute back pain reaches the stage of "chronic." Too often the physician is unaware of the changes that have occurred in the patient. A simple rule is probably the best: All patients must be treated according to the chronic, rather than the acute algorithms before they reach the 3 month stage. With rare exception, by 3 months the neurochemical, physiological, and psychosocial changes have occurred.

The first step is to be sure that both the physician and the patient are confident that there is no likely cure. Most patients by this time will have had an MRI and an EMG, but they may not be technically adequate, or they may be outdated. Other structural diagnoses might be found with bone scan, diagnostic blocks, and provocative injections. Serious considerations of immune disorder, malignancy, or metabolic cause may lead to blood tests. It is crucial that the physician proceed with an honest sense that no reasonable treatable diagnosis has been missed. Chapter 27 is a good review of the unusual diagnoses that may present as back pain.

The physician should differentiate cure from partial relief. The patient may have spent so much time and energy seeking out a cure that he or she finds it a struggle to move forward with rehabilitation plans that have a high likelihood of success in providing partial relief of pain. There are dozens of medications and other treatments that might partially relieve the pain. They might be tried at the same time as the steps proposed in the chronic pain algorithm, but the rest of the steps in the algorithm should not be delayed to pursue partial or unlikely cures.

An important value judgment to be made by the physician is whether the pain or disability are "severe." This is a qualitative decision, involving an understanding of the whole patient-not only the report of pain and disability itself, but also an understanding of how this person communicates painful or disabling experiences, and an understanding of other social, financial, medical, and other factors that may modulate the impact of pain or disability on quality of life in the present or future for this particular patient. Some of the treatments for severe pain and disability require effort and risk that simply are not appropriate for patients who are doing relatively okay.

Most patients with chronic pain will be referred to a specialist, typically a physiatrist. The patients with less severe disability and pain can often be evaluated in an office consultation with to a local physiatrist, whereas more severe pain and disability really require a multidisciplinary team approach available only in some centers.

For patients with less severe pain and disability, the physiatrist will review a number of factors as outlined in the left-hand box in Figure 25-1. More than scientific literature, substantial clinical experience (including knowledge of the quality of local resources) will dictate further treatment.

For patients with more severe pain and disability, the process is quite complex. Figure 25-2 outlines just a few of the issues involved in wisely choosing treatment. Perhaps the most important element of the assessment is the team assessment. The way in which information is gathered and processed, and the way in which the team makes decisions about treatment recommendations determines the quality and appropriateness of future therapy. Although one would hope that a physiatric team would consider all of these options and access all appropriate treatments, individual teams are commonly limited by their own protocols or ideology. Thus,

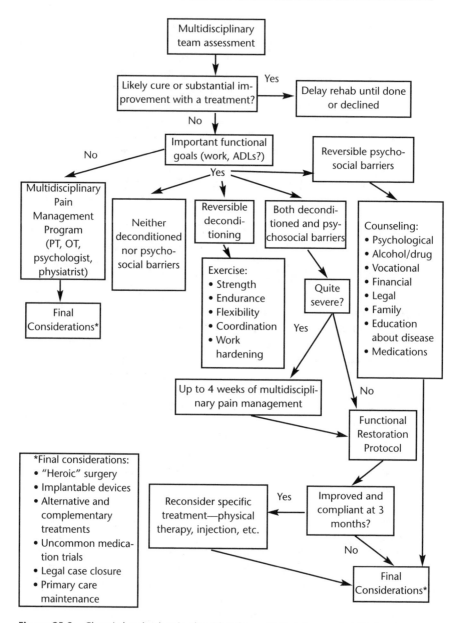

Figure 25-2   Chronic low back pain algorithm for multidisciplinary rehabilitation team.

it is helpful for the primary care physician to understand the possibilities and to continue to advise the patient of potential options.

At Michigan, we have advocated a standardized protocol for multidisciplinary assessment called the Spine Team Assessment (2,3). It has served as a model for other centers. The Spine Team Assessment is intended for persons with substantial chronic back related disability. It includes assessments by a physical therapist, occupational therapist, exercise physiologist, psychologist, and vocational counselor, followed by a physiatrist lead team meeting and a detailed plan of action for the patient. Patient demographics, physical test results, functional test results, psychological test results, and relationships between these are discussed by the team, and concrete, detailed, sequenced recommendations are provided to the patient and referral source.

In the Spine Team Assessment, the team values are that treatment of disability takes precedent over treatment of pain. Figure 25-2 is a simple summary of team decisionmaking for the Spine Team Assessment. Reversible causes (e.g., deconditioning, psychosocial factors) are commonly found. When multiple reversible causes are found, a multidisciplinary approach, such as Mayer's functional restoration protocol, is used (4).

When a patient's disability is not reversible, options include a pain management program (aimed at relief of pain, rather than improvement in function) or the numerous case closure considerations (i.e., final considerations) listed in the box on the right-hand side of Figure 25-1. These are worthy of comment.

Most good surgeons will not want to see a chronic patient, but there are a few cases where fusion or other procedure is helpful. The risk-benefit ratio for such "heroic" surgery is improved after a patient's complete psychosocial and physical status are known. Implantible devices have waxed and waned in popularity.

Alternative/complementary treatments, regardless of effectiveness, empower the patient and bring hope. Caution should be taken in recommending these therapies if the physician feels that the patient is vulnerable to emotional, physical, or financial loss out of proportion to the potential gain.

Dozens of medications and combinations of medicines have been shown to decrease chronic pain, but none cure the pain and few have been studied in the long term. Furthermore, an adequate trial of most medication involves slow titration over weeks or months. Thus rehabilitation should not be delayed on the hopes that medications will make a difference. But it may be reasonable to develop try different medications, one at a time, in a controlled fashion, when other variables (litigation, work status, rehabilitation exercises) have stabilized.

Sometimes legal case closure does amazing things to a patient. Research shows that a favorable result (e.g., qualifying for social security disability) does not improve quality of life. But when the physician makes a legal statement of case closure (different terms in different jurisdictions), the parties typically settle the case. The patient is not torn between proving disability and working to eliminate disability. The extent to which the defendant or the insurer will pay for lost wages, schooling, or medical debts is known, and the patient often emotionally is more ready to make plans for a future with chronic pain.

Primary Care Physician's Role

The primary care physician sometimes feels that the management of chronic pain is what happens in the speciality clinic. In fact, even when a specialty clinic is available, the primary care physician has a very important role. It is often the primary care physician who sees past the orthopedic or neurosurgical consultation to realize that the patient needs a multidisciplinary team approach. During the often challenging and scary process of rehabilitation, the primary care physician is the one unbiased member of the health care team who can educate and encourage the patient along a rational path. When the spine specialists have completed most of their work, the patient transitions into primary care maintenance. Good communication between the team and the primary care physicians can help the patient have realistic expectations of the primary care physician.

Other chapters deal with when a primary care physician should refer to a specialist. A checklist helps the physician judge whether the consultation accomplished its goal:

1. Has there been a significant change or relief?
2. Is there improved clarity of diagnosis?
3. What is the patient's understanding of their condition and the prognosis now?
4. Is there effective communication between the patient and te consultant?
5. Were details clarified or missed?
6. Will this be an ongoing relationship with the consultant or a short-lived one?
7. Is there a need for another opinion or a different perspective?
8. What is the short- and long-term future, and what will the plan be?
9. Was disability addressed?
10. How will pain be managed?

The primary care physician is often the one who recognizes the need for a second opinion. Sometimes the patient has worked with a non-surgeon to the point where surgery is really a better option, or conversely a surgeon has not picked up on the non-surgical opportunities. Often enough the patient struggles with a surgeon's recommendation to operate or not to operate, and a second surgical opinion is the best solution.

Especially in rural areas, patients may be referred to distant rehabilitation teams for assessment. Transportation or other factors may preclude participation in the distant program, so the primary care physician takes on the role of team coordinator. Although the primary care physician is unlikely to call a team meeting to coordinate rehabilitation, he or she is perhaps in the best position to recommend competent local therapists and counselors. The primary physician can meet with the patient occasionally to coordinate the resources and set deadlines and time frames.

In the long term, after the rehabilitation, surgery, and medication trials have ended, the patient typically returns to the primary care physician for maintenance. The physician needs to have a level of comfort with the medications he or she is continuing, develop a strong enough relationship with the patient that malignant "doctor shopping" does not harm the patient, and know when a crisis or opportunity should lead to new interventions.

Finally, the primary care physician needs to be comfortable in setting limits. Recognizing that chronic back pain is often accompanied by or preceded by significant mental health problems, the physician should stand by his or her rational approach to pain and disability management. Knowing that no medication eliminates more than perhaps half of the pain that a chronic back pain patient suffers, the physician needs to weigh function, cognition, mood, and medical side effects against escalation of medications. The primary care physician needs to be able to call it quits, or supporting the specialist's decision to close the case when medical interventions will not likely make a difference.

■   ■   ■

Recommendations

- After 3 months of work or significant lifestyle disability, all patients should be evaluated by a multidisciplinary team, regardless of whether they are currently in the care of a surgeon, pain specialist, or physiatrist.
- The primary care physician should take an active role in the subjective decision about whether pain and disability are severe enough to require more aggressive care.
- The primary care physician's role as an educated but disinterested "outsider" to the team can be of great value to the patient and team when difficult decisions are being made.

■   ■   ■

Key Points

- Effective triage is one of the most important steps in the management of chronic pain.
- Less severe pain and disability benefit from referral to a local specialist (physiatrist).
- More significant pain and disability require a multidisciplinary team.
- The primary care physician's role is to be sure the patient and specialty team are understanding goals and looking at all options as they decide on a plan.

■   ■   ▦

REFERENCES

1. **Livengood JM, Parris WC.** Early detection measures and triage procedures for suicide ideation in chronic pain patients. Clin J Pain. 1992;8(2):164-9.
2. **Haig AJ, Geisser ME, Nicholson C, Parker E, Yamakawa K, Montgomery D, et al.** The effect of order of testing on functional performance in persons with and without chronic back pain. J Occup Rehab. 2003;13(2):115-23.
3. **Haig AJ, Haig DD.** Software to Remove Barriers to Multidisciplinary Rehabilitation Assessment. Prague: International Society for Physical and Rehabilitation Medicine (ISPRM); 2003.
4. **Mayer TG, Gatchel RJ, Mayer H, Kishino ND, Keeley J, Mooney V.** A prospective two-year study of functional restoration in industrial low back injury: An objective assessment procedure. JAMA. 1987;258:1763-82.

26

■ ■ ■

Low Back Pain: Exhausting the Differential Diagnosis

Miles Colwell, MD

Management of chronic low back pain involves a huge paradigm shift for the physician and the patient, in which the goal is restoration of function and minimizing discomfort, not cure. But it is hard for the patient to accept this and sometimes even harder for the physician to let go of the wish for a miracle discharge. In fact, there are occasional odd diagnoses and unusual successful treatments for chronic low back pain. It is crucial for the physician to feel comfortable that he or she is aware of these and has reasonably eliminated their existence.

The unusual provable diagnoses can be thought of in four categories: Obscure provable causes for back pain and sciatica, difficult to prove lesions, lesions outside of the spine, and metabolic disorders.

Obscure Provable Causes

Bent Spine Syndrome

This relatively uncommon syndrome involves fatty replacement (not atrophy) of the paraspinal muscles, probably related to a mild myopathy. Patients present with fatigue on ambulation, as in spinal stenosis. Magnetic resonance imaging (MRI) shows the fatty replacement, and an astute electromyographer will note decreased insertional activity. Correction of hip flexion contractures helps these persons walk with an extended spine, thus using less of their atrophic muscle.

Cyclic Sciatica

Endometriosis of the sciatic nerve can result in a complaint of pain and even weakness on a recurrent basis related to menstrual cycles.

Bicycler's Sciatica and Other Sciatic Trauma

Pressure from a wide bicycle seat-for example, the kind often used on stationary bicycles-can result in direct trauma to the sciatic nerve. Other causes of trauma can include prolonged squatting or a direct blow.

Neurogenic Pyriformis Syndrome

In a small percentage of anatomic specimens, the sciatic nerve splits the pyriformis muscle. In the earlier parts of the twentieth century, this was thought to be the prime cause of sciatica, and thousands of operations were performed to relieve this syndrome. In fact, only a handful of well-documented cases have been described. This is in contrast to common "pyriformis syndrome," which is simply a tight muscle.

Baastrup's Disease ("Kissing Spine")

The spinous processes may contact each other in hyperextension. This results in focal tenderness and occasionally x-ray findings of a pseudoarthrosis between spinous processes. Baastrup's disease was frequently described in historical literature, but the author has only seen a handful of cases, in butterfly and breast stroke swimmers and gymnasts. Historically surgery was performed, but we have had success with a simple cortisone injection into the painful interspace and correction of the biomechanics.

Paraspinal Compartment Syndrome

Either very strenuous activity or infiltration of fluids (e.g., a misplaced postoperative epidural catheter for pain) can cause severe pain, atrophy, and myoglobulinuria. We do not know of fasciotomy for this. It often acts like the bent spine syndrome (see above) after resolution.

Difficult-to-Prove or Difficult-to-Treat Lesions

Internal Disk Derangement

Internal disk derangement often is positional with pain during loading of the spine and easing when lying down. MRI will reveal dehydrated disk, may reveal evidence for annular tears, and plain x-ray may be normal or show loss of disk height. Other etiologies are typically first ruled out. Symptoms are frequently a central burning aching pain that progresses to a radiating pain into the buttocks, sometimes in a radicular pattern, with unilateral or bilateral radiation. The patient becomes relatively comfortable when lying down. When seated or standing, they have a steady increase in central back pain, which will frequently be described as a deep ache or burning. It begins to refer laterally and radiate as the corresponding nerve root becomes irritated. Some clinicians will use diskogram to confirm. The specificity of this test is debated. If there is high certainty that this is the diagnosis, diskectomy with spinal fusion is one of the more traditional procedures performed. If total disk height loss is not severe and no significant arthritis is present, less invasive procedures are being tried at some centers. Intradiskal electrothermo coagulation (IDET) is being used. This is a percutaneous procedure in which the inventors claim a heating element coagulates the central disk, causing it to stiffen. Long-term follow-up is not available. Studies to date have mixed results.

Missed Disk Herniation

Imaging studies can miss a small percentage of disk herniations, perhaps 10%. Electromyography (EMG) including careful evaluation of the paraspinal muscles may provide evidence of dennervation and assist to focus further imaging studies to confirm a compressive lesion.

High lumbar disk (L2, 3, and 4) herniations deserve special mention. They do not cause the classic pain below the knee (the distribution of pain is typically the anterior thigh), the straight leg raise test is negative (a reverse straight leg raise test-prone hip extension with bent knee, is sometimes positive), strength examination (hip flexors) and reflex examination are often normal. About 50% of surgically proven high lumbar disks are read as normal on MRI. Indeed, far lateral herniations, which are harder to appreciate on MRI, are more common at these higher levels, although the usual limb EMG does not include L2 or L3 innervated muscles and these limb muscles may not be very sensitive. Electromyographers who use paraspinal mapping will detect these on routine examination. See Chapter 18 for more on EMG.

Focal Spinal Segmental Motion Restriction

Spinal segmental relative hypermobility is difficult to establish. It also tends to be a diagnosis of exclusion. This is not the type of instability seen on flexion-extension x-rays but might be thought of as a laxity in joint play. The patient may be relatively comfortable at rest, but when trying to increase activity level, their back pain flares. Frequently, the physical therapist may report that they are having difficulty achieving and maintaining alignment of certain spinal segments. They may also report segments that are hypomobile with compensatory hypermobility above or below. There may be compensatory muscle hypertonicity or impaired muscle firing in response to ongoing pain. There is difficulty achieving stabilization strengthening. Two physical exam techniques used to assess this are side lying segmental rotatory stretching and side lying anterior to posterior challenge across the individual spinal segments. When successful in isolating the involved segment, the patient will report that this reproduces their achiness when that segment is challenged to move to its end of joint play. A skilled manual physical therapist often will be able to release the areas of hypomobility above and below the hypermobile segment. When successful, eventually the involved segments begin to stabilize. Core strengthening about the area is essential. If at the end of these efforts, full relief is not achieved and clinically there remains the sense of hypermobilty, some clinicians may consider a trial of prolotherapy. Prolotherapy is the practice of injecting sclerosing substances into ligaments and joints in order to create scar tissue. There is substantial basic science literature on prolotherapy, but no convincing proof of effectiveness to date. The literature is limited concerning the efficacy of this intervention. In selected cases the author has seen this to be quite helpful.

Muscle Imbalance

Impaired and compensatory muscle firing can perpetuate back pain. A common pattern is inhibition of low lumbar paraspinal firing with compensatory excessively firing of the low thoracic and upper lumbar paraspinals. Consider this in the patient who has made progress and minimal pain with basic activities of daily living but is having increased low back and hip region symptoms when they try to become more active. They will often present with a complaint of deep achiness in the lumbosacral junction and buttock area when they try to do prolonged walking or the higher functioning individual will present thus when they try to get back into running activities. On the exam, one notes the early activation and hypertonicity of the compensatory paraspinals. This requires experienced palpatory skills. Referral to a skilled therapist will prove beneficial to work on reestablishing more appropriate muscle firing and then subsequent strengthening.

Hip Capsule Restriction

Hip capsule restriction may lead to impaired firing of the gluteal muscles which in turn may result in overactivity or compensation with the low thoracic and lumbar paraspinal muscles. These muscles may be painful from overuse. Therapy directed at the muscles will ease the symptoms temporarily but not provide lasting relief. It may appear that the piriformis muscle(s) continue to be tight. An experienced examiner will be able to isolate the hip capsule from the surrounding muscles. If x-rays are relatively clean of arthritis, hip capsule restriction is likely present. Successful physical therapy to release with appropriate interventions confirms the diagnosis. Stabilization strengthening should follow.

Hip Flexion Contracture

There are subtleties of the hip flexion contracture combined with hip capsule restrictions, which can perpetuate low back pain. Hip flexors originate on the lateral bodies and transverse processes of the lumbar spinal segments. Tightness of the hip flexors can impair the function and mobility of the lumbar vertebrae as well as antagonize proper back muscle firing. At times, there is increased lumbar lordosis. Often there may not be an obvious increase in lumbar lordosis secondary to the low back achiness with hypertonic paraspinal muscle guarding maintaining a relative loss of lordosis despite tight hip flexors. There may be sufficient movement in the spine above and the sacroiliac joints below that the body compensates such that one does not observe obvious hip flexion contracture. To assess for hip flexion contracture, it is recommend that the clinician use the modified Thomas position. If restricted, refer to a skilled therapist for further evaluation and treatment.

Subtle or Hard to Fully Treat Sacral and Innominate Dysfunctions

Nonresolving pain and achiness in the region of the lower lumbar spine, sacroiliac joints, and buttock may be perpetuated by impaired mobility and alignment of the sacrum, sacroiliac joint, sacrotuberous ligament tightness, or pelvic floor muscle dysfunction. A highly skilled manual physical therapist should be able to sort out these issues and treat them.

Sacrotuberous Ligament Dysfunction

Sacrotuberous ligament tightness can in tether the sacrum and limit joint play. This can perpetuate dysfunction resulting in back and buttock pain. To test the sacrotuberous ligaments, with the patient prone, slide your thumbs along the hamstring muscles to their origin at the ischial tuberosity. Proceed slightly medial and superior from this along the sacrotuberace ligaments. At approximately the midpoint between the initial tuberosity and the inferior aspect of the sacrum, put tension simultaneously on the ligaments by taking your thumbs in a superior lateral direction. When hypertonic, they may actually feel as if the examiner is palpating bone. The patient may note tenderness and discomfort in the region.

Nonspinal Disorders

Rib Cage Dysfunction

Rib cage dysfunction can lead to or perpetuate back pain. The author believes this is mainly due to its interaction on muscle inhibition and compensation for inhibition. Hypertonic thoracic paraspinal muscles may be perpetuated due to restricted mobility of the corresponding rib cage. The hypertonicity can progress inferior to involve the lumbar paraspinals.

The overactive thoracic parapspinals may substitute for the lumbar paraspinals leaving them with poor firing and endurance perpetuating an achy back. Clinically, it has been observed that releasing the rib cage will finally allow the paraspinals to normalize their tone and function. Lower rib cage restriction, once released has been a big key to allowing the lumbar paraspinal muscles to finally release their hypertonicity. Treatment consists of referral to a physical therapist to perform myofascial release and rib cage rolling to restore the mobility. The skilled therapist will also know how to evaluate the ribs during inhalation and exhalation for restrictions.

Pelvic Floor Dysfunction

Pelvic floor muscle impairment can also lead to imbalance and secondary low back or buttock region pain. To evaluate pelvic floor muscle dysfunction, one will need to perform a rectal exam. At the same time, palpation of the distal tips of the coccyx can be performed to see if they may be part of the painful situation. Once feeling internally, start by palpating and sweeping of the pelvic floor muscles lateral to the sacrum. Work your way superior-inferior and lateral-medial. End by palpating the joint play of the distal coccygeal segments.

Low Level Cholecystitis

Cholecystitis can result in low level discomfort and muscle guarding in the right lower rib cage. The rib cage and paraspinal muscles become tight and the patient presents with back achiness. Physical therapy provides temporary relief but the tightness returns. Consider ultrasound to evaluate for sludge, stones and evidence for low level inflammation.

Low-Level Gastroesophageal Reflux Disorder

Gastroesophageal reflux may be low level and present as mid back achiness with muscle guarding and tightness. This can cause paraspinal hypertonicity and imbalance that secondarily results in mechanical back pain. Physical therapy provides temporary relief but the same pattern recurs. A trial of evening antacid, H^2 blocker, diet modification, and elevating the head of the bed may provide evidence pointing to this as a factor.

Renal Disease

Kidney stones and kidney infections often cause a complaint of back pain, although the examination shows both signs of infection and no specific location for pain.

Aortic Aneurysm

Sudden onset low back pain can be the result of an aortic aneurysm. These may occur more commonly in people with connective tissue disorders, who are also prone to multiple disk herniations.

Psychological Problems

Stress, fear, and more serious psychiatric disorders, as discussed elsewhere, remain common causes of continued back complaints after reasonable treatment. (See Chapter 27 for a discussion of psychological status assessment.)

Systemic and Metabolic Disorders

There are numerous systemic disorders that can cause back pain. Many of them also cause the patient to act irrationally, making the exclusion of mechanical and psychiatric disorders difficult. Complete discussion is not possible here, but the physician may consider the following:

- Acute intermittent porphyria
- Sickle cell crisis
- Vasculitis
- Coagulation disorders with retroperitoneal bleeding
- Myopathies
- Cramping disorders
- Paraneoplastic neuromuscular syndromes
- Venom (snake, fish, or spider)
- Tetanus
- Meningitis
- Narcotic or other drug withdrawal
- Metastatic cancer
- Calcium or potassium disorders
- Retroperitoneal fibrosis
- Endometriosis
- Mittleschmertz
- Undetected pregnancy
- Ectopic pregnancy

Key Points

- Partially treated musculoskeletal imbalances may perpetuate back pain.
- A physical therapist with extra postgraduate training in the evaluation and treatment of biomechanical dysfunctions will be needed to fully delineate and treat subtle or stubborn musculoskeletal dysfunctions.
- Occasionally, a rare, provable spinal disorder can be detected and treated.
- Pain may be from a nonspinal cause, either musculoskeletal or an abdominal organ.
- Numerous systemic disorders can present as back pain, often along with mental status changes.

27

■   ■   ■

Rehabilitation Diagnostic Assessments

Mark A. Harrast, MD

Many patients with chronic pain have complex physical, psychological, and social barriers that prevent them from regaining a functional life (1). In order to even attempt to treat their chronic pain, we need a better understanding of these complex physical and psychosocial issues. Assessments of these barriers can take many forms, such as physical testing and psychological interviews and questionnaires.

Whenever a patient is disabled for more than 3 months, it is safe for the primary care physician to assume that a complex multidisciplinary look at the problem will be key to success. The primary care physician's role is to diagnose the chronicity and seek out a competent multidisciplinary plan. Almost every community has physical therapy and most these days even have a physiatrist or an anesthesiologist "pain program" consisting of a "doctor and a needle" or a therapist, but such a simple approach is not sufficient. The knowledgeable primary care physician will have the name of a truly interdisciplinary pain program that can deal with the patient's complex needs.

This chapter presents the various forms of assessment of the physical and psychosocial barriers of patients with chronic pain. By understanding the diagnostic tools that rehabilitation teams use to determine their treatment plans, the primary care physician can better understand the factors that are important in successful rehabilitation. The exact type of rehabilitation provided, as discussed in Chapter 28, can vary in relationship to the patient's needs, but also in terms of availability. Here at the University of Michigan, we have worked extensively on the Spine Team Assessment, an assessment protocol that customizes multidisciplinary treatment to the patient, rather than the program. The Spine Team Assessment can serve as a model and comparison to rehabilitation assessments available in the community.

Psychological Status Assessment

An assessment of the psychological status of the patient with chronic pain is of utmost importance. Depression, anxiety, and fear are common psychological factors that significantly contribute to patients' chronic pain. A multitude of tests and questionnaires are quite effective to assess these psychological factors:

Center for Epidemiological Studies Depression Scale (CES-D) is designed to measure self-report of depressive symptoms. The CES-D is a 20-item scale where patients rate the frequency of there depressive symptoms on a 0-3 scale over the past week. A total score is obtained by summing the responses to all of the items (2).

McGill Pain Questionnaire (MPQ) is designed to measure subjective pain experience in a quantitative manner. Used to obtain a self-report of pain intensity. The MPQ consists of twenty groups of single word pain descriptors with the words in each group increasing in rank order intensity. The sum of the rank values for each descriptor results in a score termed the Pain Rating Index (PRI) (3).

Multidimensional Pain Inventory (MPI) is another means of measuring subjective pain. It is a 3-part inventory, composed of 12 scales, designed to examine the impact of pain on the patients' lives, the response of others to the patients' communications of pain, and the extent to which patients participate in common daily activities (4).

Quebec Back Pain Disability Scale (QBPDS) is designed to measure functional disability due to pain. The QBPDS asks patients to rate their degree of difficulty, ranging from 0 "not difficult at all" to 5 "unable to do," in performing twenty various activities, such as getting out of bed, riding in a car, carrying two bags of groceries, and climbing one flight of stairs (5). Results on the Quebec are helpful in both understanding the magnitude of the effect of the back problem on the patient and the areas in life that are specifically impacted. The Quebec is a useful program outcome measure, as well.

Short Form-36 Health Survey (SF-36) is designed to measure overall health status in the context of life function. The SF-36 includes a scale that assesses eight health areas: 1) limitations in physical activities because of health problems; 2) limitations in social activities because of physical or emotional problems; 3) limitations in usual role activities because of physical health problems; 4) bodily pain; 5) general mental health (psychological distress and well-being); 6) limitations in usual role activities because of emotional problems; 7) vitality (energy and fatigue); and 8) general health perceptions (6).

Tampa Scale of Kinesiophobia is designed to measure subjective fear of physical movement or activity. It consists of 13 items that patients are asked to rate their level of disagreement or agreement with in a 1 "strongly disagree" to 4 "strongly agree" scale. Sample items include "pain always means I have injured my body" and "it's really not safe for a person with a condition like mine to be physically active" (7).

Visual Analog Pain Scale (VAS) is designed to measure subjective pain experience in a quantitative manner. It is used to obtain a self-report of pain intensity. The VAS is a scale comprising of a 10-cm-long line that is anchored by the statement "no pain" on the left and "the worst possible pain imaginable" on the right (8). The visual analog scale is a useful simple measure of the patient's pain status and improvement in pain over time.

Physical Status Assessment

An assessment of the physical status of the patient with chronic pain is just as imperative as assessment of the psychological status in determining the optimal rehabilitation program. It is well-known that the majority of patients with chronic pain are deconditioned and deactivated. They have poor cardiovascular fitness and thus poor endurance for any sustained activity. Many also tend to demonstrate poor effort when it comes to attempting a functional task. It is obvious that all these factors will contribute to disability in patients with chronic pain. Physical status assessment therefore includes the measurement of the patient's cardiovascular fitness level, flexibility, strength, ability to perform certain basic functional tasks, as well as the effort expended in performing such tasks. A team-based approach is used for this assessment. This team should consist of a physical therapist, an occupational therapist, and an exercise physiologist. The physical therapist is trained to perform a detailed manual examination of the entire spine and appendicular skeleton, looking for osteopathic lesions, contracture, motor firing pattern abnormalities, and trunk endurance. Trunk endurance tests include examination of both flexor(abdominal muscles) and extensor (back muscles). One such useful test is the Sorenson test of trunk extensor strength (9).

The occupational therapist is trained in assessing patient performance in functional tasks, such as those designed to simulate work or home conditions. Two useful functional tests for this assessment are:

Functional Assessment Screening Test (FAST) is a group of five time-limited, self-paced tests which include two minutes of static kneeling, stooping, and squatting, a five minute test of repeated stooping and overhead reaching, and five minutes of repeated reaching and twisting while standing. The test is scored in terms of completion or noncompletion, but the OT can record patient performance in seconds (10).

Progressive Isoinertial Lifting Evaluation (PILE) is an exercise in which patients lift a weight from the floor to waist level and then back to the floor four times within 20 seconds and also from waist to shoulder level. The weight is progressively increased until a predetermined lift limit is reached, safety limits of heart rate and blood pressure are exceeded, or the patient requests to stop (11).

The final step in the assessment of physical status is best performed by an exercise physiologist who has expertise in analyzing cardiovascular endurance. The cardiovascular endurance or aerobic fitness level is typically very poor in the population of patients with chronic pain; as they are markedly deconditioned and deactivated. To quantify this, an exercise physiologist can monitor the patient as he undergoes a submaximal exercise stress test, say on an ergonomic bicycle, in order to determine cardiac fitness level recorded as VO_2 and MET level.

Functional Capacity Evaluation

Functional capacity evaluations (FCEs) are essentially work capacity evaluations, or vocational functional capacity evaluations. Their prime focus is to determine if a patient can return to the workforce in the routine performance of a specific job. Commonly, they are viewed as legal documents. FCEs are typically performed by physical or occupational therapists. The therapist methodically tests the worker through simulated job tasks in order to determine the workers' capacity to perform such a job task. After the evaluation it is usually determined whether the patient can return to the workforce or not (12).

This form of evaluation is better used as a triage tool, as opposed to a final determinant, when evaluating a patient with chronic pain. The information that an FCE provides is only one step in the overall assessment of such patients for proper placement into a functional rehabilitation program.

Putting It All Together: Spine Team Assessment

One example of a format that uses the diagnostic assessment protocol presented in this chapter is the Spine Team Assessment (STA) (13, 14). The STA is a codified, multidisciplinary, single-visit assessment intended for persons with chronic back pain-related disability. It includes assessments by a physical therapist, occupational therapist, exercise physiologist, psychologist, and vocational counselor followed by a physiatrist-lead team meeting where a detailed plan of action for the patient is formulated. Patient demographics, physical test results, functional test results, psychological test results, and the relationship between these are explored to choose an individualized treatment program, which are described and further explored in Chapter 28. The following case study is drawn from the experience of the Spine Team Assessment. Table 27-1 summarizes the components of the Spine Team Assessment.

Table 27-1   Spine Team Assessment Components and Purposes

	Component	Purpose
Patient questionnaires	Health/social history	Comprehensive team understanding without duplication of effort
	Center for Epidemiologic Studies Depression Scale	Screen for depression
	Tampa Kinesiphobia Scale	Detect pain avoidance tendencies
	Visual Analog Pain Scale	Baseline pain perception
	Multidimensional Pain Inventory	Determine impact of pain on life and coping strategies
Quebec Back Pain	Quantify amount and areas of Disability Scale	perceived disability
	Short Form 36	Quantify health-related quality of life
Physical therapy	Manual physical examination	Detect treatable mechanical causes
	Knee extension test	Test lower limb strength
	Bench press test	Test upper limb strength
Occupational therapy	Patient interview	Detect functional deficits and work and home barriers
	Progressive isoinertial lifting evaluation	Detect conditioning, effort, and functional ability
	Functional activity screening test	Detect effort, pain behavior, minimal functional ability
Exercise physiology	Patient interview	Detect unhealthy lifestyle habits
	Submaximal stress test	Detect deconditioning and effort
Psychologist	Patient interview/ test interpretation	Detect psychopathology and personality strengths and weaknesses
Social worker	Patient interview	Understand social, financial, legal, and vocational status
Physician	History and physical examination	Determine diagnosis, prognosis, medication, and invasive treatment options, and therapy precautions and limitations
Team meeting	Reports	Promote group understanding of the issues
	Discussion	Promote transdisciplinary problem-solving
	Documentation	Share with all stakeholders the comprehensive case summary and plan with goals, time frames, and persons responsible
	2-week follow-up	Promote patient understanding and acceptance of plan

Case Study 27-1

A 43-year-old man presented for the first time to a primary care physician. He had been out of work for more than 2 years due to a work-related low back injury. The physician ascertained that appropriate medical diagnostic tests had been done, and the patient was not a surgical candidate. He was referred for a half-day Spine Team Assessment.

The social worker found that the patient had not contacted his supervisor in more than a year and was unsure of his status with his employer. The psychologist noted major depression on the CES-D depression scale, more fear of movement and avoidance of movement than most chronic pain patients on the Tampa scale, and a dysfunctional profile on the Multidisciplinary Pain Inventory.

The physical therapist found that the patient had failed multiple attempts at individual therapy. On bicycle ergometry his estimated aerobic capacity was 4.5 METS, putting him in the lowest 1 percentile for men of his age. His actual heart rate did not go over 70% of predicted maximum for age, suggesting less than full physiologic effort on the test. The Sorenson test of trunk extension endurance was 20 seconds, well below the 2-minute cut-off for norms. A squat test, bench press test, and others confirmed poor performance.

In occupational therapy the patient failed 3 of the 5 components of the 15-minute FAST, suggesting that a more extensive Functional Capacity Evaluation would not be useful. On the PILE, he only lifted 20 pounds from floor to waist and 10 pounds from waist to shoulder, again showing poor physiologic effort as measured by a heart rate of 65% of maximum.

At the team meeting, it was concluded that the patient was not in need of more hands-on physical therapy, that he did need aggressive conditioning, but that he was not capable of participating in therapy or a health club gym program without substantial psychological support. The team recommended that he participate in a 3-week intensive multidisciplinary functional restoration program (see Chapter 28), but that a month prior to the program be used to gradually acclimatize him to exercise, begin antidepressants, and start counseling. On completion of the program, physical performance was substantially improved primarily because of increased physiologic effort (he attained a heart rate of 85% on the PILE). Although his MET level had increased to 7.5, it was recognized that cardiovascular fitness would be a long-term project. Depression was much less, and he had negotiated a graduated return to work schedule. At 6 month follow-up he was still in some pain, but employed and quite happy with his situation.

Conclusion

A rehabilitation-based diagnostic assessment of patients with chronic back pain-related disability needs to include a quantified assessment of disabling comorbidities. This requires the assessment of psychological status (depression, anxiety, fear, coping skills, etc.), physical status (strength, flexibility, endurance, etc.), and functional status (ability to perform home activities, work activities, and avocational pursuits) of these patients. Once these assessments have been made by an expert multidisciplinary team, the patient can be more appropriately triaged to a proper treatment program which can be optimized to successfully lessen their disability.

▪   ▪   ▪

Key Points

- Patients with chronic back pain-related disability have complex physical and psychosocial issues that compound their disability and greatly contribute to the difficulty seen in returning to a functional life.
- Assessment strategies that quantify the patient's disabling comorbidities are the basis for designing the most appropriate treatment program for patients with chronic pain.
- Physical status assessment is carried out through a team-based approach: a physical therapist performs a detailed manual examination of the spine and appendicular skeleton, and an occupational therapist assess the patient's ability to perform functional tests.
- Functional capacity evaluations are used to determine the patient's capacity to perform a job task.
- A multidisciplinary assessment team is a useful approach for such a diagnostic assessment of chronic pain-related disability.

▪   ▪   ▪

REFERENCES

1. **Mayer TG, Gatchel RJ, Mayer H, Kishino ND, Keeley J, Mooney V.** A prospective two-year study of functional restoration in industrial low back injury. JAMA. 1987;258:1763-7.
2. **Radloff L.** The CES-D scale: a self-report depression scale for research in the general population, J Appl Psychol Meas. 1977;1:385-401.
3. **Melzack R.** The McGill Pain Questionnaire: major properties and scoring methods. Pain. 1975;1:277-99.
4. **Kerns RD, Turk DC, Rudy TE.** The West Haven-Yale Multidimensional Pain Inventory (WHYMPI). Pain. 1985;23:345-56.

5. **Kopec JA, Esdaile JM, Abrahamowicz M, Abenhaim L, Wood-Dauphinee S, Lamping DL, et al.** The Quebec Back Pain Disability Scale: measurement properties. Spine. 1995;20:341-52.

6. **Ware JE, Sherbourne CD.** The MOS 36-item Short Form Health Survey (MOS SF-36): I. Conceptual framework and item selection. Med Care. 1992;30:473-81.

7. **Clark ME, Kori SH, Brockel J.** Kinesiophobia and chronic pain: psychometric characteristics and factor analysis of the Tampa Scale. Am Pain Soc Abstr. 1996;15:77.

8. **Huskisson EC.** Visual Analogue Scales. In: Melzack R, ed. Pain Measurement and Assessments. New York: Raven Press; 1983:33-7.

9. **Novy DM, Simmonds MJ, Olson SL, Lee CE, Jones SC.** Physical performance: differences in men and women with and without low back pain. Arch Phys Med Rehabil. 1999;80:195-8.

10. **Ruan CM, Haig AJ, Geisser ME, Yamakawa K, Buchholz RL.** Functional capacity evaluations in persons with spinal disorders: predicting poor outcomes on the Functional Assessment Screening Test (FAST). J Occup Rehabil. 2001;11:119-32.

11. **Mayer TG, Barnes D, Nichols G, Kishino ND, Coval K, Piel B., et al.** Progressive isoinertial lift evaluation. I. A standardized protocol and normative database. Spine. 1988;13:993-1002.

12. **Kraus J.** The independent medical examination and the functional capacity evaluation. Occup Med. 1997;12(3):525-56.

13. **Haig AJ, Theisen M, Geisser ME, Michel B, Yamakawa K.** Team Decision Making for Spine Team Assessment: Standardizing the Multidisciplinary Assessment for Chronic Back Pain. American Academy of Physical Medicine and Rehabilitation Annual Assembly, San Francisco, CA, 2000.

14. **Haig AJ, Geisser ME, Theisen M, Michel B, Yamakawa K.** The Spine Team Assessment: Physical and Psychosocial Performance of 429 Adults with Chronic Low Back Pain Disability. American Academy of Physical Medicine and Rehabilitation Annual Assembly, San Francisco, CA, 2000.

28

■　■　■

Rehabilitation Treatments for Chronic Back Pain

Michael E. Geisser, PhD

Mary E. Theisen-Goodvich, PhD

Chronic back pain is diagnostically complex and difficult to treat. Proposed pathophysiological causes of chronic back pain vary, but in general the vast majority of persons with chronic back pain are believed to have no specific underlying organic pathology to explain their symptoms. Although many of these persons are believed to have some evidence of musculoskeletal dysfunction, systematic empirical study of the diagnosis and treatment of musculoskeletal pain among persons with chronic back pain has been rare. Consequently, there has been much debate in the scientific community regarding whether specific treatments for chronic back pain are beneficial. This has led to the emergence of interventions for chronic back pain such as functional restoration, in which the primary goal of treatment is to achieve improvements in physical fitness and function, and not to reduce pain.

Clinicians treating chronic back pain who choose to have patients pursue rehabilitative treatments for the disorder must decide between various unimodel treatments, such as physical therapy, or multidisciplinary treatment. Current trends in chronic pain care and research suggest that the preferred intervention for chronic back pain is a multidisciplinary treatment program. Although the specific components and treatment philosophies of multidisciplinary treatment programs differ, these programs generally include 1) ongoing medical care or supervision; 2) exercise or specific physical therapy intervention; 3) psychosocial intervention; and 4) occupational therapy or other services related to increasing daily functioning and/or vocational rehabilitation. Some programs also offer specialty treatment involving pharmacology, dietetics, nursing, and case management. Programs are offered in both inpatient and outpatient settings, although the trend has been shifting toward providing services through less costly, outpatient settings.

A meta-analytic review of multidisciplinary pain treatment for chronic back pain conducted by Flor et al. (1) concluded that persons with chronic pain treated in multidisciplinary programs were functioning better than 75% of persons who either received no treatment or were treated with unimodal approaches such as conventional physical therapy. The benefits of multidisciplinary treatment appear to persist over time and extend beyond pain relief and include increased return to work and decreased use of health care.

Recent studies have focused on attempting to subgroup persons with chronic pain in order to match them with interventions that optimize outcome with the least cost. For example, Turk et al. (2) demonstrated that multidisciplinary treatment tailored for patients with temporomandibular disorder who had a dysfunctional profile type on the Multidimensional Pain Inventory produced the best outcomes. This study suggests that certain subgroups of persons with chronic back pain may require more intensive multidisciplinary treatment, whereas some may respond well to less intensive and less costly interventions. Hopefully, future studies will shed more light on this issue. Studies on treatment outcome for chronic back pain suggest that patients with a high degree of disability and/or psychological distress may benefit more from multidisciplinary treatment, whereas persons who appear to be coping well with their pain may do well with unimodal interventions such as physical therapy.

This chapter will focus on rehabilitative treatments for chronic back pain. Individual treatments for chronic back pain will be reviewed first. Readers should keep in mind that many interventions for back pain reviewed in other chapters (such as injections) may also be appropriate for chronic back pain, either alone or as an adjunct to other treatments. Multidisciplinary treatment will then be presented, followed by a discussion of the important issues to consider in the rehabilitation of chronic back pain.

Individual Treatments

Exercise

Exercise is believed to be an important component of chronic back pain, as deconditioning and muscle weakness and atrophy due to disuse may contribute to chronic back pain disability. For example, decreased strength in the abdominal and spine extensor musculature has been shown to be associated with the recurrence or persistence of low back pain (3-5). Similarly, diminished cardiovascular fitness has been found to be associated with a higher incidence of back pain disability as well as more frequent episodes of low back pain (4). Research examining whether poor physical fitness is a cause or consequence of chronic back pain suggests that there is evidence to support both relationships.

Rodriquez et al. (6) reviewed the role of exercise in the treatment of chronic neck and back pain and concluded that general exercises such as nonspecific strengthening and aerobic conditioning appear to decrease the intensity of chronic back pain and protect against recurrence. They indicated that little research has been done to examine the effectiveness of specific types of exercises on pain, and that it is unknown whether improvements are related to stretching, strengthening, increased endurance, and/or improved coordination. In addition, the optimal frequency and duration of exercise is unknown. The issue of compliance with exercise for pain, particularly on a long-term basis, has not been adequately addressed. Empirical studies addressing strategies for increasing compliance, such as simplifying prescribed regimens, would be very beneficial. In addition, strategies that have been proved to be beneficial for increasing long-term compliance with exercise in the general exercise literature may be useful in increasing adherence to prescribed exercise regimens among persons with chronic back pain.

Manual Therapy

Manual therapy involves the application of specific interventions, such as muscle energy techniques, myofascial release, and thrust techniques to minimize or eliminate musculoskeletal dysfunctions (7,8,9). Descriptions of these interventions and the mechanisms by which they relieve pain is given elsewhere in this text (see Chapters 20 and 24). In addition to manipulation, there is some suggestion that education on proper body mechanics and posture and exercises specifically tailored for the patient with chronic musculoskeletal pain and dysfunction are an important part of treatment (10). These exercises might include specific stretches for shortened muscles and self-mobilization exercises. Ideally, these techniques can be used by the patient as specific pain management tools to improve function and to decrease dependence on ongoing medical care.

Although manual therapy is often employed in the management of chronic back pain, there is scarce literature to support its use. Recently, we have completed a randomized, controlled trial of manual therapy and specific adjuvant exercise for chronic low back pain (11). In summary it did show that manual therapy is effective in managing pain, but not disability. Importantly, the effect of manual therapy was much greater when the patient was given lesion-specific exercises compared with general exercise. The implication is that whomever is performing the manual therapy must instruct, not just passively treat. Further studies need to be conducted to examine long-term benefits of this approach and additional interventions that may have a greater impact on disability.

Cognitive Behavioral Therapy

Cognitive behavioral therapy has been found to be beneficial for many psychological disorders and for patients coping with various medical conditions. Although the various components of cognitive behavioral therapy vary across studies, the elements commonly included are 1) biofeedback and/or various forms of relaxation; 2) the use of operant principals to produce desired changes in behavior (e.g., exercise or functional activity); 3) cognitive reframing to alter beliefs that may lead to increased pain or distress; and 4) coping skills training to increase the repertoire and use of different behavioral or cognitive coping skills to reduce pain or emotional distress. A recent meta-analytic study conducted by Morley et al. (12) examining the impact of cognitive behavioral therapy on nonheadache pain indicated that cognitive behavioral therapy appeared to be beneficial in reducing the experience of pain, increasing positive coping behavior, and decreasing expressions of pain. These interventions, however, did not appear to alter mood, negative cognitive appraisals, or social role functioning. Some have suggested that biofeedback may change muscle activity patterns that contribute to pain.

Recent studies suggest that cognitive behavioral therapy aimed at specific co-morbid problems that arise in persons with chronic pain may be beneficial. For example, high rates of psychopathogy have been reported among persons with chronic back pain, and interventions designed to decrease comorbid conditions such as depression and post-traumatic stress disorder might be particularly beneficial. As pain-related fear and avoidance of situations that are believed to cause pain have been shown to be highly-related to disability among persons with back pain, exposure to feared or avoided activities may be highly beneficial in decreasing disability. For example, a recent study by Vlaeyen et al. (13) demonstrated that exposure to feared daily activities while simultaneously challenging persons' maladaptive beliefs about that activity significantly reduced disability in a sample of persons with chronic back pain observed over time.

Work Hardening

Work-hardening programs generally attempt to assist clients with achieving a level of work productivity that allows them to participate in the competitive labor market (14). Work-hardening programs may be either an isolated therapist or may involve a team of physical and occupational therapists. The procedures employed generally include gradually increasing involvement in functional activities, providing feedback regarding ergonomic issues, encouraging the patient to employ various pain management strategies such as posture breaks, and assisting the patient with work adaptation including the use of adaptive devices. Some work-hardening programs are part of a larger, multidisciplinary pain program, whereas others may initiate vocational rehabilitation once initial pain management treatment has been completed. Few controlled outcome studies have examined work hardening among chronic pain patients, but these services, along with vocational counseling, are an important aspect of the rehabilitation of the chronic back pain patient.

King (14) examined data collected from 928 clients from 22 work-hardening programs in Wisconsin. Most clients were males, and the most frequent condition treated was lumbar spine injury (47%). Of patients with lumbar injury, 59% returned to their usual job, some with modifications, and 12% returned to an alternative job with the same employer. It is unclear, however, how many of these individuals had ongoing pain, for what duration, or of what intensity.

Multidisciplinary Treatment

It is estimated that there are more than 1000 multidisciplinary pain clinics and pain centers in the United States (15). Given the complexity and multidimensional nature of pain, multidisciplinary treatment is often viewed as the preferred treatment for a number of chronic pain conditions. Although the orientation and composition of multidisciplinary treatments vary, specific programs have emerged in the literature. For example, Feuerstein et al. (16) presented data from a program they term Multidisciplinary Rehabilitation, and indicated that 71% of patients who completed the program were working or in vocational rehabilitation at 12 month-follow-up, compared to only 44% in corresponding comparison groups. Case Study 28-1 describes the treatment of a patient treated in a multidisciplinary program.

Case Study 28-1

A 48-year-old female with a history of polio at age 3, bicycle accident at age 16, and a motor vehicle accident at age 28 presented with chronic musculoskeletal neck, arm, head, and back pain with fibromyalgia and degenerative joint disease. Despite multiple individual treatments, she had ongoing pain and disability from life activities and reduced her work hours to half time. She presented with moderate levels of depression and anxiety and a significant sleep disturbance. She was enrolled in a multidisciplinary program where she received ongoing medical management and physical, occupational, and psychological therapies. Over the course of her 8-week program, the patient received manual physical therapy and specific instruction in a home exercise program including stretching, self-corrections, and strengthening and cardiovascular exercise. She learned pacing and energy conservation techniques and proper body mechanics and posture in occupational therapy. Psychological treatment included instruction on relaxation and used cognitive behavioral techniques to assist the patient in decreasing catastrophic thoughts and to reframe maladaptive pain beliefs, and increase her sense of control over the pain. She was also placed on nortriptyline 20 mg qhs for her sleep disturbance. The patient made significant improvements, reporting decreased pain, increased range of motion, and improved function. She was diligently working on her home exercise program, joined a health club, and was increasing her work hours at discharge. She also reported that she was sleeping and managing her pain much better.

Given the lack of knowledge regarding "treatable" organic pathology in many chronic pain patients, functional restoration methods have been proposed as an alternative treatment paradigm. Typically, the goal of treatment in a functional restoration program is not to "treat" the etiology of pain or guide treatment by pain reports, rather, the focus is on increasing function despite pain. This treatment suggests that activity progression may be crucial among patients with musculoskeletal pain as improving their strength and conditioning may ultimately decrease pain. Further, patients who are fearful of certain activities because they overestimate the amount of pain they will experience may benefit from the exposure to feared activities, as performing them without experiencing unmanageable pain will likely decrease their fear of movement and increase their functioning. Hazard (17) outlines the crucial elements of a functional restoration approach, including an interdisciplinary staff, quantification of function to monitor patient status and progress, physical training, and counseling. Two initial studies (18, 19) reported that more than 80% of patients treated in a functional restoration program were able to return to work following treatment, and a high percentage were still working at 1-year follow-up. Case Study 28-2 describes a patient who completed a functional restoration program.

Case Study 28-2

A 40-year-old male presented with a 4-year history of low back and leg pain that began after his second lithotripsy treatment for nephrolithiasis. Multiple individual treatments, including spinal cord stimulator, were ineffectual in relieving his pain. At the time of his evaluation, he was on multiple medications, including MS-Contin, baclofen, MSIR, and Klonopin. X-rays demonstrated mild degenrative joint disease, and electromyogram (EMG) demonstrated mild right peroneal mononeuropathy without axon loss. He had been out of work for 2 years, on long-term disability, and was having significant functional difficulties, including completion of his activities of daily living. He presented with depression and anxiety, concentration and memory problems, and a significant sleep disturbance. He was fearful of reinjury and did not have a good understanding of his pain problem. He also demonstrated deconditioning and some biomechanical abnormalities. The patient received 3 weeks of manual physical therapy and psychological treatment while weaned from his narcotic analgesics. He then entered the Functional Restoration Program. After treatment, he returned to work and reported increased activity level and ability to perform activities of daily living and improved mood and sleep. At discharge, the patient had joined a health club to continue his home exercise program, was off of all narcotics, and was scheduled to have his spinal cord stimulator removed.

Historically, functional restoration programs have focused on chronic pain patients who are middle aged and disabled from work. We developed a Senior Functional Restoration Program (senior functional restoration program) directed toward patients with disabling back pain who are 60 years and older, whose goals are not typically to return to work and for whom the standard functional restoration program is too intensive and fast paced. Similar to the traditional functional restoration program, the primary goals of the program include improved functional status and quality of life. Unlike functional restoration program, the senior functional restoration program includes manual physical therapy and the goal to improve pain/treat the specific lesion. The program also focuses on other issues important to the elderly such as fall risk, community reentry/resources, and adaptive equipment and home adaptations for maximizing function and safety. The program is still in its infancy and outcome research is underway. Customer satisfaction surveys reveal that patients are happy with improvements made in the program and are quite willing to recommend the program to others.

Conclusion

Although the underlying pathophysiology of chronic back pain is largely unknown, there is increasing evidence that musculoskeletal dysfunctions may contribute to pain in the majority of persons with chronic back pain. Therefore, specific treatments for and education regarding the nature of musculoskeletal pain may be useful interventions. There is some initial evidence that manual therapy may be beneficial in reducing chronic back pain, although pain reduction may not lead to improved function in this population.Numerous other individual interventions, including exercise, biofeedback and cognitive-behavioral therapy, appear to have some efficacy for reducing or altering a person's experience of pain. The issue of compliance with exercise for pain treatment has not been adequately addressed, and empirical studies related to strategies for increasing compliance, such as simplifying prescribed regimens, would be beneficial.

In practice, many of these individual therapies are employed as part of multidisciplinary treatment programs. In general, multidisciplinary treatment appears to be superior to unimodal or no treatment. Nevertheless, there is some preliminary evidence that persons with chronic back pain who have little disability or psychological distress may benefit from individual interventions such as exercise or physical therapy. It is not really known which elements of multidisciplinary treatment are most beneficial, and therefore, further study is needed to determine the most desired elements of these programs. Optimal treatment length also needs to be determined.

Many programs differ in their emphasis on managing pain versus increasing daily functioning despite pain. Although strategies such as activity pacing may decrease pain, they also may encourage patients to avoid activities that they believe cause pain, which may actually then inhibit rehabilitation. Exposure-based interventions seem to hold some promise in terms of decreasing disability due to chronic back pain by reducing pain related fear and avoidance. It would be interesting to examine the relative impact of each interventional strategy on pain and function among persons with chronic back pain. It is possible that coping strategies that emphasize pain avoidance might be beneficial for some patients, while others may benefit from directly confronting painful situations. In addition, pain avoidance strategies may be beneficial early in treatment, while having patients confront feared situations may be a beneficial addition to treatment in the latter stages. Little is known about how to best balance progression of activity with managing pain. It would be useful to compare the long-term outcomes of these different treatment paradigms.

In practice, many persons who are offered a rehabilitation program as an intervention for their chronic back pain may have beliefs about their situation which are not compatible with rehabilitation. Patients who strongly believe that specific interventions exist to cure their pain, or who do not necessarily see the therapeutic benefits of exercise, will possibly do poorly in rehabilitation settings. The patient's beliefs and their willingness to undergo rehabilitation needs to be addressed prior to treatment. For persons who are not a good match for rehabilitation, education and counseling to address the appropriateness of their beliefs may be beneficial.

■   ■   ■

Recommendations

- The patient's beliefs (e.g., that specific treatments do exist that will "cure" the pain) and willingness to undergo rehabilitation need to be addressed before treatment.

- Education and counseling should be offered or recommended to patients with beliefs that are incompatible with rehabilitation.
- Patients with little disability or psychological distress may benefit from individual interventions such as exercise or physical therapy.
- For more distressed or disabled persons, multidisciplinary treatment should be considered.
- Patients older than 60 years with disabling back pain may benefit by a Senior Functional Restoration Program.
- Choosing a rehabilitation treatment may depend on local resources and expertise as well as the patient's presentation.

Key Points

- Multidisciplinary programs for pain management are effective. The benefits appear to persist over time and extend beyond pain relief to include return to work and decreased use of health care.
- Some programs emphasize pain management, whereas others stress restoration of function.
- Individual or multidisciplinary treatments may be used, depending on the patient's degree of disability and psychological distress.
- Because of the complexity and multidimensional nature of pain, multidisciplinary rehabilitation is often considered the preferred treatment for chronic pain.

REFERENCES

1. **Flor H, Fydrich T, Turk DC.** Efficacy of multidisciplinary pain treatment centers: a meta-analytic review. Pain. 1992;49:221-30.
2. **Turk DC, Rudy TE, Kubinski JA, Zaki HS, Greco CM.** Dysfunctional patients with temporomandibular disorders: evaluating the efficacy of a tailored treatment protocol. J Consult Clin Psychol. 1996;64:139-46.
3. **Biering-Sorensen F.** Physical measurements as risk indicators for low-back trouble over a one-year period. Spine. 1984;9:106-19.
4. **Cady LD, Bischoff DP, O'Connell ER, Thomas PC, Allan JH.** Strength and fitness and subsequent back injuries in firefighters. J Occup Med. 1979;21:269-72.
5. **Troup JD, Martin JW, Lloyd DC.** Back pain in industry: a prospective survey. Spine. 1981;6:61-9.
6. **Rodriquez AA, Bilkey WJ, Agre JC.** Therapeutic exercise in chronic neck and back pain. Arch Phys Med Rehabil. 1992;73:870-5.

7. **Mein EA.** Low back pain and manual medicine: a look at the literature. Phys Med Rehabil Clin North Am. 1996;7:715-29.

8. **Simons DG.** Myofascial pain syndrome due to trigger points. Int Rehabil Med Assoc Monogr Ser. 1987;1:1-39.

9. **Greenman PE.** Principles of Manual Medicine. Baltimore: Williams and Wilkins; 1989.

10. **Bookhout MR.** Exercise and somatic dysfunction. Phys Med Rehabil Clin North Am. 1996;7:845-62.

11. **Geisser ME, Wiggert EA, Haig AJ, Colwell MO.** A randomized, controlled trial of manual therapy and specific adjuvant exercise for chronic low back pain. J Pain. 2002;3(Suppl. 1):53.

12. **Morley S, Eccleston C, Williams A.** Systematic review and meta-analysis of randomized controlled trials of cognitive behavior therapy and behavior therapy for chronic pain in adults, excluding headaches. Pain. 1999;80:1-13.

13. **DeJong JR, Vlaeyen JW, et al.** Fear of movement/(re)injury in chronic low back pain: education or exposure in vivo as a mediator to fear reduction. Clin J Pain. 2005;21:9-17.

14. **King PM.** Outcome analysis of work-hardening programs. Am J Occup Ther. 1993;47:595-603.

15. **Crue BL.** Multi-disciplinary pain treatment programs: current status. Clin J Pain. 1985;1:31-8.

16. **Feuerstein M, Menz L, Zastowny T, Barron BA.** Chronic back pain and work disability: vocational outcomes following multidisciplinary rehabiliation. J Occup Rehabil 1994;4:229-251.

17. **Hazard RG.** Spine update: functional restoration. Spine. 1995;20:2345-8.

18. **Hazard RG, Fenwick JW, Kalisch SM, Redmond J, Reeves V, Reid S, et al.** Functional restoration with behavioural support: a one year prospective study of patients with chronic low back pain. Spine. 1989;14:157-61.

19. **Mayer TG, Gatchel RJ, Mayer H.** A prospective two year study of functional restoration in industrial low back injury: an objective assessment procedure. JAMA. 1987;258:1763-7.

■   ■   ■

KEY REFERENCES

Flor H, Fydrich T, Turk DC. Efficacy of multidisciplinary pain treatment centers: a meta-analytic review. Pain. 1992;49:221-30.
A review of a number of different approaches. The authors find that multidisciplinary pain treatment is effective.

Hazard RG. Spine update: functional restoration. Spine. 1995;20:2345-8.
Hazard, one of the first to use this approach, performs a critical review of the literature.

29

■ ■ ■

Medications for the Management of Chronic Back Pain

Carolyn R. Zaleon, PharmD

By the time patients are diagnosed with chronic back pain, many have either tried and failed various treatment regimens, including nonsteroidal anti-inflammatory drugs (NSAIDs), or are currently using the prescribed regimens with suboptimal pain control. At this point, other medication options need to be considered including combination regimens. In addition, for optimal pain control, it is important to identify and treat comorbid conditions that may contribute to the perception of pain, including anxiety, depression, and disordered sleep (1-3).

Opioid (Narcotic) Analgesics

In the author's opinion, opioids are the mainstay of pharmacologic treatment of chronic back pain. Generally, unless the pain is entirely neuropathic, a long-acting opioid given with a short-acting agent for breatkthrough pain will achieve pain relief (4).

Precautions and Barriers to Use

There are often barriers on the parts of the practitioner (5,6) and the patient to use opioid analgesics (opioids) on a chronic basis (7). The practitioner must initially determine the existence of substance abuse/misuse, including alcohol or illicit drugs. Patients with chronic pain and a *current* substance abuse problem should concurrently be enrolled in and supervised by a substance abuse rehabilitation program if possible; opioids should be used with caution. If the patient has a *history* of substance abuse, the practitioner may cautiously prescribe opioids but must be alert

Table 29-1   Selected Examples of Drug-Seeking Behaviors

- "Lost" or stolen opioid medication(s)
- "Lost" or stolen opioid prescription(s)
- Request(s) for early refills
- Use of pain relievers belonging to friends, family members, et al.
- Self-titration of opioid dosage

Data from Refs. 2, 4, and 8.

to behaviors and symptoms that may indicate a recurrent problem (Table 29-1) (3). The practitioner must also determine if the patient is currently depressed and suicidal or has a history of attempted suicide (1). Opioids should cautiously be used with a history of suicide attempts; patients with current suicidal ideation should be treated by a mental health provider prior to, or in conjunction with, cautious outpatient treatment with opioids. Persons with liver or renal disease may need dosage adjustment, especially with opioids combined with acetaminophen or non-steroidal anit-inflammatory medications.

It is not uncommon for the patient to be reluctant to take opioid analgesics (7). Fears often include potential for addiction, stigma, or the inconvenience of monthly hand-written prescriptions. The apprehension in younger to middle-aged adults often also includes issues surrounding adverse effects from chronic opioid use, employment status while taking opioids, the ability to operate a motor vehicle, and the fear of having no future alternatives for pain control. The provider should spend time with each patient frankly and honestly addressing all concerns. The answers will vary with the patient and the situation. The time in most situations will be well spent.

Regardless of substance abuse/misuse status, all patients receiving chronic opioids should agree to and sign a standard "Narcotic Contract" (Figure 29-1) (6). With the initial narcotic prescription, the practitioner and the patient should discuss each point of the contract, address questions and concerns, and the appropriate comments should be written directly onto the contract. When both parties agree, the contract should be signed and dated. It should become a permanent part of the medical record and re-viewed and re-signed periodically (e.g., annually).

Selecting an Opioid Analgesic

Consider the following points in the initial selection of an opioid for chronic therapy:

1. *Previous opioid use:* If a particular agent worked in the past, it will likely work again. If it failed *and* the dose and duration were adequate, choose another opioid to initiate treatment.

Figure 29-1   Policy on Narcotic Drugs for Noncancer Pain

It is our policy to discourage the use of narcotic, i.e., strong, pain-killers, for the management of noncancer pain. In the few instances that we will prescribe these types of medications on a regular basis, the following policy will be strictly enforced.

1. If there is evidence of narcotic medications being obtained or requested from more than one source, we will NOT write any further narcotic prescriptions.
2. Narcotic prescriptions will be written on a monthly basis and the patient must expect to be seen each month in the clinic.
3. Each prescription will be for a fixed amount of medication sufficient to last until the next visit (no more than 1 month); this will not be increased or renewed early.
4. It is the responsibility of the patient to prevent loss of prescriptions or medicines. They cannot be expected to be replaced regardless of the circumstances.
5. Prescriptions will not be renewed over the telephone. Doses will not be adjusted over the telephone. Phone calls regarding prescriptions will only be entertained in the event of an adverse reaction.
6. Patients must show signs of appropriately improved function and increased daily activities.
7. The patient must adhere to all prescribed therapy such as physical therapy, psychological counseling, and other medications.
8. Appointments must be kept, or cancelled 24 hours prior to the scheduled time, for medications to be extended. However, repeated cancellations or failing to show for appointments will result in discontinuation of the narcotic medication.

Any deviation from this policy will be solely at the discretion of the physician and does not guarantee future deviations. Consequences for future violations should be expected to apply.

Violation of any of the above can result in immediate discontinuation of the narcotic prescription with no further prescriptions being written.

I have read and understand the above policy and agree to abide by these conditions:

_____
Patient signature   Date

_____
Witness signature   Date

Adapted from Department of Veterans Affairs, Ann Arbor Healthcare System. Ann Arbor VA Healthcare System Pain Clinic. Policy on narcotic drugs for non-cancer pain. Ann Arbor, Michigan.

Figure 29-1   Sample narcotic contract.

2. *Drug allergies/intolerances:* Always differentiate a true allergy from intolerance. Intolerance may be manageable; true opioid allergies are rare (10). In the truly allergic individual, an opioid from a different opioid class is *less likely* to precipitate an allergic reaction (Table 29-2) (10).

3. *Patient age:* Older adults are often more sensitive to the therapeutic and adverse effects of the opioids (11). Initiate at a lower dose, titrate more slowly, consider fall risk and consider comorbid medical conditions (11). The dose may be titrated to the usual adult dose based upon clinical status (Table 29-3).

Table 29-2   Opioid Analgesic Classes

- Morphine-like (phenanthrenes)

    Morphine (MSIR, MS Contin, Oramorph, Roxanol, etc.)

    Codeine (codeine sulfate, acetaminophen with codeine, etc.)

    Hydromorphone (Dilaudid)

    Hydrodocone (Lorcet,* Lortab,* Vicodin,* etc.)

    Oxycodone (oxycodone HCl, Oxycontin SR, Percocet,* Percodan,* Tylox,* etc.)
- Methadone-like (phenylheptylamines)

    Methadone (Dolophine)

    Propoxyphene (HCl salt = Darvon; napsylate salt = Darvocet*)
- Meperidine-like (phenylpiperidines)

    Meperidine (Demerol)

    Fentanyl (Duragesic, etc.)

*Product also contains acetaminophen.
Adapted with permission from Way WL, Fields HL, Schumacher MA. Opioid analgesics and antagonists. In: Katzung BG, ed. Basic and Clinical Pharmacology, 8th ed. New York: McGraw-Hill; 2001;512-31; and Nissen D, ed. Mosby's Drug Consult. St. Louis: Mosby; 2002.

Table 29-3   Recommended Doses for Initiating Opioid Therapy*

Drug	Oral Starting Dose
Morphine	Long-acting: 15 mg twice daily
	Short Acting: 5-10 mg every 4 hours for breakthrough pain only
Codeine	15-30 mg every 4-6 hours scheduled or as needed
Hydrocodone	5-10 mg every 4-6 hours scheduled or as needed; do not exceed 4000 mg acetaminophen per 24 hours (from all sources)
Hydromorphone	2 mg every 4-6 hours for breakthrough pain only
Oxycodone	IR: 5 mg every 4-6 hours, scheduled or as needed basis
	SR: 10 mg up to twice daily as scheduled doses
Methadone	Not recommended for initiation of pain control
Fentanyl	Not recommended for initiation of pain control
Tramadol	50-100 mg every 4-6 hours as needed; not to exceed 400 mg per 24 hours†
Propoxyphene	65 mg of HCl salt (= 100 mg of napsylate salt) 4 times a day, scheduled or as needed basis; do not exceed 4000 mg acetaminophen per 24 hours (from all sources); no more than 390 mg per 24 hours of propoxyphene HCl, 600mg per 24 hours of propoxyphene napsylate

IR = immediate release; SR = sustained release.
*Opioid-naive, otherwise healthy adults, approximately 18 to 65 years old.
†If older than 75 years or if renal and/or hepatic insufficiency present, decrease starting dose and maximum daily dose (11,16).

4. *Renal/liver status:* All opioids are metabolized primarily by the liver (12). Morphine is metabolized in the liver to several active compounds, one of which, morphine-6-glucuronide (M6G) is more active than morphine (12). M6G is renally eliminated, accumulates in renal insufficiency, and is associated with adverse effects. Morphine should therefore be avoided or used with caution these patients. It should also be used with caution in patients with hepatic dysfunction, with the dose reduced accordingly. This is also true of meperidine (13).

5. *Drug duration of action:* The advantages of using long-acting opioids, compared with short-acting opioids include the following: improved medication compliance, less fluctuation in pain control (less difference between plasma opioid concentration peak and trough levels) (2), and possibly less abuse potential (lack of fast onset, high plasma concentration peaks). All opioid analgesics except methadone are inherently short acting compounds. Morphine, oxycodone and fentanyl are available as immediate release *and* as extended release formulations. Methadone is inherently longer acting and therefore maintains a longer duration of action regardless of the formulation (tablet or liquid) (2). Longer duration usually means longer time to onset of effect and longer time for elimination after the last dose.

6. *Pain component (nociceptive and/or neuropathic):* Opioids tend to be more effective for nociceptive than neuropathic pain (14). Methadone and propoxyphene additionally block *N*-methyl-D-aspartate (NMDA) receptors (17) and therefore may provide neuropathic pain relief as well.

7. *Drug cost to patient/healthcare system:* Drug costs vary widely based on numerous factors. Be aware of the relative costs in your particular practice setting.

8. *Abuse potential/street value:* One may need to consider the potential for opioid abuse and/or drug diversion in the patient and possibly in a significant other or family member.

If the patient is opioid-naive, it is reasonable to begin with a less potent opioid (e.g., combination acetaminophen with codeine or hydrocodone, propoxyphene, tramadol) and titrate to pain control, tolerability or maximal recommended doses. If the patient has a history of opioid use, it is reasonable to begin with a more potent opioid and titrate upwards as described below.

Initial Dose Selection

Consider age, renal/hepatic status, previous opioid use/tolerance, comorbid medical conditions and level of pain with initial dose selection. The objective of successful pain management is 24-hour pain control; try to avoid "chasing" pain; that is, waiting until the pain returns before treating it. This can best be achieved using scheduled doses of long-acting morphine or oxycodone, or methadone, or fentanyl patches; often a short-acting opioid is prescribed on an as needed (prn) basis for breakthrough pain. Monitior the patient's use of the shorter acting opioid; a significant increase in use for breakthrough pain indicates that the dose of the maintenance opioid needs to be increased. In selected patients, one may use scheduled doses of the shorter acting agents (oxycodone, propoxyphene, hydromorphone, hydrocodone). Those patients may include those at higher risk for falls, those with relatively minor pain syndromes or those with renal or hepatic insufficiency. However, the duration of relief from immediate-release morphine is often too short for adequate coverage in chronic pain. Recommended intial doses for opioid therapy are shown in Table 29-3.

Long-acting morphine and oxycodone require approximately 36-48 hours of around-the-clock dosing for onset, with maximal effects at approximately 1 week. For this reason, neither of these products should be use on a prn basis. Fentanyl patches usually require 1-3 patch changes (every 3-day dosing) for effects and often require approximately 5 patch changes for maximal effects. Fentanyl patch dose changes should occur no more frequently than every 2 weeks. Fentanyl is not recommended for initiation of pain control.

Meperidine should not be used for chronic pain (13). It has significant anticholinergic effects and may have negative inotropic effects on the heart. It is associated with a potential for inducing seizures due to the accumulation of its active metabolite (primarily associated with higher doses, renal and/or hepatic insufficiency) (2,12). Hydromorphone should be used for breakthrough pain control only due to its short duration of action.

Methadone is not recommended for initiation of pain control; it is usually best saved as a second or third option. Methadone's half-life approaches 48 hours with repeated dosing and therefore requires approximately 2-3 days of scheduled (2-3 times daily) dosing for onset, with maximal effects generally seen in 4-5 days. Because methadone accumulates in tissues, a dose reduction within the first couple of weeks may be necessary. Methadone should not be used on a prn basis and dosage increases should occur no sooner than every 4 days (15).

Tramadol is a centrally acting analgesic that binds to the mu receptors similarly to the opioids; its active metabolite binds to the mu receptors but is also a weak norepinephrine (NE) and serotonin (5HT) reuptake blocker. Tramadol is associated with a risk of seizures which is increased in the following situations: individual doses greater than 100 mg; dosing intervals sooner than every 4 hours; greater than 400 mg per day; increased patient age; concomitant use of: tricyclic antidepressants (TCAs), selective serotonin reuptake inhibitors (SSRIs), opioids, cyclobenzaprine, promethazine, MAO-inhibitors or other medications that lower the seizure threshold. Tramadol may also contribute to precipitation of the serotonin syndrome when combined with other medications that increase 5HT such as the

TCAs, the SSRIs, trazodone, etc. Consult prescribing information for complete information prior to initiating this medication (2,16).

Calculating Dose Conversions

Refer to Table 29-4 for approximate dose conversions when switching from one *oral* opioid to another *oral* opioid. Rule of thumb:

1. Calculate the current 24-hour opioid requirement (for *each* opioid if using more than one).
2. Convert *each* 24-hour total obtained in step no. 1 to the 24-hour equivalent of the new opioid using the conversions in Table 29-4. Add the values together (if currently using more than one).
3. Decrease the total value obtained in step no. 2 by 30-50% (or by 70-80% if switching TO methadone) due to incomplete cross-tolerance.
4. Divide the new total daily dose requirement obtained in step no. 3 by the desired dosing interval for the new opioid.
5. Monitor the patient closely during the first several weeks. Do not allow unsupervised self-titration of the opioid (2).

A word about methadone dosing: Many dosing strategies have been used when converting *to* methadone. Instead of the 3:2 (morphine: methadone) conversion in Table 29-4, ratios ranging from 3:1 to 10:1 have been used. No matter which dosing strategy is used, individual dose titration is often necessary (17). Maintain close communication with the patient during the initial titration phase. Converting *from* methadone *to* another opioid is much like any other opioid conversion and does not require any special precaution.

When converting from an oral opioid to the fentanyl patch, refer to Table 29-5 for dosage recommendations. For a safer conversion, use *one-half of the fentanyl dosage recommended in the table* and titrate upward as needed no more frequently than every 2 weeks. Note that to calculate the fentanyl dose, the 24-hour dose of the current opioid(s) must first be converted to the 24-hour oral morphine equivalent.

Table 29-4   Approximate Equianalgesic Oral Doses

Drug	Dose
Morphine IR, SR	30 mg
Methadone	20 mg
Oxycodone IR, SR	20 mg
Codeine	200 mg
Hydrocodone	20 mg
Hydromorphone	7.5 mg
Meperidine	300 mg

IR = immediate release; SR = sustained release.
Adapted from Department of Veterans Affairs. Analgesic Pocket Card. Veternas in Partnership. VISN 11 Healthcare Network.

Table 29-5   Conversion for Fentanyl Patches in Chronic Use (Do Not Use for Acute Pain Conversions)

24-Hour Oral Morphine Use (mg)*	Fentanyl Patch (mcg/h)
24-66	25
69-111	50
114-156	75
159-201	100
204-246	125
249-291	150
294-336	175
339-381	200
384-426	225
429-471	250
474-516	275
519-561	300

*Assumes use of morphine SR.
Adapted from Department of Veterans Affairs. Analgesic Pocket Card. Veterans in Partnership. VISN 11 Healthcare Network.

Adverse Effects

The most common opioid-induced adverse effects include CNS effects (sedation, respiratory depression, miosis, euphoria, nausea and vomiting) and peripheral effects (cardiovascular and gastrointestinal) (12).

CNS Effects

Sedation: Sedation is a common, often dose-related effect. Tolerance occurs rapidly. Persons who drive, fly, operate heavy equipment or work in dangerous or challenging environments often cannot use opiates because of legal or functional problems. Elderly persons are at more risk of cognitive impairment and the risk of falling is increased in elderly patients on opioids.

Respiratory depression: Opioids inhibit brain stem respiratory mechanisms and, among other effects, causes a dose-related decreased response to increases in carbon dioxide concentrations (12). Respiratory depression is not a common occurrence in cases in which the opioid dose has been slowly titrated since tolerance to the respiratory depressant effects usually occurs (18). However, patients with increased intracranial pressure, asthma, COPD, obstructive sleep apnea or other severe respiratory disorders may not tolerate a decrease in respiratory function; use opioids with caution, if at all, in these patient populations.

Miosis: Tolerance rarely develops to this opioid effect.

Nausea/vomiting: This dose-related adverse effect results from the direct activation of the chemoreceptor trigger zone and the vestibular apparatus (19). Tolerance often occurs within days.

Peripheral Effects
Cardiovascular effects: Hypotension and peripheral edema are possible, due to potential for both venous and arterial dilatation (12).

Gastrointestinal effects: Constipation occurs via both direct and indirect effects of the opioids on the local enteric nervous system (19). Constipation, therefore, can occur when non-oral formulations of opioids (e.g., parenteral, transdermal) are used. Tolerance rarely, if ever, develops. Be aggressive with prophylaxis and treatment of constipation; daily laxatives (e.g., senna) are often required. Opioids decrease gastrointestinal emptying time (19), which may result in *gastroparesis.* This may be especially problematic in predisposed patients (e.g., diabetes, concomitant medications with strong anticholinergic effects). Tolerance rarely develops.

Other Effects
Histamine-release: The naturally occurring (codeine and morphine) and the semisynthetic (hydrocodone, hydromorphone, oxycodone, etc.) opioids may cause an endogenous *release of histamine* (10). Symptoms may include sneezing, pruritis, flushing, urticaria or an asthma attack in susceptible individuals (10,12). This is often mistaken for an allergic reaction.

Tolerance to the analgesic effects occurs at varying rates: One may use "opioid rotation" strategies for the management of many of the opioid-induced adverse effects or analgesic tolerance, based upon the concept of incomplete cross-tolerance (2,19). Stop the current opioid and start another for a couple of months; switching back to the original or to another agent may be made at any time.

Case Study 29-1

An obese (300-pound) 54-year-old diabetic male with bilateral SI joint dysfunction, s/p 4 surgeries, and several SI injections has taken propoxyphene/acetaminophen for more than 10 years; 3 months ago he was switched to immediate release oxycodone 5 mg four times daily. With continued poor control at 30 mg/day, he was switched to methadone. According to the conversion approximation, this is equivalent to 30 mg/day of methadone. The methadone dose was initiated at 10 mg twice daily (the dose was decreased due to incomplete cross-tolerance, but it was also taken into consideration that oxycodone 30 mg was ineffective and some tolerance likely developed from years of opioid use). Oxycodone was continued for breakthrough. After 6 months, he was taking methadone 40 mg/day and oxycodone 30 mg/day with fair pain control. The methadone was increased to 60 mg and then to 80 mg daily, the oxycodone was decreased to 20 mg/day but he continued to take 30 mg daily. With pain control still suboptimal, he was switched to sustained release morphine. Switching from methadone *to* morphine does not require the special care that switching *to* methadone requires. The methadone and the oxycodone doses were converted to 24-hour morphine equivalents and added together (165 mg using a 2:3 methadone:morphine ratio, 285 mg using a 1:3 ratio). The morphine was initiated at 240 mg/day and later titrated to 300 mg/day. No initial dose reduction of 30-50% was made in this instance due to persistent lack of pain control and years of opioid use. After one month, the morphine was changed to the fentanyl patch. According to the table, 300 mg/day of morphine is equivalent to 175 mcg/h of fentanyl. The dose was reduced due to incomplete cross-tolerance and the fentanyl was initiated at 100 mcg/h every 3 days. The patient felt some pain relief without substantial side effects on this regimen.

Antidepressants

Selecting an Antidepressant

Antidepressants are now part of many chronic pain treatment regimens. They are adjunctive in nociceptive pain, and primary treatment in neuropathic pain (3). Opioids are less effective for neuropathic pain and are often not first-line for pain control (14). The SSRIs are not consistently useful unless there is a significant component of depression involved in the perception of pain. The only SSRI that *may* be useful, based upon limited information, is paroxetine (20).

Tricyclic antidepressants (TCAs) are often considered first-line treatment for neuropathic pain (14,21) and are used in doses lower than typical antidepressant doses (22). The exact mechanism of action is unknown, but all TCAs, in varying degrees, block the reuptake of both NE and 5HT to potentiate the inhibitory pain pathway. In addition, they may also block the sodium (Na) channel to potentiate the inhibitory pain pathway and may block the NMDA receptor as well. As an exploitation of the side-effect profile (anticholinergic effects), the TCAs are also often helpful in the management of sleep disorders. The TCAs most often used include amitriptyline (AMT) and its active metabolite nortriptyline (NTP); also imipramine (IMI) and its active metabolite desipramine (DES). Doxepin is also an option.

In addition to NE and 5HT reuptake inhibition, TCAs block other receptors, many of which contribute to the often dose-limiting side effect profile. Amitriptyline and NTP are more widely studied and more widely used than IMI and DES. Relative receptor blockade activity and their consequences are provided in Tables 29-6 and 29-7, respectively.

It is important to note that the TCAs may be fatal in overdose situations. Additionally, TCAs are associated with a prolongation of the QTc interval

Table 29-6   TCA Relative Receptor Blockade Profile

Drug	Muscarinic	Histamine 1	Alpha 1
Amitriptyline	4+	4+	3+
Nortriptyline	2+	1+	1+
Imipramine	2+	1+	3+
Desipramine	1+	1+	1+
Doxepin	3+	4+	2+

Adapted with permission from Kando JC, Wells BG, Hayes PE. Depressive disorders. In: DiPiro JT, Talbert RL, Yee GC, et al, eds. Pharmacotherapy: A Pathophysiologic Approach, 4th ed. Stamford, CT: Appleton & Lange; 1999:1141-60.

Table 29-7   Effects of Receptor Blockade (at "Therapeutic" Concentrations)

Muscarinic	Sedation, dryness of mucous membranes, constipation, urinary retention, memory impairment, blurred vision, decreased GI motility
Histamine 1	Sedation, weight gain
Alpha 1	Orthostasis, sedation, weight gain

and therefore must be used with caution in selected patients or when combined with various other drug regimens. Consider obtaining an ECG prior to and periodically (e.g., change in medical status, TCA dose increase, addition of other medications with similar cardiac effects) during TCA therapy. All TCAs are hepatically metabolized; use with caution in patients with severe liver dysfunction.

Venlafaxine has also been used in situations when TCAs are not an option (14). Venlafaxine blocks the reuptake of NE and 5HT similarly to the TCAs but does not bind to muscarinic, histamine1 or alpha1 receptors. It has a "cleaner" side effect profile, is better tolerated than the TCAs and seems to be without the TCA-associated cardiotoxicity. It *is,* however, associated with a dose-related idiosyncratic elevation of blood pressure.

Bupropion sustained-release (150 to 300 mg daily) is also an option for the treatment neuropathic pain (24). Bupropion blocks the reuptake of NE and dopamine but does not affect 5HT reuptake. It has a low affinity for muscarinic, histamine, or alpha-adrenergic receptors and is associated with fewer cardiovascular effects or sexual dysfunction. Common adverse effects include restlessness, anxiety, insomnia, dry mouth, weight loss, and dizziness. Bupropion is associated with a dose-related risk of seizures; use with caution if at all in patients with a history of seizures, those on concomitant medications that lower the seizure threshold, those with alcohol or illicit drug abuse and those with severe hepatic impairment. It is contraindicated in patients with seizure disorders or eating disorders (e.g., anorexia nervosa, bulimia).

The muscle relaxant cyclobenzaprine is chemically related to the TCAs and carries the same monitoring parameters. Adverse effects, including QT prolongation, are additive and therefore TCAs should not be used concurrently with cyclobenzaprine.

Dosing and Side-Effect Management

The onset of pain relief with all of the antidepressants is usually described in terms of weeks; the adverse effects may, however, occur within days.

The dose of paroxetine for adjunctive pain control is 30-70 mg daily (20). In older adults, initiate paroxetine at 10 mg/day and titrate upwards based upon clinical and adverse effects. Due to its short half-life (approximately 24 hours), withdrawal symptoms may emerge upon abrupt discontinuation. Nausea and diarrhea are common side effects associated with all SSRIs. Tolerance to these side effects usually develops. Dry mouth, drowsiness or restlessness (patient-specific), increased sweating and sexual dysfunction are side effects that may or may not resolve with continued dosing.

The TCAs should be initiated at a low dose (10 mg at bedtime) and depending upon the age and comorbid medical conditions of the patient, titrated to at least 50 mg or 75 mg (but usually no more than 150 mg) at bedtime. Younger adults (18-65 years old) often tolerate a titration of 25 mg every 5 days, older adults often require a week between dosage changes (22).

Venlafaxine should be started at 25-37.5 mg 1-2 times daily and may be titrated to 75 mg once or twice a day (14). Bupropion sustained release should be started at 150 mg per day for approximately one week, then increased if tolerated to 150 mg twice daily with at least 8 hours between administration times (24).

With any of the antidepressants, initiate a slower dose titration if side effects are bothersome. Additionally, the lowest effective dose can be more readily discovered with smaller incremental dose changes. Consider monitoring TCA blood concentrations if noncompliance, over-compliance or toxicity is suspected. Lab supplied target ranges are better correlated with antidepressant and toxic effects rather than pain effects.

Several of the TCA-associated side effects deserve special mention and may preclude use in certain patient populations. Constipation should be treated aggressively, as with the opioids; constipation potential with opioids and TCAs is additive. TCAs are often associated with a dose-related weight gain; patients should receive nutrition counseling and be encouraged to increase activity as appropriate for the condition. Meticulous dental hygiene is essential due to the anticholinergic effects on the mucous membranes; dental caries and infection may be consequences of neglect in this situation. Orthostasis may be dangerous and precipitate falls, especially upon arising during the sleeping hours. Counseling is essential. Urinary retention is also common and may be especially problematic in older males with benign prostatic hyperplasia. Never underestimate the associated car-diotoxicity or potentially lethal effects in an overdose situation.

Trazodone as adjunctive therapy for the treatment of insomnia is given in low doses of 25-100 mg. It is associated with priapism; appropriate coun-seling must be provided to the patient.

Selected Agents for Neuropathic Pain

A very large number of medications designed to treat other disorders from hypertension to seizures to schizophrenia have been shown in animals or humans to have at least short-term effect on pain. Some of the more com-monly used and more studied ones will be mentioned here. There is a dearth of information about how to prioritize prescription of these medica-tions. Most physicians choose medications based on side effects, familiarity, and cost. Others try the medications based on some theoretical sense of what pain pathway is most important, and still others will add one to an-other for a combined blockade of pain signals. Physicians are challenged to decide when the risk-benefit of the infinite number of drugs and drug com-binations is no longer in favor of the patient. In general titrating dosage of one medication at a time is the best plan.

Gabapentin

Originally studied and marketed as an adjunct to seizure control, gabapentin is now commonly used in the treatment of neuropathic pain, despite the lack of FDA approval for this indication. Gabapentin may be used in addition to or as a substitute for the use of antidepressants. Its mechanism of action is unclear. It appears to increase GABA synthesis and release but does not bind to GABA receptors, does not alter GABA reup-take or the metabolism of GABA, and has no apparent Na-channel block-ing effects. It may interact with NMDA receptors and appears to increase plasma 5HT concentrations. Gabapentin is not metabolized by the liver and therefore associated with fewer drug interactions. It is eliminated renally therefore the dose should be decreased in renal insufficiency. The most common dose-related side effects include drowsiness, edema, GI upset, dizziness, fatigue, and ataxia; the most common idiosyncratic reaction is weight gain. The dose should be titrated upwards, initiated at 100-300 mg daily (depending upon age and renal function) and titrated to *at least* 900 mg/day (depending on renal function) over a period of as little as a week, or as tolerated. The dose of gabapentin may be titrated as high as 3600 mg per day (depending upon renal function). Gabapentin displays saturable absorption kinetics, therefore single doses should be limited to approxi-mately 800 mg. Onset of effect is in weeks rather than days once a stable dose has been achieved. Abrupt discontinuation may precipitate seizures regardless of previous seizure history (16,21).

Other antiseizure medications have also been used in neuropathic pain but are beyond the scope of this chapter; the reader is referred to a thorough review by Tremont-Lukats et al. (25).

Case Study 29-2

A 45-year-old male with chronic lower back pain, and s/p several surgeries complains of severe burning pain radiating into both legs. He has no other medical problems and has normal renal and hepatic function. He took gabapentin (1800 mg/day) in the past that was stopped due to sedation. He currently takes long-acting morphine tablets 30 mg 3 times a day with little effect on the burning pain. The decision was made to add a low dose TCA to his morphine regimen. Although he is relatively young, he feared daytime sedation, so the drug was chosen and titrated as follows: NTP (less anticholinergic and antihistaminergic than AMT) 10 mg at bedtime (hs) for 1 week, 20 mg hs for 1 week, then 30 mg hs. At his next visit 1 month later, the patient refused to continue with the NTP due to the dry mouth and sedative effects. He was quickly tapered off the NTP over 1 week and started on a low dose of gabapentin, as it had previously provided relief. The dose was titrated upwards very slowly: 100 mg hs for 1 week, 200 mg hs for 2 weeks, 300 mg hs for 2 weeks, and increased by 100 mg every 2 weeks until therapeutic or adverse effects occurred. The dose was divided into 2 daily doses after 400 mg hs was reached. The patient achieved "good" pain control with no adverse effects at a dose of 400 mg morning and hs, a lower dose than his original 1800 mg/day.

Antiarrhythmics

Lidocaine and mexiletine are the two antiarrythmic agents most studied for neuropathic pain (22). Both block the Na channel and act as a membrane stabilizer to decrease abnormal neuronal firing. Lidocaine is not absorbed when given orally and parenteral administration is not practical for the management of chronic pain. It is, however, available as a patch to be applied topically to the skin for local absorption. It is most studied in acute postherpetic neuralgia, but has been used in selected situations on a chronic basis for other types of neuropathic pain. Up to 3 patches may be applied at one time (the patches may be cut) for a maximum of 12 hours within any 24-hour period. One must choose the patient wisely based upon comorbid medical conditions; monitor for signs and symptoms of systemic lidocaine toxicity (e.g., confusion, dizziness, drowsiness, vomiting, nervousness) (16).

Mexiletine is an oral agent chemically related to lidocaine. A baseline ECG is recommended prior to initiating mexiletine. This agent must be used with caution, if at all, if ECG abnormalities are present; it is contraindicated in patients with second or third degree heart block. The dose should be initiated at 150-200 mg once or twice daily and titrated slowly to a maximum of 1200 mg per day. Plasma concentrations should remain below 2 mcg/ml. Adverse effects include nausea, vomiting, heartburn, dizziness, tremor, headache and dose-related seizures. Mexiletine should be taken with food to minimize GI discomfort (22).

Drug-Drug Interactions

In addition to the well-known drug interactions with opioids (e.g., other CNS depressants, alcohol), many opioids are metabolized by the hepatic cytochrome P450 (CYP450) isoenzyme system and therefore are subject to interactions with other medications/substances that induce or inhibit these enzymes. The discussion of CYP450 drug interactions is beyond the scope of this chapter; the reader is referred to a complete review for more information (26). A brief comment follows.

The consequences of CYP450 inhibition can occur in two distinct fashions best shown by examples. Codeine, oxycodone, and hydrocodone exemplify the first and less common situation. Codeine's primary analgesic effects are due in part, to its hepatic metabolism by CYP450 2D6 to morphine (12); hydrocodone is metabolized by 2D6, in part, to hydromorphone (27); oxycodone is metabolized by 2D6, in part, to oxymorphone (12). In individuals with a genetic deficiency of 2D6 (e.g., 5-10% of the caucasian population), or in patients concurrently taking a medication that inhibits 2D6 (e.g., fluoxetine, paroxetine, sertraline, bupropion), the metabolism of codeine to morphine (or hydrocodone to hydromorphone or oxycodone to oxymorphone) cannot occur. Consequently, the patient may not achieve the expected clinical analgesic response.

In the second and more common situation, rather than decreased effects, one may see *increased* effects in the form of drug toxicity or the emergence of side effects. The interaction between TCAs and SSRIs provide an example. Again, if the patient is genetically deficient in CYP450 2D6 or if a 2D6 *inhibitor* is added to a regimen containing AMT, the metabolism of AMT is likely to decrease. As a result, the plasma concentrations of AMT may increase up to 4-fold and the patient may show clinical symptoms (ranging from discomfort to toxicity) not anticipated at this dose. This drug combination does not need to be avoided, but it must be considered in the following situations: when dosing the TCA , if the patient complains of side effects when least expected (may be isoenzyme deficient), or when other medications in the regimen are added or discontinued.

Enzyme *inducers* enhance the metabolic capability of a given isoenzyme. Drugs which are metabolized by this isoenzyme are metabolized much more rapidly, resulting in a decrease in plasma concentration and a decrease in clinical effects. For example, carbamazepine (cbz) induces the 3A4 enzyme, which is responsible for metabolizing methadone. If cbz is added to a stable methadone regimen, methadone plasma concentrations may fall resulting in a clinical loss of pain control.

Comorbid Conditions

Many other conditions affect pain perception. Depression is commonly present in chronic pain patients, not necessarily as a cause/effect relationship. Increased anxiety, regardless of cause, or disordered sleep also contribute to an increased perception of pain. These issues should be addressed concurrently to most efficiently and effectively provide optimal pain management. Chapters 27 and 28 describe the diagnosis and treatment of these conditions in the context of chronic pain. Pharmacological treatments of anxiety, depression, and sleep disorders are quite successful in chronic pain patients, but are beyond the scope of this book. The reader is referred to the ACP publication, *Depression* (28).

Recommendations

- *Above all, get to know your chronic pain patient.* Be honest in your expectations and be aware of the patient's expectations.
- From the beginning, set realistic target levels as goals for pain control and monitor frequently.
- Do not forget to have the patient sign the narcotic contract, and stay alert for drug-seeking behaviors.
- Opioids are the mainstay of pharmacologic treatment of chronic back pain, and although no one opioid is superior, optimal treatment will likely include a long-acting scheduled opioid with a short-acting opioid for prn use.
- For neuropathic pain components, add a TCA (unless contraindicated), preferably NTP (or AMT) and titrate.
- Venlafaxine or bupropion are also options for neuropathic pain. One may add gabapentin or substitute gabapentin for the antidepressant.
- A "trial and error" approach may be required to find the best medication/combination of medications for optimal pain control.

- Antidepressants and anticonvulsants should not be discontinued abruptly.
- Stay aware of potential drug interactions prophylactically and address comorbid conditions.

■   ■   ■

Key Points

- Make one change in drug therapy at a time to determine what change caused what effect.
- The objective of successful pain management is 24-hour pain control.
- Unless the pain is entirely neuropathic, start with a long-acting opioid analgesic dosed on a scheduled basis plus a short-acting opioid dose as needed for breakthrough pain.
- Methadone is usually best saved as a second or third option.
- Increase the dose of the maintenance opioid when use of the breakthrough opioid increases significantly.
- Add/use an antidepressant (TCA, venlafaxine, bupropion) or gabapentin (or other anti-seizure medication) for control of neuropathic pain.
- Be aware of all other drugs that the patient may be taking, tomonitor for drug and/or herbal interactions.
- Be aware of and treat comorbid conditions that affect pain perception, such as depression, anxiety, and sleep disorders.
- Monitor for drug seeking behaviors; intervene as needed.

■   ■   ■

REFERENCES

1. **Thornton D.** Psychological syndromes. In: Kanner R, ed. Pain Management Secrets. Philadelphia: Hanley and Belfus, Inc.; 1997:145-52.
2. **Savage S.** Opioid use in the management of chronic pain. Med Clin North Am. 1999;83:762-87.
3. **Marcus DA.** Treatment of nonmalignant chronic pain. Am Fam Phys. 2000;61:1331-8, 1345-6.
4. **Kaplan HI, Saddock BJ.** Substance-related disorders. In: Kaplan HI, Saddock BJ; eds. Synopsis of Psychiatry, 8th ed. Baltimore: Lippincott, Williams & Wilkins; 1998:375-456.
5. **Cooper E.** Regulatory issues. In: Kanner R, ed. Pain Management Secrets. Philadelphia: Hanley and Belfus, Inc.; 1997:242-6.
6. **Krames ES.** Rational use of opioids for nonmalignant pain. J Pharmaceutical Care Symptom Control. 1997;5:3-15.

7. **Joranson DE, Ryan KM, Gilson AM, Dahl JL.** Trends in medical use and abuse of opioid analgesics. JAMA. 2000;283:1710-14.

8. **Vaillancorut PD and Langeuin HM.** Painful peripheral neuropathies. Med Clin North Am. 1999;83:627-42.

9. **Department of Veterans Affairs, Ann Arbor Healthcare System.** Ann Arbor VA Healthcare System Pain Clinic, Policy on narcotic drugs for non-cancer pain. Ann Arbor, MI.

10. **Micromedex Healthcare Series.** Opioid Analgesics—Cross Allergenicity. Vol. 110. Drug Consults; 2001. Expires December 2001.

11. **American Geriatrics Society Panel on Chronic Pain in Older Persons.** The management of chronic pain in older persons. Clinical Practice Guidelines. J Am Geriatr Soc. 1998;46:635-51.

12. **Way WL, Fields HL, Schumacher MA.** Opioid analgesics and antagonists. In: Katzung BG; ed. Basic and Clinical Pharmacology, 8th ed. New York: McGraw-Hill; 2001: 512-31.

13. **Baker DE.** Meperidine: a drug past its prime. Hosp Pharm. 2001;36:1131-2.

14. **Sumpton JE, Moulin DE.** Treatment of neuropathic pain with venlafaxine. Ann Pharmacother. 2001;35:557-9.

15. **Department of Veterans Affairs.** Analgesic Pocket Card. Veterans In Partnership. VISN 11 Healthcare Network.

16. **Nissen D, ed.** Mosby's Drug Consult. St Louis: Mosby, Inc.; 2002.

17. **Manfredi PL, Gonzales GR, Cheville AL, Kornick C, Payne R.** Methadone analgesia in cancer pain patients on chronic methadone maintenance therapy. J Pain Symptom Manage. 2001;21:169-74.

18. **Kanner R.** Opioid analgesics. In: Kanner R; ed. Pain Management Secrets. Philadelphia: Hanley and Belfus, Inc.; 1997:172-5

19. **Herndon CM, Jackson III KC, Hallin PA.** Management of opioid-induced gastrointestinal effects in patients receiving palliative care. Pharmacotherapy. 2002;22:240-50.

20. **Sindrup SH.** Concentration-response relationship in paroxetine treatment of diabetic neuropathy symptoms: a patient-blinded dose-escalation study. Ther Drug Monit. 1991;13:408-14.

21. **Lackner TE.** Strategies for optimizing antiepileptic drugs therapy in elderly people. Pharmacotherapy. 2002;22:329-64.

22. **Guay DRP.** Adjunctive agents in the management of chronic pain. Pharmacotherapy. 2001;21:1070-81.

23. **Kando JC, Wells BG, Hayes PE.** Depressive disorders. In: DiPiro JT, Talbert RL, Yee GC, et al., eds. Pharmacotherapy: A Pathophysiologic Approach, 4th ed. Stamford, CT: Appleton & Lange; 1999;1141-60.

24. **Semenchuk MR, Sherman S, Davis B.** Double-blind, randomized trial of bupropion SR for the treamtnet of neuropathic pain. Neurology. 2001;57:1583-8.

25. **Tremont-Lukats IW, Megeff C, Backonja MM.** Anticonvulsants for neuropathic pain syndromes: mechanisms of action and place in therapy. Drugs. 2000;60:1029-52.

26. **Michalets EJ.** Update: clinically significant cytochrome P450 drug interactions. Pharmacotherapy. 1998;18:84-112.

27. **Otton SV, Schadel M, Cheung SW, Kaplan HL, Busto UE, Sellers EM.** CYP2D6 phenotype determines the metabolic conversion of hydrocodone to hydromorphone. Clin Pharmacol Ther. 1993;54:463-72.

28. **Levenson JL, ed.** Depression. Philadelphia: American College of Physicians; 2000.

30

■ ■ ■

Invasive Treatments for Chronic Pain

Oren Sagher, MD

A mong the most difficult decisions in the management of chronic low back pain is when to consider invasive treatments for intractable symptoms. Patients whose pain has failed to resolve with noninvasive measures and who continue to be disabled by it are among the most difficult patients to treat. The relevant questions in treating these patients are, therefore, not only which invasive measures to take, but whether to take them and when to take them. The following chapter will attempt to summarize some of the key points in invasive management of intractable pain. It is noteworthy that these surgical interventions are generally reserved for persons with very chronic pain, at least more than 6 months, both because of the invasiveness, expense, and permanence of some surgical treatments and because patients have seldom explored all reasonable noninvasive options before this time.

Case Study 30-1

A 45-year-old electrical engineer began to experience severe low back and flank pain 6 months ago. His pain was episodic and responded to oral opiates. A spine MRI revealed multilevel disk degeneration without frank herniation or nerve compression. A spinal cord stimulator was placed, and the patient did not achieve any benefit. Three months after placement of the stimulator, the patient was found to have nephrolithiasis. Upon treatment of his kidney stone, his pain completely resolved.

Case Studies 30-2 and 30-3

Neuropathic Pain

A 45-year-old electrician was severely shocked by a high-voltage line. Since his injury, he has been complaining of bilateral foot and leg pain, radiating to the buttocks. He characterizes his pain as "burning" and "stabbing" and likens it to a severe sunburn. His skin is sensitive to touch, and he is unable to wear socks due to painful hypersensitivity.

Nociceptive Pain

A 48-year-old woman with a history of gallbladder disease is diagnosed with chronic pancreatitis. She complains of severe epigastric pain radiating to the back. She characterizes the pain as "deep," "boring," and "aching."

Procedure Types in Invasive Management of Pain

Invasive treatments for managing chronic pain can be classified as either anatomic, ablative, or augmentative procedures. Anatomic procedures are those in which the cause of the pain can be successfully addressed. For example, in the setting of a lumbar radiculopathy due to herniated disk, surgical diskectomy carries with it a 90-95% chance of success. Decompressive laminectomy for spinal stenosis carries with it a similar success rate for neurogenic claudication. Similarly, pain due to major spinal instability is best dealt with using a spinal fusion. These anatomical procedures typically have the highest rate of success, but in the setting of chronic pain may not be applicable. By the time patients have become chronic, they have often either had a procedure or have been determined not to be a candidate for a procedure. Furthermore, chronic pain causes chemical and structural changes in the brain and spinal cord that may not respond to treatment of the mechanical cause as well as acute pain does.

Although anatomic procedures for relief of pain are clearly preferred when possible, one major caveat does exist. When pain has been present for a significant period of time, anatomic procedures have a significantly lower success rate. The lower rate of success in chronic pain may be related to changes in the central nervous system that sometimes accompany injury. (A detailed discussion of these surgical procedures is given in Chapter 22.)

Ablative procedures comprise those procedures that intentionally destroy nerves or other neurologic pathways thought to be involved in pain generation or transmission. These range in complexity from a simple nerve block to a cordotomy. The common thread of ablative procedures is the assumption that pain generated in a certain region is transmitted uniquely by the nerve or pathway being intentionally destroyed. In addition, success in ablative procedures depends on lack of return of the pain via other pathways. Ablative procedures, by and large, are thought to be irreversible. However, return of pain following such procedures is almost inevitable in the long term. The reason for late recurrences of pain following ablative procedures is believed to be related to elasticity within the nervous system.

Augmentative procedures comprise the third type of invasive treatment for chronic pain. These are procedures that modulate rather than destroy nervous tissue. Also called neuromodulation, these interventions attempt to alter the pain signal generated by injured tissue or nerves. Such procedures neither destroy nor repair nervous tissue and do not address the cause of the pain. In general terms, augmentative procedures consist of either electrical stimulation or intrathecal drug delivery. These procedures have gained prominence in the treatment of chronic pain in the past decade. Because of the variable course of pain syndromes and the frequent inability to treat its cause directly, augmentative procedures are often considered the most attractive options for treating patients with chronic, medically intractable pain.

Invasive procedures to treat pain must take into consideration the characteristics of the pain. For example, nociceptive pain syndromes are typically best treated by either ameliorating the tissue injury or disease (e.g., repairing a compressed vertebral body, removing a cancerous growth) or by use of intraspinal opioids. On the other hand, neuropathic pain syndromes are best treated by reducing the pathological, neural transmission. This may be accomplished using electrical stimulation. Mixed pain syndromes (pain syndromes that have both nociceptive and neuropathic components), which may be caused by failed back surgery syndrome, spinal fractures with spinal cord injury, and cancer invasion of the spinal column and nerves, may respond to intrathecal therapy. For mixed pain syndromes, choice of procedure type depends on the predominance of axial or appendicular pain.

Electrical Stimulation

Electrical stimulation of the nervous system arose as a direct consequence of the gate control theory of pain neurotransmission in 1965. In Melzack and Wall's gate control theory, there are postulated "gating" mechanisms located within the dorsal aspect of the spinal cord. In addition, Melzack and Wall postulated that the supraspinal centers have a direct modulating influence upon these gates, perhaps through dorsal column pathways. Two years after the initial publication of the gate control theory, Norman Shealy reported clinical trials of attempts to reduce pain using artificial stimulation of the dorsal aspect of the spinal cord (1). Believed to work via antidromic stimulation of the dorsal columns, spinal cord stimulation soon became popular in the treatment of many different types of pain. However, initial results were mixed and spinal cord stimulation fell out of favor. A resurgence in interest followed the observation that spinal cord stimulation is quite effective in the treatment of neuropathic pain.

Although the physiological mechanisms underlying spinal cord stimulation remain somewhat controversial, it is generally believed that electrical stimulation alters ascending output from the dorsal horn. There is evidence that stimulation may work through a conduction block via A-beta fiber stimulation. There is also evidence for activation of fibers outside the dorsal columns or sympathetic fiber activation. In addition, there is evidence for supraspinal mediation of the effects of spinal cord stimulation. It is generally agreed, however, that there is no known role for endogenous opioid release induced by spinal cord stimulation. For example, administration of the opioid antagonist, naloxone, does not diminish the analgesic effect of spinal cord stimulation (2). Taken together, these lines of evidence suggest that, while electrical stimulation alters central processing of pain signals, as of yet there is no known single physiological mechanism underlying this effect (3).

Despite the questions and controversies concerning the mechanisms of electrical stimulation, a few practical considerations are worthwhile noting. First, in order for electrical stimulation to work, there is need for intact A-beta fibers. In other words, a complete neurologic injury will not permit successful spinal cord stimulation to be performed. Therefore, a completely anesthetic but painful extremity will not generally respond to electrical stimulation of the nerves or spinal cord. In addition, stimulation is best performed rostral to the level of injury, in order to allow modulation of the neural signals from the dorsal horn to higher centers. Another practical consideration is that appendicular pain is most likely to be effectively addressed. Axial stimulation is difficult to achieve, possibly due to the size and location of those nerve fibers subserving sensation around the spine. The third and most important practical consideration is that stimulation in general works best on neuropathic pain rather than nociceptive pain. The reasons for this are not clear and largely experiential. However, this predilection may have to do with the possible amelioration of aberrant neuronal signaling that accompanies nerve injury. The nature of electrical stimulation is that it does not completely eliminate pain sensation, but a more pleasant sensation may substitute for much of the pain.

Clinical series of spinal cord stimulation have reported success rates averaging approximately 55% over the long term (4-14). Table 30-1 summarizes the results of several large studies performed over the past decade.

Outcomes from spinal cord stimulation have recently been compared to reoperation for back and lower extremity pain. Bell et al. in 1997 conducted a prospective study of 45 patients with symptoms recurrent following lumbar diskectomy. All patients were found to have new, operable lesions on their imaging studies. These patients were then randomized to either spinal cord stimulation or re-operation, and were followed over a mean of three years. At six months, the patients were afforded the opportunity to voluntarily cross over to the other treatment group. The crossover rate from reoperation to spinal cord stimulation was 54%, whereas crossover from spinal cord stimulation to reoperation occurred in only 21% of patients. In those patients who primarily underwent spinal cord stimulation, 47% reported significant relief over a mean of three years. Those reoperated primarily had significant relief only 12% of the time. Of those who crossed over to a secondary treatment group, 33% experienced pain relief

Table 30-1   Spinal Cord Stimulation Series

Series	Year	% of Patients with Failed Back Surgery	No. Patients	F/U (Years)	% Success
Probst	1990	100	112	4.5	67
Kumar	1991	55	121	3.3	52
Simpson	1991	12	60	2.4	47
LeDoux	1993	100	19	2	74
North	1993	75	171	7.1	52
Broggi	1994	45	410	2	58
Kupers	1994	Not specified	70	3.5	52
Meglio	1994	100	33	3.8	40
Lazorthes	1995	44	692	10	53
Lang	1997	89	200	4	53
Kumar	1998	49	235	6.5	59

using spinal cord stimulation, but no patient experienced sufficient pain relief after crossing over into the re-operation group. The study also examined cost data for both treatment groups. Spinal cord stimulation fared favorably in this analysis as well, costing $31,655 per patient, whereas re-operation cost $40,490 per patient in medical care (15). This important study underscores the potential usefulness of electrical stimulation in treatment of low back pain as much as it does the apparent futility of reoperation.

Although we have been using spinal cord stimulation as a primary example of electrical stimulation therapy, it is worthwhile noting that other forms of electrical stimulation do exist. Peripheral nerve stimulation functions with many of the same patients. However, it is usually reserved for pain due to injury to a specific peripheral nerve. Deep brain stimulation is also a form of electrical stimulation therapy. Although no longer routinely performed in the United States, thalamic and periventricular stimulation may hold promise in the treatment of some of the most intractable of deafferentation pain syndromes, such as central post-stroke pain. With recent favorable experience using deep brain stimulation for movement disorders, it is likely that deep brain stimulation for pain will eventually find a role in the treatment of chronic pain once again.

Case Study 30-4

A 54-year-old auto worker was injured on the job 5 years ago. He experienced low back pain and left leg pain and was found to have a herniated L5/S1 disk. After his surgery, he began to experience a burning sensation in his left leg and foot. His back pain was somewhat improved, but his left lower extremity discomfort overwhelmed any efforts at rehabilitation. He found TENS helpful, but could not cover the entire region of his pain. Medical treatment with gabapentin and amitryptiline was complicated by side effects. MRI of his spine demonstrated postoperative scar. He underwent insertion of a spinal cord stimulator lead, which provided him with a vibrating sensation in his left leg, and was associated with a 70% reduction in his pain.

Intrathecal Drug Therapy

Although electrical stimulation offers a great deal of potential benefit to those patients with neuropathic appendicular pain, a significant number of patients would not benefit from such therapy because of the prominent nociceptive component to their pain or overwhelming axial pain. In such patients, systemic opioids may be used, but may be complicated by central side effects, such as sedation. Intrathecal therapy using permanently implanted pumps may offer patients a delivery mechanism for morphine with a greater therapeutic window. Implanted pumps were first devised for treatment of patients with pain due to cancer. However, in recent years, use of these pumps has increased dramatically in the treatment of non-malignant pain syndromes such as low back pain. The mechanisms underlying intrathecal therapy consist of a localized delivery of the medication into the lumbar subarachnoid space, bypassing the blood-brain barrier and offering a concentration gradient of medication near the tip of the catheter. This is particularly useful for the treatment of low back pain, where the presumed generator of pain lies within the lumbar enlargement of the spinal cord. The ability of this therapy to bypass processing via the blood-brain barrier for its effect allows medications delivered using this therapy to be administered at much lower doses and to reduce concentrations of these potentially sedating medications in the brain.

The advantages and disadvantage of delivery of medications via implanted intrathecal pumps are shown in Table 30-2.

Table 30-2　Advantages and Disadvantages of Intrathecal Medications

Advantages Versus Systemic Delivery	*Advantages Versus Epidural Delivery*
• Around-the-clock dosing	• Totally implanted technology
• Direct delivery	• Long-term infusions
• Low systemic concentrations	• Predictable concerntration gradients
• Wide therapeutic window	

Disadvantages
- Need for a surgical procedure
- Placement of a foreign body
- Need for maintenance and reoperation
- Expense of therapy

In general, intrathecal therapy is indicated primarily for nociceptive or mixed pain syndromes. In addition, intrathecal therapy should be limited to those patients who have experienced significant side effects with adequate systemic administration of opioids. Patients undergoing intrathecal therapy should first have a successful trial of intraspinal administration of morphine. Since intrathecal pumps are purely delivery mechanisms, they are subject to the same issues of tolerance seen in systemic administration. Therefore, conerns regarding tolerance and addiction are as relevant with intrathecal therapy as they are with systemic opioids.

It is common practice to screen patients for psychological disturbances prior to implantation of intrathecal pumps. Although it is generally agreed that active, major psychopathology contraindicates intrathecal pump placement (as well as any other invasive therapies), it has never been shown that minor psychopathology has any influence on outcomes in intrathecal therapy. In general, however, major depressive illness or untreated psychopathology are contraindications for intrathecal therapy.

Intrathecal morphine therapy has generally been associated with success rates in the neighborhood of 60-70%, when success is defined as greater than 50% relief of pain (16-21). There is a significant reduction in success rate over time, however, and it is clear that tolerance plays a major role in long term failures of this therapy. It should be no surprise, therefore, that cancer pain continues to be the more promising of indications for intrathecal therapy. Table 30-3 summarizes the results from major clinical series over the past decade.

Intrathecal drug therapy is a rather expensive treatment for patients with chronic pain. The cost-effectiveness of this therapy has been examined in two studies. Bedder et al. looked at the cost of intrathecal morphine therapy compared to the cost of an external epidural pump for patients with cancer pain. This study found that the intrathecal pump cost averaged $1300/month, whereas epidural delivery costs were $2900/month. De Lissovoy et al. examined the issue in a mathematical model that took into consideration complication rates of the therapy, as well as the cost of medical care either with or without the intrathecal pump. This study concluded that even in the absence of repeat spine surgery (which many patients with

Table 30-3   Intrathecal Pump Series

Series	Year	% Relief/Success
Paice	1996	62
Winkelmuller	1996	58
Tutak	1996	77
Angel	1998	67
Anderson	1999	50
Kumar	2001	58

chronic back pain undergo), intrathecal drug therapy proved less expensive over the long term ($1382/month vs. $1420/month in health care costs with and without the pump, respectively). These studies suggest that intrathecal drug delivery, though expensive, does provide a cost-effective solution for patients with intractable pain.

As of the writing of this book, only morphine is approved by the U.S. Food and Drug Administration for use in intrathecal pumps for treatment of pain. Despite this, off-label use of other opioids such as hydromorphone and the use of adjunct analgesics such as bupivacaine and clonidine are rather commonplace. The use of secondary agents has been fueled by long-term failures using morphine monotherapy. However, the role of these medications is, as yet, unclear.

Case Study 30-5

A 70-year-old woman has had severe osteoporosis and a history of multiple vertebral compression fractures. She had severe low back pain and was unable to tolerate oral narcotics due to sedation. She underwent a trial intraspinal injection of morphine and experienced near-total relief of her pain for a period of 12 hours. Following placement of an intrathecal pump, she has been receiving intrathecal morphine. Her dose requirement has escalated from 1 mg/day to 5 mg/day now 2 years after implantation. She states that she obtains greater than 50% reduction in her pain and is able to be more active since her pump was implanted. She still takes occasional low-dose oral opiates for breakthrough pain.

Ablative Procedures

The role of ablative procedures in the management of chronic low back pain is rather limited. The tendency for pain to recur following ablation is troublesome, and ablation of major sensory nerves carries with it morbidity many would find unacceptable. In addition, chronic pain is rarely limited to the distribution of a single nerve. Neurectomies of large nerves, therefore, have no significant role in the management of chronic pain.

Unlike the morbidity associated with ablation of large nerves, the morbidity of ablation of smaller nerves may have therapeutic benefit in the management of chronic back pain. Ablation of the small, sensory rami to the facet joints (facet rhizolysis) is a useful intervention in the management of low back pain related to facet arthropathy. Facet rhizolysis is usually accomplished percutaneously using radiofrequency current. The success rate of facet rhizolysis in the relief of chronic low back pain reportedly ranges from 40% to 70% (22,23,24).

Case Study 30-6

A 67-year-old farmer has had insidious onset of low back pain over the past 5 years. His pain has been fairly positional and is greatly relieved by lying down. Physical examination disclosed tenderness over the right paraspinous region, exacerbated by turning. A CT scan of the lumbar spine demonstrated hypertrophic L4/5 facet joints, with no evidence of malalignment or instability. A facet injection provided him with temporary, near-total relief of his pain. Facet rhizolysis was performed, and his pain has been significantly improved.

Conclusion

The most important step in successful treatment of pain is an accurate diagnosis of the cause. Regardless of whether of the cause of pain is treatable, simply stating that a patient has pain is not sufficient for adequate treatment. The treatment that ensues should then follow an orderly progression of rationally chosen interventions. The three most important questions in considering invasive treatment are as follows.

1. *Should invasive treatments be used?* When conservative treatments for low back pain fail to provide adequate relief, invasive treatments may be appropriate. It is not appropriate, however, to consider these treatments as an alternative to less invasive measures such as physical therapy and medical treatment. Patients who have untreated, major psychopathology are also poor candidates for invasive treatments. Finally, since many invasive treatments require active patient participation (e.g., programming of electrical stimulation), they should be reserved for patients who are able to understand and participate in the treatment regimen.

2. *Which invasive treatment should be used?* The answer to this question hinges on the cause and characteristics of the pain. Nociceptive pain is usually responsive to opioids, but does not usually respond to electrical stimulation. Therefore, intrathecal morphine therapy is best suited for this type of pain. On the other hand, neuropathic pain responds best to electrical stimulation. In patients who have mixed (nociceptive and neuropathic) pain, the choice of procedure type usually depends on the predominance of axial or appendicular pain. Ablative procedures are rarely performed for chronic low back pain. The use of facet rhizolysis should be reserved for those patients who exhibit facet pain and who have obvious facet arthropathy.

3. *When should invasive procedures be used?* These treatments should be undertaken for chronic pain only when more conservative interventions

(such as medical therapy, TENS unit, physical therapy) have failed to provide adequate relief.

■   ■   ■

Recommendations

- Invasive procedures should be considered only when more conservative measures have failed.
- Electrical stimulation therapy may be considered for patients with neuropathic pain. This therapy is most effective in those with appendicular pain.
- Electrical stimulation should not be used in patients without intact A-beta fibers (i.e., a complete neurologic injury), those with predominantly axial pain, and those with nociceptive pain.
- Intrathecal drug therapy is indicated primarily for nociceptive or mixed pain syndromes. This therapy should be reserved for patients with nociceptive, opioid-sensitive pain who have dose-limiting systemic side effects.
- Patients who are to undergo intrathecal therapy should first have successful trial of intraspinal administration of morphine.
- Intrathecal drug therapy should not be used in patients with active, major psychopathology, major depressive illness, or untreated minor psychopathology.
- In patients with mixed pain syndrome, the choice of procedure usually depends on whether the pain is predominantly axial or appendicular.
- For low back pain related to facet arthropathy, facet rhizolysis (an ablative procedure) may be helpful.

■   ■   ■

Key Points

- Successful invasive therapy for pain relies on an accurate diagnosis.
- Pain should be clearly chronic before considering invasive treatments.
- Classification of pain into neuropathic and nociceptive types guides invasive therapy.
- Invasive treatments for chronic pain may be classified as anatomic, ablative, or augmentative (e.g., electrical stimulation therapy and intrathecal drug therapy).
- Anatomic procedures thave a lower success rate in patients with chronic pain than in those with subacute pain.

- Electrical stimulation therapy works by altering (rather than eliminating) the pain signal that is generated. This therapy is best used in neuropathic pain syndromes.
- Intrathecal therapy offers localized delivery of the drug, bypassing the blood-brain barrier, widening the therapeutic window.
- The role of ablative procedures in treating chronic low back pain is limited.

■   ■   ■

REFERENCES

1. **Shealy CN, Mortimer JT, et al.** Electrical inhibition of pain by stimulation of the dorsal columns: preliminary clinical report. Anesth Analg. 1967;46:489-91.
2. **Freeman TB, Campbell JN, Long DM.** Naloxone does not affect pain relief induced by electrical stimulation in man. Pain. 1983;17:189-95.
3. **Stanton-Hicks M, Salamon J.** Stimulation of the central and peripheral nervous system for the control of pain. J Clin Neurophysiol. 1997;14:46-62.
4. **Probst, C.** Spinal cord stimulation in 112 patients with epi-/intradural fibrosis following operation for lumbar disc herniation. Acta Neurochir. 1990;107:147-51.
5. **Kumar K, Nath R, Wyant GM.** Treatment of chronic pain by epidural spinal cord stimulation: a 10-year experience. J Neurosurg. 1991;75:402-7.
6. **Simpson BA.** Spinal cord stimulation in 60 cases of intractable pain. J Neurol Neurosurg Psychiatry. 1991;54:196-9.
7. **LeDoux MS, Langford KH.** Spinal cord stimulation for the failed back syndrome. Spine. 1993;18:191-4.
8. **North RB, Kidd DH, Zahurak M, James CS, Long DM.** Spinal cord stimulation for chronic, intractable pain: experience over two decades. Neurosurgery. 1993;32:384-94, discussion 394-5.
9. **Broggi G, Servello D, Dones I, Carbone G.** Italian multicentric study on pain treatment with epidural spinal cord stimulation. Stereotact Funct Neurosurg. 1994;62:273-8.
10. **Kupers RC, Van den Oever R, Van Houdenhove B, Vanmechelen W, Hepp B, Nuttin B, et al.** Spinal cord stimulation in Belgium: a nation-wide survey on the incidence, indications and therapeutic efficacy by the health insurer. Pain. 1994;56:211-6.
11. **Meglio M, Cioni B, Visocchi M, Tancredi A, Pentimalli L.** Spinal cord stimulation in low back and leg pain. Stereotact Funct Neurosurg. 1994;62:263-6.
12. **Lazorthes Y, Siegfried J, Verdie JC, Casaux J.** Chronic spinal cord stimulation in the treatment of neurogenic pain. Cooperative and retrospective study on 20 years of follow-up. Neurochirurgie. 1995;41:73-86, discussion 87-8.
13. **Lang P.** The treatment of chronic pain by epidural spinal cord stimulation—a 15 year follow up; present status. Axone. 1997;18:71-3.
14. **Kumar K, Toth C, Nath RK, Laing P.** Epidural spinal cord stimulation for treatment of chronic pain—some predictors of success. A 15-year experience. Surg Neurol. 1998;50:110-20, discussion 120-1.

15. **Bell GK, Kidd D, North RB.** Cost-effectiveness analysis of spinal cord stimulation in treatment of failed back surgery syndrome. J Pain Symptom Manage. 1997;13:286-95.

16. **Paice JA, Penn RD, Shott S.** Intraspinal morphine for chronic pain: a retrospective, multicenter study. J Pain Symptom Manage. 1996;11:71-80.

17. **Tutak U, Doleys DM.** Intrathecal infusion systems for treatment of chronic low back and leg pain of non-cancer origin. South Med J. 1996;89:295-300.

18. **Winkelmuller M, Winkelmuller W.** Long-term effects of continuous intrathecal opioid treatment in chronic pain of nonmalignant etiology. J Neurosurg. 1996;85:458-67.

19. **Angel IF, Gould HJ Jr, Carey ME.** Intrathecal morphine pump as a treatment option in chronic pain of nonmalignant origin. Surg Neurol. 1998;49:92-8, discussion 98-9.

20. **Anderson VC, Burchiel KJ.** A prospective study of long-term intrathecal morphine in the management of chronic nonmalignant pain. Neurosurgery. 1999;44:289-300, discussion 300-1.

21. **Kumar K, Kelly M, Pirlot T.** Continuous intrathecal morphine treatment for chronic pain of nonmalignant etiology: long-term benefits and efficacy. Surg Neurol. 2001;55:79-86, discussion 86-8.

22. **North RB, Han M, Zahurak M, Kidd DH.** Radiofrequency lumbar facet denervation: analysis of prognostic factors. Pain. 1994;57:77-83.

23. **Cho J, Park YG, Chung SS.** Percutaneous radiofrequency lumbar facet rhizotomy in mechanical low back pain syndrome. Stereotact Funct Neurosurg. 1997;68:212-7.

24. **Tzaan WC, Tasker RR.** Percutaeous radiofrequency facet rhizotomy—experience with 118 procdedures and reappraisal of its value. Can J Neurol Sci. 2000;27:125-30.

■   ■   ▓

KEY REFERENCES

Anderson VC, Burchiel KJ. A prospective study of long-term intrathecal morphine in the management of chronic nonmalignant pain. Neurosurgery. 1999;44:289-300.

Bell GK, Kidd D, North RB. Cost-effectiveness analysis of spinal cord stimulation in treatment of failed back surgery syndrome. J Pain Symptom Manage. 1997;13:286-95.

Stanton-Hicks M, Salamon J. Stimulation of the central and peripheral nervous system for the control of pain. J Clin Neurophysiol. 1997;14:46-62.

31

Alternative and Complementary Therapies

Susan Schmitt, MD
Kimberly Ivy

lternative therapies have gained increasing popularity in the past decade. In 1993, the *New England Journal of Medicine* published a study showing that one out of three Americans uses some form of alternative health care (1). As many as one third of medical schools now offer courses in alternative medicine (2). In 1992, the National Institutes of Health (NIH) formed the Office of Alternative Medicine (OAM) for purposes of researching the benefits of alternative medicine (3). For many physicians and nonphysicians alike, however, alternative medicine is still considered experimental, and of these, several view alternative treatment with suspicion and skepticism. This is despite the fact that numerous research studies have now shown the benefit of chiropractic, massage therapy, acupuncture, therapeutic touch and many other methods of alternative care. As recently as 1971, the American Medical Association (AMA) had a "Committee on Quackery" that declared as one of its missions to "contain" and then "eliminate" the practice of chiropractic. It was not until 1991 that a U.S. District Court in Illinois, ruling on *Wilk et al. v. the American Medical Association*, forced an end to this mission (4). Fortunately, times are slowly changing due in part to the rising health care costs and the public demand for alternative methods and greater freedom of choice. Today, alternative medicine treatments are becoming increasingly popular and are being used for almost every health condition.

Before one can understand how alternative methods might offer relief for back pain, it is imperative to understand a few fundamental differences between conventional medicine and alternative medicine. Conventional medicine today views disease as a biochemical phenomenon that can be diagnosed through technological means and then treated, where possible, through standardized and objective means (5). Two important intellectual currents contributed to this viewpoint: Newtonian physics and Cartesian dualism (5). Newtonian physics breaks the entire universe into building blocks that follow basic laws. Cartesian dualism asserts that the mind and body exist and function separately. This assertion splits the outer (objective) world from the inner (subjective) world. The biochemical model discounts the individual's mental, emotional and spiritual realities from disease and health (5). This is fundamentally different from most alternative approaches whereby the entire individual (mind and body) is taken into consideration. The biochemical model relies on a scientific explanation for disease and its treatment. Disease is viewed as an "outside" invader that attacks some part of the body. Treatment is then aimed at the invader.

The hallmark of alternative medicine is the viewpoint of holism. In this paradigm, disease is viewed as having multiple causes that are amenable to multiple therapeutic interventions that include many systems of care including biochemical, environmental, social, psychological, behavioral, and spiritual (5). The mind and body are not separate but integrally connected. A condition such as chronic pain or arthritis is viewed as having many causes and amenable to many different interventions, all of which have the common goal of restoring balance to the whole person on many levels (mental, emotional and psychological). Many alternative methods share common assumptions: something within the body is constricted or blocked, the body is not fixed and rigid but rather is changeable and can be educated, and the body is the place for transformation (6).

A report from the NIH on alternative systems of care concluded that there are seven major fields of holistic care:

1. Mind-body interventions (biofeedback, yoga, prayer)
2. Bioelectromagnetics (electroacupuncture, Reiki, polarity therapy)
3. Alternative systems (traditional Chinese medicine, acupuncture, Native American medicine, homeopathic medicine)
4. Manual healing methods (osteopathic, chiropractic, massage)
5. Pharmalogical and biological treatments (chelation therapy, cartilage products)
6. Herbal medicine (Native American herbs, Chinese herbs, Ayurvedic herbs)
7. Diet and nutrition.

Worldwide, 70-90% of individuals use holistic or alternative methods, whereas only 10-30% use biochemical methods (7).

The number of different alternative practices is extensive and to fully understand a particular method is beyond the scope of this chapter. However, the following paragraphs will provide a brief overview of several of the more popular alternative methods that have been commonly used in the treatment of low back pain. This list is by no means exhaustive and the reader is encouraged to learn about other methods of alternative care-not only from other material but also by actively inquiring of patients about what is working. After all, holism emphasizes the role of the patient including his or her beliefs in health and healing. It is important when reading this chapter to remember that these methods view the body and the mind from a different paradigm. Back pain is not viewed as an anatomical deviation from the normal such as a slipped disc or lumbar strain. Rather, the entire person is taken into consideration including lifestyle, habits, diet, stress level, sleep patterns, pain patterns, perception of self, emotional state, spiritual beliefs, and so on. The holistic model searches for an imbalance among these variables that contributes ultimately to the pathological process. And in some cases like acupuncture, the paradigm includes entirely different systems of belief that include meridians and organ systems for which there is no counterpart in the biochemical models.

Manipulative Medicine

The movement of vertebrae and other bones has been an integral part of therapeutic systems in many cultures for thousands of years, including those of Chinese and Ayurvedic medicine. Interestingly, it was also a part of Hippocratic practice in the fourth century BC (8). Andrew Taylor Still is considered the father of osteopathic medicine, and Daniel David Palmer is considered the father of chiropractic. From the Greek, *osteo* means "bone" and *pathos* means "suffering" or "disease." Andrew Still, who lost several family members to meningitis and pneumonia, was deeply disturbed by the inadequacies of contemporary medicine. Initially, he turned to magnets (popularized by Mesmer's work) where he learned about magnetic imbalances. He later expanded these ideas and came to believe that the body's imbalances came from impeded blood flow. By flexing, extending and realigning the spine, he observed that blood flow could be restored to restricted areas. He founded, in 1892, the American School of Osteopathy in Missouri (8).

David Palmer was a grocer and magnetic healer. He discovered that by using thrusting maneuvers of the thoracic spine, he was able to restore the hearing of a janitor by the name of Harvey Lillard. Thus he founded chiropractic and eventually Palmer College, the first chiropractic school (from the Greek *cheir,* "hand," and *praxis,* "practice"). Palmer believed that by correcting imbalances in the spine called subluxations or partial displacements, pressure could be relieved from nervous tissue (8).

Over the years, osteopathy and chiropractic have fought hard to distinguish themselves from one another in their philosophy and techniques. However, both believe that structural abnormalities in the spine and joints affect nerves and blood flow, which in turn affects the internal organs and the musculoskeletal system. Osteopathic training today, unlike the past, is very similar to allopathic training except that students also learn the art of manipulation. Chiropractic training takes four years and today includes a basic science curriculum (anatomy, physiology and so on); however, the clinical training is quite different. Chiropractors are not licensed to perform surgery or prescribe medication. Numerous research studies have found spine manipulations to be helpful for a variety of back conditions (8).

Osteopathic and chiropractic manipulations are used in a variety of back conditions. It has become common practice for chiropractors to combine massage therapy prior to chiropractic manipulations in order to reduce muscle tension. For acute conditions, patients typically undergo chiropractic manipulation 3-5 times per week for several weeks, then tapering to 1-3 times per week. For spine maintenance, chiropractors advocate at least one time per month. To date, studies are lacking which could guide the referring practitioner to know how many visits per week are optimal or how best to combine such manipulations with physical therapy.

Touch/Massage

Touch is an integral part of life and, it can be argued, even essential to survival. Studies by Rene Spitz in the 1930s, and others, have shown the effects on growth and development in young infants deprived of touch. It has been documented that infants denied a period of initial contact by their mothers after delivery develop more childhood illnesses (8). Massage is one of the best known and most widely used of the touch therapies. Like chiropractic, massage was considered suspect for many years and in addition was often associated with sex parlors. Swedish massage is the best known of the massage styles and is done primarily for relaxation. Per Ling of Sweden developed this style, which consists of five basic strokes that he borrowed from similar approaches of the ancient Chinese methods (8). Massage includes many different styles such as sports massage, lymphatic massage, and pregnancy massage. However, there are numerous other techniques, which include Western contemporary therapies (trigger point therapy, craniosacral therapy, Trager Integration) and structural techniques (Rolfing, Hellerwork, Aston-Patterning, myofascial release). Rolfing, founded by Ida Rolf (whose backround includes biochemistry, yoga and osteopathic manipulations), developed a technique for manipulating the fascial or connective tissue layers. Photographs are routinely taken of the client before and after a series of ten basic sessions to show the remarkable changes in posture (9). Joseph Heller, a longtime student of Ida Rolf and former president of the Rolf Institute, devised his own system for rebalancing the whole body. This system combines his knowledge of connective tissue manipulation with movement reeducation and verbal dialogue (which assists the client in recognizing the relationship of body, emotions and attitudes) (9). Other hands-on therapies combine different elements of touch and energy work such as Shiatsu. Shiatsu is a Japanese technique of finger pressure which combines Western anatomy, Buddhist philosophy, and acupoint therapy (9). Only recently have clinical studies of these many different techniques come out. Although some do show favorable outcomes for some of the techniques, it is exceedingly difficult to standardize the treatment, obtain a homogenous subject population, and provide an alternative or placebo treatment that has a similar attention effect.

Acupuncture

Thousands of years older than all of Western medicine is acupuncture. Curiosity about acupuncture first appeared in the United States in the early 1970s when the political relationship between the United States and China began changing and there was an increasing exchange of information. At that time, the press reported anecdotal stories of surgery being performed without the use of general anesthesia (10). In the past 30 years, acupuncture has become increasingly popular as a valid means of medical care for a variety of diseases and conditions. The NIH has reported that studies on acupuncture produce measurable physiological changes. These include release of endogenous opiates, counter irritant, autonomic, and other effects that lend credibility to the use of acupuncture in the Western world. There are many different styles of acupuncture (with different philosophies), but the most common style in the United States is TCM, or traditional Chinese medicine.

Philosophy of Traditional Chinese Medicine

Critical to understanding this style of acupuncture is to understand the philosophy of traditional Chinese medicine, which emphasizes the nature of the symptom to the whole person. A case of shingles on the trunk is treated differently in Chinese medicine than a case of shingles on the face, although both are from the same virus (10). A perplexing question asked by most Westerners is: How could both systems of medicine be clinically effective when both are so radically different in their assessment and treatment approach (10)?

Chinese medicine is deeply rooted in fundamental principles of Taoist philosophy and yin/yang theory. This theory is based on the construct of two complementary opposites. Yin and yang also represent a system of thought in which all things are seen as parts of a whole. Nothing exists separate from itself but is integrally connected to the whole. Thus disease is not seen as an isolated invader to the body but rather as having a relationship to the whole person. Chinese medicine does not focus on a particular disease that, in linear progression, leads to an illness. Instead, it focuses on the relationship between symptoms and the individual (10).

The highly developed disciplines of biology, physiology, and biochemistry that make up the foundation of the biochemical model have little to do with Chinese medicine. Instead, the Chinese have an elaborate system of organizing signs and symptoms. They look for imbalances of yin and yang which make the body susceptible to environmental influences. To understand their model of disease, it is important to have a brief understanding of their concepts of body substances, meridians and organ systems (10).

Chinese medicine views anatomy differently than does the West. Organs are not seen as fixed structures but instead as dynamic functions. For example, the Chinese describe the liver by the functions that go with it and not as an organ located in the abdomen. The Chinese believe there are five fundamental substances: Qi, Blood, Jing, Shen, and Fluids. Qi is fundamental to Chinese thought and has no counterpart in Western medicine. Qi resides in everything but it is not material nor is it merely energy (although it is often translated as such). The understanding of Qi is complex as there are many forms and it has many functions. When Qi is out of balance such as deficiency of Qi or stagnation of Qi, a person's health suffers (10).

Chinese medicine describes Blood as the fluid that circulates continuously throughout the body in blood vessels and meridians to provide nourishment to the body. Blood disharmonies include either Blood deficiency (which can lead to pale or dry skin and dizziness, among other things) or congealed Blood (which can lead to sharp, stabbing pain) (10).

Jing (translated as essence) is the substance that underlies all organic life and is derived from parental Jing and from food. Jing plays an integral role in development from conception to death. Shen is described as spirit. It is the vitality behind Qi and Jing. Meridians are the pathways in the body that carry Qi and Blood. They are not physical entities such as blood vessels. Meridians are the link between the five fundamental substances and the organs (10).

When the body is out of balance or when yin and yang are in disharmony, the body becomes susceptible to environmental factors known as the six pernicious influences, which can invade the body and create illness. These factors are wind, cold, heat, dampness, dryness and summer heat. According to Chinese medicine, several common causes of low back pain include kidney deficiency, Qi and Blood stagnation, liver Qi stagnation, spleen Qi deficiency and wind-cold-damp invasion (10). A diagnosis is made after a thorough history including an exhaustive review of systems and a physical exam. The most important parts of the physical exam include an inspection of the tongue and palpation of the twelve different pulses (six from each wrist). The mainstay of treatment is combination of acupuncture and herbs. It is only in the West that we have separated the two. Physicians who have taken acupuncture courses over a period of 2-3 years are often taught only acupuncture and not the use of herbs.

Techniques

Acupuncture includes many different techniques; needling, moxibustion (the burning of herbs on the affected area of the body), cupping, scraping, massage known as "tu ina" (which includes chiropractic in China), nutrition and Qigong. Other styles of acupuncture include Korean, Vietnamese, Japanese, 5-Elemental acupuncture, and electroacupuncture.

TCM training in the United States takes 4 years and includes study in both acupuncture and herbs followed by a national board exam in some states. Acupuncture sessions typically last 45-60 minutes. A practitioner may defer on prescribing herbs if a patient is taking coumadin, seizure medication, lanoxin, or other medications that require blood level monitoring. Side effects are usually minimal and include needle discomfort, local needle bruising, vasovagal response and minimal local skin bleeding. The depth of needle insertion depends on the style of acupuncture and the site to be needled. Acute conditions are felt to be easier to treat than chronic conditions. For an acute condition, treatment may be recommended every 1-3 days. Chronic conditions are often treated once a week. Acute sciatica is typically treated with acupuncture, massage and herbs. Rheumatoid conditions are often treated with moxabustion, acupuncture and herbs.

Several insurance carriers now cover acupuncture but some require that it be performed by a licensed MD. Due to insurance reasons, the frequency of sessions is often less than in China.

Case Study 31-1

A 40-year-old male strained his lower back while helping a friend move furniture 3 days ago. When he awoke the next morning, he reported extreme difficulty getting out of bed and difficulty straightening up. On day 3, he went to his primary care physician who recommended short-term rest, ice, muscle relaxants, and an x-ray (which was normal). By the sixth day, his back was not appreciably changed and he went to see his friend who practices traditional Chinese medicine.

He was tender on exam over the lumbosacral junction and across the iliac crest. Lasègue's sign was negative but it did increase his low back pain. His tongue showed a thin white coating (felt to be fairly normal) and his pulse was wiry (a finding consistent with pain). He was tender over several points on the Bladder meridian (B-23, B-25, and B-26) which correspond to L2-L4 on the lumbar spine. The finding of tender points indicated stagnation of Qi and Blood and it was felt that the specific location of pain obstructed flow in the Bladder channel (11).

Based on these findings, acupuncture points were chosen primarily along the Bladder channel. A type of needle manipulation was done to help "drain" the stagnation and stimulate flow of Blood and Qi. After the first treatment, the pain subsided enough to allow straightening of the back. Treatment was continued on successive days for a total of five visits by which time the pain had completely disappeared. He was advised to avoid heavy lifting for 1 month (11). Although the natural history of back pain suggests that many persons will recover in this time period, Joe felt that the process was greatly speeded by the acupuncture treatments.

Movement/Functional Approaches

Recognizing the inseparability of the mind-body connection, there are many healing modalities that are based on function, movement, breathing and posture. These include the Indian traditions of yoga and meditation, the Chinese traditions of Qigong and Tai Chi, the martial arts, Pilates, Continuum, Alexander technique, Feldenkrais, and Hanna Somatic Education. If a muscular contraction or particular pattern of movement is repeated enough, it will soon become an unconscious reflexive habit. One Spanish proverb states, "Habits at first are silken threads, then they become cables" (12). When a postural or muscular pattern that is faulty becomes habitual, this can lead to discomfort and disease such as tendonitis, stress fractures, muscular strains, arthritis and pain. F.M. Alexander, the originator of the Alexander technique, called it "debauched kinesthesia" when the body perceives a faulty muscular habit as feeling right (12).

Alexander Technique

Australian-born Frederick Matthias Alexander (1869-1955), a Shakespearean orator, discovered his functional approach after he cured himself of recurring voice loss. For years he went to different doctors, but not one was able to offer a cure for his problem. Through self-observation, he was able to sense his unconscious propensity to pull his head back and down while reciting, which put unnecessary pressure on his neck and throat. By correcting his habit, he was also able to heal himself of years of respiratory and nasal difficulties since childhood. Gradually he developed a method for correcting faulty use and improving coordination. Initially he worked with actors who flocked to see him in London. Among his best known pupils were George Bernard Shaw, Aldous Huxley, Virginia Woolf, and the Nobel prize-winning scientist Nikolaas Tinbergen (12).

Alexander's work has become the most popular in the performance world. Learning takes place either as one-on-one session or in a group in which an Alexander teacher uses his hands and verbal directions to guide the pupil through basic movements: bending, sitting, and walking. Alexander felt that the head-neck relationship was extremely important in correcting faulty patterns, lengthening the spine and creating fluid movement. The intention of each lesson is to help the client feel kinesthetically what he or she is doing wrong so that it can be corrected. Other areas of emphasis include letting the neck be free, letting the head go forward and up, lengthening and widening the trunk, and freeing the legs from the trunk. There is no forcing, only the intention of letting it happen. Alexander teachers train at least 1600 hours over a minimum of 3 years at recognized institutes. The Alexander technique can be found worldwide (12).

Feldenkrais Method

The Feldenkrais method of somatic education offers another functional approach to health and healing. Named after its founder, Moshe Feldenkrais (1904-1984), this approach shares many similarities in its understanding of human function to the Alexander Technique; however, it is quite different. Moshe Feldenkrais was a Russian-born Jew with degrees in chemistry and physics and a passion for judo and soccer. After a knee injury left him unable to pursue recreational interests, he discovered a unique and comprehensive perspective on sensory-motor function and how it relates to thought, intention, emotion, and action.

There are several fundamental principles that set the work apart from other functional approaches. Feldenkrais practitioners emphasize that the method is not an "alternative health practice" but instead an educational process (13). Feldenkrais practitioners consider themselves educators. They do not focus on making diagnoses or curing pain. Moshe believed that a properly organized skeleton is felt as weightlessness and he emphasized the importance of freedom of movement. He defined good posture as being organized in such a way that one is able to move in any of the six cardinal directions at any moment and with great ease. However, he felt strongly that good posture is unique for each individual and thus there is not a single correct way to move or be. Good posture can only be discovered by the individual through his or her own explorations in moving and living. There exists no perfect picture for what is right. The student, as the individual is called by the Feldenkrais practitioner, learns to refine his or her posture and movement by first learning to kinesthetically sense how he or she moves. Moshe felt that most people have a poor picture of how their bodies work. The method emphasizes observing and feeling differences in sensation. Lessons, as the sessions are called, can be done one on one (Functional Integration lessons), which involve hands on guidance, or as a group (Awareness Through Movement lessons), which involves verbally directed movements. Movements are often explored in a sitting or lying down position, which helps the student discern how he or she initiates actions and how much effort he or she expends. Done in this manner, the habitual use of the antigravity musculature is reduced and students slowly learn to distinguish between moving with effort and moving with efficiency (13).

To become a Feldenkrais practitioner, one trains more than 800 hours over a 4-year period after which time he or she is tested by the educational director and then certified by the Feldenkrais Guild. There have been a handful of small-scale research papers that have documented such benefits as increased range of motion, reduction in pain, ease of movement and increased body awareness after weeks of Awareness Through Movement lessons. The Feldenkrais method has been shown to be beneficial as an educational method in working with a variety of diagnoses including low-back pain, neck-shoulder pain, cerebral palsy, rheumatoid arthritis, Parkinson's, and multiple sclerosis (14). Guild certified trainings take place worldwide.

Case Study 31-2

Mary is a 70-year-old female with mid back and low back pain of many years' duration. She states that as a child, she developed a bad habit of slouching. Even now, she finds it difficult to sit up straight and after 30 minutes of playing bridge with her friends, she has to change positions in order to be comfortable.

She tried physical therapy for 3 weeks and states that she didn't see much of a difference and thus she stopped attending.

On inspection, the Feldenkrais practitioner notices that Mary sits with slouched posture and that she sits back on her ischium. With hands placed on the ASIS (or front of the pelvis), the Feldenkrais practitioner visually observes and kinesthetically feels (through very minimal movements) that Mary does not know how to sit forward and into her hip joints. She cannot bend through the hips. The practitioner invites Mary to make the same observation through kinesthetic touch and through a few verbal cues.

After an hour of movement exploration with her Feldenkrais practitioner, Mary has learned, through gentle touch and minimal verbal guidance, where her hips are and how she can rotate her pelvis over her ischium. At the conclusion of the session, Mary is asked to sit at the edge of the table and observe how she sits. She is then asked to walk and notice any additional changes. After three sessions, Mary reports that she is sitting up straighter with less pain in her mid and low back. Over time, she learns how to extend through her upper thoracic spine and how to breathe more fully through her ribs. Two months later, she reports almost complete resolution of her back discomfort and she is sitting with greater ease for the first time in 10 years. She decides to sign up for once-a-week ATM classes (Awareness Through Movement) to learn more about how to feel comfort and ease in her body.

Taijiquan (T'ai Chi Ch'uan)

Taijiquan ("grand ultimate fist") is a movement practice that has become very popular in the past 20 years. The most common image of Taiji (as it is more commonly known) is that of large groups of elderly people moving in a slow graceful dance-like fashion early in the morning throughout the parks of China. Taiji is a martial art that has a traceable history more than

400 years old. Today, people practice Taiji all over the world, and practitioners of the art find it beneficial for developing martial arts skills, a calm mind, and superior health.

There are many different styles of Taiji. The most popular are Chen, Yang, Sun, Wu, and Fu. These systems include choreographed routines of varying length, the use of weapons, and one-on-one interactive practice. Each has its root in the family lineage that bears its name and has a distinct style reflective of the philosophy and environment from where it was cultivated. Taiji is a living art and continues to evolve in style and form. Though it originated in China, some of the most skilled practitioners are found in America and Europe.

Taiji is becoming well-known for its health benefits. Studies have shown Taiji to positively enhance the immune and endocrine systems, reduce stress, lower blood pressure, and to help relieve arthritis pain. The most visible study regarding Taiji was in collaboration with Emory University showing the superior benefits of Taiji in relationship to balance for the elderly. The National Institutes of Health has also funded a study to examine Taiji, among other methodologies, in relationship to lower back pain.

Practicing Taiji is unlike practicing conventional exercises. With weightlifting or aerobics the individual strives to build up muscle or develop speed. However, in Taiji the practitioner or student strives to relax the body and move deliberately. In this way, he or she develops the skill of relaxing muscles, tendons, and joints. Over time, the student is able to continually refine his posture based on the organic nature of his skeleton uninhibited by muscular tension.

In Taiji, the fundamental core of movement takes place from the waist and hip area. This involves gentle rotation of the waist, release of the lumbosacral vertebra and hip flexors, and relaxation of the hip joints. As the student's skills develop, this part of the body becomes more supple. It is believed that energy can then flow through the legs and into the ground for support. Movement serves to organically bring about relaxation and correct posture. There is an emphasis on lower abdominal breathing which enhances flow of blood and Qi to this important region of the body. The practitioner learns to develop "internal power" which is expressed outwardly by improved coordination. This internal power takes longer to develop than conventional strength but is considered more durable. Perhaps most importantly, over time, the student develops a high level of self-awareness about movement and the ability to coordinate all parts of the body efficiently.

Case Study 31-3

A physically fit woman in her late 40s came to Taiji during her recovery from breast cancer. She had heard that Taiji was useful for boosting her

immune system and wanted to learn a form of movement that was med-
itative. Becky also suffered from lower back pain and sciatica stemming
from a long-standing injury. Becky attended Taiji classes twice per week
for 1½ hours and practiced an additional one to two sessions per week at
home. Six months into this routine, Becky reported that her lower back
pain and sciatic were completely gone. Throughout the next 5 years of
her study, her symptoms never returned.

Qigong (Ch'i Kung)

Qigong predates Taiji and is considered to be as old as 5000 years. Qigong
means simply "the study of Qi." Qi being the idea of vitality or life force. It
is the art and science of using breath, movement, visualization and meditation to cleanse, gather and circulate Qi. Taiji is considered a form of
Qigong, but Qigong encompasses a much broader range of exercises than
does Taiji. Currently, there are approximately 5000-7000 different forms and
styles of Qigong that can be categorized as Medical, Martial Arts, Buddhist,
Taoist, and Confucius. Qigong is considered one of the important branches
of Traditional Chinese Medicine along with herbs, acupuncture and Tui Na
(Chinese Massage). Based on the principles of Traditional Chinese
Medicine discussed earlier, Qigong is considered both a practice for health
and for spiritual insight.

The Chinese use Qigong for health maintenance, sports training, martial arts and medical treatment. In one study out of a hospital in Shanghai
in 1958, thousands of hypertensive patients were able to reduce their blood
pressure, lower their pulse rate and improve oxygen demand with Qigong.
Qigong exercises range in form and include: stillness and meditation, visualization, slow movements, and quick movements. The use of the intentional breathing is very important in developing Qigong skill.

Though older in origin, Qigong has been a bit more obscure than Taiji
and somewhat slower to gain popularity. Unfortunately because of the spiritual nature of the practice, it is often misunderstood and thought to be
cult-ish in nature. However, as with Taiji, Qigong is being studied for its
health benefits in endocrine and immune function, arthritis conditions,
stress and blood pressure. Highly skilled practitioners can also learn the
skill of emitting their own Qi for healing others.

For individuals with back pain, the use of Qigong is similar to Taiji.
The student practices relaxation first and then learns slow non-impact
movements that gently stretch and massage the body. This process is slow
enough to allow the student time to develop self-awareness and to learn
what movements are comfortable and how to make proper adjustments.
These skills can also be applied to daily life activities. With time, the internal

energy and blood flow of the body become the guiding and supporting mechanism for movement. Skilled practitioners often say that the "Qigong moves them."

Case Study 31-4

David is a physically fit man in his mid-40s. He came to Qigong after a car accident in which he lost a great deal of function. He had surgery to relieve damaged disks in his lumbar spine and then re-injured himself one week out of surgery. When David began the practice of Qigong, he was in constant pain and had difficulty bending over. The Qigong teacher recommended that David do all movements within a comfortable range of motion and to visualize or imagine any movements that he was unable to perform. Within 2 weeks, David's range of motion increased and within 1 month, he was able to bend over without pain. Additionally, David's mood improved and he began applying Qigong principles toward enhancing his quality of daily life.

Conclusion

Although this chapter has provided a brief overview of some of the alternative practices available for pain management, the reader is encouraged to experience as many methods first-hand in order to have a better understanding of them. Many alternative practitioners are willing to offer complementary sessions to health care providers and the public. Almost all of the alternative methods and their associated organizations have Web sites. Hopefully, in the near future, alternative methods will be more fully integrated into Western practices. Some insurance plans cover massage, chiropractic, and acupuncture; however, most alternative methods are fee for service. There is great controversy whether insurance should cover many of the alternative methods. At the same time, many alternative practitioners do not want to become subject to the rules and regulations of insurance systems, which are often thought to be too stringent. In fact, it is for this reason that many practitioners choose to practice alternative care rather than traditional methods.

Key Points

- The hallmark of alternative medicine is holism.
- Osteopathic and chiropractic manipulations are used for a variety of back problems. The basis of both of these forms of manipulative medicine is the concept that structural abnormalities in the spine and joints affect the internal organs and musculoskeletal system.
- The philosophy of traditional Chinese medicine is crucial to the acupuncture style used most commonly in the United States.
- Movement/functional approaches such as Qigong, Tai Chi, the Alexander technique, and the Feldenkrais method are based on function, movement, breathing, and posture to promote healing.

■   ■   ■

REFERENCES

1. **Eisenberg DM.** Unconventional medicine in the United States: prevalence, costs, and patterns of use. N Engl J Med. 1993;328(4):246-52.
2. **Daly D.** Alternative medicine courses taught at United States medical schools: an ongoing list. J Altern Complement Med. 1997;3:405-10.
3. **Cohen M.** Complementary & Alternative Medicine: Legal Boundaries and Regulatory Perspectives. Baltimore: The Johns Hopkins University Press; 1998.
4. **Gordon J.** Manifesto for a New Medicine. Reading, MA: Perseus Books; 1996.
5. **Cohen M.** Complementary & Alternative Medicine: Legal Boundaries and Regulatory Perspectives. Baltimore: The Johns Hopkins University Press; 1998.
6. **Knaster M.** Discovering the Body's Wisdom. New York: Bantam Books; 1996.
7. Complementary & Alternative Medicine: Legal Boundaries and Regulatory Perspectives. Baltimore: The Johns Hopkins University Press; 1998.
8. **Gordon J.** Manifesto for a New Medicine. Reading, MA: Perseus Books; 1996.
9. **Knaster M.** Discovering the Body's Wisdom. New York: Bantam Books; 1996.
10. **Kaptchuk T.** The Web That Has No Weaver: Understanding Chinese Medicine. Chicago: Congdon & Weed; 1983.
11. **Jirui C, Wang N.** Acupuncture Case Histories from China. Seattle: Eastland Press; 1988.
12. **Knaster M.** Discovering the Body's Wisdom. New York: Bantam Books; 1996.
13. **Haller J.** The Feldenkrais method of somatic education and lumbar instability. Orthopaed Phys Ther Clin North Am. 1999;Sept:415-25.
14. **Schmitt S, Nichols J, et al.** Clinical and Electromyographic Outcomes in a Pilot Study of the Feldenkrais Method vs. General Reconditioning for Chronic Low Back Pain. Presentation at the Association of Academic Physiatrists, San Diego; March 2000.

32

Back Pain Laws and Disability

Andrew J. Haig, MD

Oh, yeah, doc, I almost forgot. Will you fill out these forms for me?" The legal aspects of medicine are the least fun for most health care providers. It is probably because our personalities, training, and experience have taught us to keep our minds open to all the possibilities. We do not like the idea of making a final answer when all the facts are not in. And with back pain, all the facts are almost never in.

But the legal system has to make final answers. On a certain date in a certain courtroom, a judge makes a final and irrevocable decision. Disabled or not. Culpable or not. Restricted or not. If we, as treating physicians, do not play in this game, it goes on despite us. For the patient, the judge's decision can mean the difference between living on the street and gainful employment. The defendant—an insurer, a second person, or the government—deserves justice as well.

A good doctor cannot ignore the legal ramifications of back pain. Just as a history of smoking puts one at increased risk for surgical failure, so does the presence of active litigation. Legal action or compensation are predictors of disability. Any good rehabilitation program involves counseling about the conflict between the need to prove one is disabled and the greater need to become able. The testimony of the treating physician is also important, whether by deposition or more commonly through forms. As we shall see, if the treating physician does not stake a claim regarding what is just and reasonable, then more polarized and biased players make the decision-often to the detriment of the patient.

Both lawyers and patients wittingly and unwittingly may alter health care decisions. Patients may be instructed to "do everything the doctor tells you," leading them to go along with suggestions about surgery, medications, prolonged therapy, and so forth, in the belief that they have no choice in the matter. Lawyers in compensation cases thrive on the appearance of fact, so gimmicks, gizmos and irrelevant medical tests are often a part of the game. (I once heard an attorney say, "If you want to win the case, show an x-ray. It doesn't have to be an x-ray of the involved part. Jury's love x-rays.") Likewise, they may counsel their clients to be absolutely sure that you understand their pain (sometimes leading to exaggeration). More health care visits are better for the plaintiff's case, as each visit implies that the person is in need of care. As a result, the patient may return to the doctor again and again with a goal of documenting his or her suffering, rather than care seeking.

Getting Paid for Disability

Many different parties may be held liable for our patient's pain experience. Each has different stature with the law and different payment obligations.

The Defendant

This one seems obvious. If someone else is the cause or partial cause of a person's pain, expense, and suffering, that person may be held liable for restitution. The other party may be another person (as in a car accident), a business (as in product liability), or a combination, as in a malpractice suit against a hospital and a doctor or a suit against a company and the driver of its vehicle that injured a patient. Class action lawsuits, where a person represents a group of persons harmed by the same company, fit into this category. "No fault" policies in some states (e.g., Michigan) are designed to avoid litigation by paying for basic needs such as lost wages and health care. In general, the injured person can sue for all reasonable damages-lost wages, health care benefits, repair of damaged property, and "pain and suffering."

The Workers' Compensation Insurer

The workers' compensation insurer is *not* the patient's insurance company. The insurance case manager who visits your office to help move the case along does *not* work for the patient. In essence, they insure the folks who, by default, have lost a lawsuit to the worker. Every state in the United States has a different law regarding compensating workers for work-related injuries. But they share a common theme. By state law, the employer agrees that the worker does not have to prove that they are negligent, and in exchange, the worker agrees to be compensated only for lost wages and health care. Contrary to popular belief, for the patient with severe disability compensation is seldom a windfall. Future wages never include opportunities for promotion, retirement benefits, or family health insurance. And the lawyer takes a chunk.

Usually any injury that occurs at work is simply settled in an uncontested manner. But there are controversies, thus there is posturing. Workers' compensation does not cover medical problems that likely would have happened anyway. (Is disk degeneration a genetic fate or a work related problem?) Compensation does not cover injuries outside of work, but does cover occupational illnesses detected outside of the work environment. (How about the guy who spent 20 years lifting heavy iron at the foundry and finally moved on to a desk job. When his back goes out, who's responsible?) Different states do or do not cover injuries in the parking lot or on the way home from work. There are rules related to alcohol, drugs, and commission of a crime at work. Rules about who is employed versus contracted, whether overtime pay is used in determination of compensation, and so forth.

Determination of case closure is often based on a physician statement that there has been a "healing plateau," "end of treatment," or similar statement. Until then, the insurer is often required to hold substantial amounts of money in low-interest rate escrow accounts. Payment for disability may be on a scale (e.g., $5000 for carpal tunnel syndrome), based on a physician rating of disability (The AMA Guides to the Evaluation of Physical Impairment [1] is used as a rule for determining a "% disability" in some states, whereas others specifically require that this guide not be used), or based on legal arguments regarding the potential for future employment and advancement given the injury sustained.

Each state has its quirks. Some states do not pay for time lost until 2 or 7 days have elapsed-so patients may beg to be kept off work more days than otherwise. In Wisconsin, there is an unintended bias toward surgical treatment in the law. If a person successfully recovers from a disk herniation without surgery, there is no payment for future lost wages, but if there was successful recovery with surgery, 5% of current wages times the number of years to retirement age is paid. State departments of labor are surprisingly proworker in most cases, to the point where an attorney is often not necessary. States typically have pamphlets or websites for injured workers. It is worth reading your state's rules.

There are sometimes permutations of the worker's compensation rules. Shipboard workers and rail workers have special federal rules, as do government employees. Law enforcement personnel may have additional protection if they are unable to perform the key duties of their work.

The Patient's Insurers

The patient may have any number of insurers who pay for various aspects of back pain disability. Personal disability insurance, insurance on credit cards, auto, home, boat, and car. Back pain often cancels or delays payment (only after the physician fills out numerous forms on a monthly basis . . .). There may be litigation regarding health care coverage, as well. On occasion a patient is in so much debt that he or she literally cannot afford to go back to work. Without financial counseling, this kind of patient may continue to fight against return to work.

Government Disability

Social Security disability is supposedly for persons who are unable to work at any gainful employment whatsoever. But the strictness of the rule has lead to different interpretation in different states. Social security disability for back pain increased 2500% in the decades after World War II, implying a substantial shift in society's opinion of whether pain is disabling. Patients will apply, be denied, apply again, and so forth, for years. They may feel that return to work interferes with their chances of getting Social Security and the Medicare insurance benefits that come along with it. Unfortunately, most research shows that when the goal is attained, quality of life actually decreased. States welfare programs may have similar issues.

Case Study 32-1

A 35-year-old male presented with 6 months of back pain disability. He wants to get back surgery, but his findings are not definitive. At the end of the visit, he hands you proof of disability forms for his work, his home mortgage, his car payment, and his credit card debt. With further discussion, you realize that he had been overspending his budget prior to the injury. Essentially, he couldn't afford to return to work because these debts would come due.

After pointing out the conflict of interest, you help him contact a financial counselor, and set reasonable restrictions and timelines for return to work based on the medical aspects of the case. He cancels his appointment with the surgeon and returns to work.

Discussion

In this case, the premorbid financial situation was the predominant force behind the work disability. It is also common for people who have back pain disability to accumulate substantial debt from health care and other expenses. The physician must be aware of these circumstances, as they may be very strong hidden motivators. An offer to help find solutions, combined with a frank discussion of the physician's obligation to honestly report the level of disability, often helps.

Permanent versus Temporary Disability

The time frame of disability is often a challenging concept. An individual may have expenses, pain and suffering, but no lost work or compensible disability. He or she may have temporary partial disability, temporary total disability, permanent partial disability, or permanent total disability.

Medically it is almost always best in the short term to minimize the amount of disability the physician gives the patient. Seldom is return to work at some limited capacity dangerous, and seldom does it interfere with the physician's treatment plan. I've often advocated, though, that the physician seek substantial advice from the patient (who is the only one who knows how much it hurts, and who is almost always more expert on the job and work environment than the physician) in determining temporary restrictions (2,3). The few patients who are "taking advantage of the situation" usually declare themselves quite early, while the vast majority of patients learn from this experience that their role is that of an active problem solver, not just a victim of the system. Chapter 23 deals with temporary disability in some detail.

At some time the treatment is ended, and some type of long-term restriction may be appropriate. Different jurisdictions may call this a healing plateau, an end of treatment, a medical end, or case closure. Such closure typically does not preclude further treatment (e.g., ongoing exercise in a health club, continued use of counseling or medications).

At this time, a "permanent" restriction is given. It is important to tell the patient that this restriction is a best guess used to help the insurer and patient come to closure on the money issues and to allow the patient to plan for vocational rehabilitation if needed. The patient who takes a job knowing that the requirements are beyond the restrictions may be committing fraud. The patient who violates these restrictions at work and is injured may not be covered for the second injury. The patient should know that there is nothing to preclude the physician from changing this restriction at a later date if circumstances or health change. It is not uncommon for a patient to come to me 3 or 4 years after an injury, with a new job opportunity that requires a change in their "permanent" restrictions. If appropriate and safe, I will change their restrictions.

Restrictions for back disorders can be highly varied. Permanent total disability is exceedingly uncommon. The few patients I've declared permanently and totally disabled may have had severe psychiatric sequellae or multiple operations to the point where spine stability is in question. The social circumstances may come into play-an illiterate 50-year-old cannot reasonably be expected to find a desk job, for instance, so restriction to that kind of job is often not realistic.

It is quite common that a patient is given no permanent restrictions-even when he or she had been on temporary restrictions for months or years. The temporary restrictions may be a judicious way to not "flare things up" during treatment or assessment, or may have been a pragmatic response to the employer's work policy, or may have been placed by an early treating physician, and never challenged. Permanent restrictions need to truthfully reflect the physician's best judgement about the foreseeable future, not about past performance.

In the midground are the many patients who will have some restriction, but not total. There is no formula for correct restrictions. Many surgeons are in the habit of arbitrary restriction (e.g., giving a 10-lb lifting restriction to all patients they operate on). This can be seen as quite self-serving (protecting "their" operation, rather than looking to the long-term need of the patient to earn a living, the social burden of disabling people who are physically able, and the ethical obligation to the defendant as well as the plaintiff). There is no support for such a generic approach. The treating physician needs to take into account the pathology (nerve damage, surgical scarring, bony deformity, soft tissue changes) and other patient factors (stature, other disability, psychiatric illness).

Physicians often incorrectly rely heavily on "functional capacity evaluations" to determine permanent restrictions. Obviously functional capacity evaluations do not take into account intrinsic pathology-the danger to the patient in performing work tasks. These tests often do not accurately measure capacity (depression, motivation, fear, and lack of familiarity are many reasons why a person may test out at less than his or her physiologic capacity). Where they do measure some physiologic capacity, the limit is most often a reversable, not a permanent one. For example it is very common for people to stop a lifting task because of cardiovascular or muscular endurance limits-which are readily reversible with exercise. The results are often very specific to the test, and not generalizable. For instance, the majority of patients tested with the standard Progressive Isoinertial Lifting Evaluation were able to lift more weight when given a short break between lifts in a test called the SlowPILE. Actual work tasks may require repeated performance daily for decades, not a simple half hour of a task. Most importantly, there is no evidence that these tests have any predictive value.

In the end, while information from functional assessments might be integrated into the decision making, the final work restriction is not based on one test, but on the overall judgement of the treating physician.

Disease, Impairment, Disability, and Handicap

These words are the key to understanding much of what happens in the legal world. *Disease* implies any departure from health. But any disease can be more or less severe. The severity can affect an individual's performance variably, and the effect of the performance deficit on life role depends greatly on social circumstances. The words impairment, disability, and handicap are defined by these differences.

Impairment implies the inability to perform a bodily task that typical persons can do or that the individual had previously been able to do. For example, the inability to straighten out one's knee is an impairment.

Disability is the functional result of impairment. For example, a person who cannot straighten out a knee is disabled from walking without aids like crutches. *Handicap* is the inability to perform a life role. In this case, the person might be handicapped in relation to a job as a forest ranger, but not from a job as a computer programmer.

Various jurisdictions reward impairment, disability, or handicap. In fact, some use the words incorrectly in their statutes. But the concepts are useful regardless in determining what the physician will say about a person's ability. Where does pain fit in? It doesn't. At least not directly. At least not usually. Although research does show that people with chronic pain have a worse quality of life than those without pain, it also shows that the extent of pain does not relate to the ability to perform.

To those who do not treat chronic pain routinely, this is hard to comprehend. They tend to take their personal experience with acute pain. So the physician with a backache thinks, "If my back would hurt more than it does now, I won't be able to lift this box." But in fact, she probably could, if sufficiently motivated. She is presumably being honest with herself. She must realize that her pain limits may not be the same as others, as people of different cultures, family upbringing, and life experience may be able to tolerate the pain more or less than she can. She will further realize that the pain she "reports" to herself may not be the same as the pain she reports to her spouse, her colleagues, or her patients. Certainly her patients' reports of pain to a judge, jury, or insurance claims agent would be highly variable. It is important for the physician to realize that, again and again, the literature points out little to no relationship between the *chronic* back pain patient's report of pain and the functional abilities or activities of the patient.

Basically, doctors and the legal system cannot get a handle on how much pain is worth how much limitation. It is crucial for physicians to understand this concept, and not use pain as a substitute for impairment, disability, or handicap.

What's Legal and What's Fair

There are many ethical flaws in the legal and compensation process. It is important for the treating physician to be aware of these. Conflict of interest can be discussed in terms of specific players in the process.

The Patient

Health is only one of our patients' life goals. The patient in a litigious situation wants to get better, but is being paid for being disabled. There may be social pressures to act disabled or to return to work before medically optimal. The patient may use health care providers to document, rather than to simply treat, disabling illnesses.

The Insurer

The insurance company probably makes more money from investments than from premiums. State legislation often requires placement of substantial sums in low-interest secure accounts until it is clear that an individual is not going to be disabled for life, so case closure at any cost is often a goal. Insurers have a lot of money and expertise for litigation, and patients are often naïve to the law. So, ethics and laws aside, it is in the interest of the insurer to fabricate or exaggerate reasons for denial of payment. Insurers of the loosing party (e.g., in worker's compensation) frequently portray the aura of being an insurer of the plaintiff, using words such as denial or approval of payment when in fact they are not in a position to deny payment.

It is not uncommon for multiple insurers to share some aspect of responsibility for a case. For example, the delivery man hurt in a car accident at work has primary health insurance, workers' compensation insurance, and litigation against the other vehicle owner's insurance. These carriers may "pass the buck," with none paying for health care or lost wages until years after the injured party has missed needed treatment and become financially destitute.

The Case Manager

Insurance case managers, often nurses or social workers by background, have no legal stature in the treatment process. They are not legally or ethically allowed to alter or suggest treatment to the patient, but this rule is frequently violated, as they often spend hours with patients, counseling, transporting, and so forth. They have no restrictions in coercing treating physicians-encouraging or discouraging referrals, restrictions, or treatments. Case managers paid by the hour, by the case, or via a contract may behave differently to optimize their personal income (4).

The Employer

Employers who are liable for compensation costs may be highly motivated to return an injured worker to work. At a more specific level, though, the immediate supervisor often has a visceral response to the burden of dealing with a back disabled worker. Supervisor performance is often judged on output with no regard for the cost savings resultant from accommodating an injured worker. Supervisors know the worker well, but do not understand psychological concepts such as depression. Employers worry that "recurrence" of an outside injury at work can turn it into a workers' compensation case.

The Attorney

An attorney's obligation is to win the court case, not to ensure the best health care or the best quality of life for the client. Even ethical attorneys will be biased in favor of more rather than less disability. It is not uncommon for attorneys to cross the line and coach plaintiffs on how often to see their doctor, how to present themselves, and so forth. Attorneys make money from turning around more cases. Although many states put limits on attorney fees, ancillary or additional expenses can add up. Attorneys may accept or decline cases more on the basis of potential settlement than on merit. For example, a fractured spine in an 80-year-old may not be as lucrative a case as the same fracture in a 25-year-old.

The Doctor

Payment for litigated cases is typically 100% of usual and customary fees—much better than for HMOs or most other insurance contracts. So there is a temptation to order excessive treatment and tests. Unfortunately, because many ethical physicians see this legal process as essentially corrupt, they refuse to participate in the legal system. This leads to more use of biased experts. Qualified experts can be paid very high fees to testify in court. In almost any community, there are physicians known as "insurance whores" whose testimony invariably supports the defendant. The reward for such testimony is more referrals and more high-paying deposition or testimony fees. On the other hand, treating physicians invariably identify more with the plight of their patient than that of the anonymous large employer or insurer. Ethical treating physicians are encouraged to endure the frustrations of the legal system to provide balanced testimony on cases where they have been involved.

Although tort reform laws have sought to place caps on many types of lawsuits, in general the amount awarded can be a gamble-dependant substantially on the skill of the attorney, the inclinations of the jury (thus the culture of the community in which the lawsuit is filed) and the leanings of the judge. Even when a case is settled out of court, the solution is typically the results of opposing attorneys taking these nonmedical factors into account. Like the lottery, this gamble attracts people who are least able to take a loss. As time drags on and the person looses work and accrues expenses, personal injury becomes a high stakes game in which our patients may sacrifice their health.

Treating doctors should be aware that, because they "happened" to see the patient-not for legal purposes, but for care purposes-their records and testimony hold great weight with a jury. Complete documentation, including the circumstances of the injury, the patient's statements, the physician's impressions of impairment and disability, and so forth, can clarify the situation for all involved, thus leading to a more just solution and fewer depositions and other hassles for the physician.

Conclusion

In our culture, back pain disability cannot be separated from the legal framework in which it is contained. To obtain optimal medical outcomes, the physician must have a sophisticated knowledge of the political, legal, and economic pressures that drive treatment and outcomes. The physician must come to grips with the fact that the legal system does not revolve around the viewpoint of physicians. Furthermore, even some of the basic constructs that physicians assume to be true—such as the idea of a linear relationship between pain and disability—are not scientifically valid in the chronic back pain population. The competent back pain physician will take these factors into account in planning treatment and in closing a case after care has been optimized.

Recommendations

- Read your state's pamphlet or booklet on workers' compensation (in some states, there is a special pamphlet for physicians). These are often available on the Web.
- Discuss compensation issues with a trial lawyer.
- Include inquiry into the legal/compensation status as part of the routine intake information on follow-up visits.

Key Points

- Litigation for back injury creates a conflict between the need to prove disability and the need to become well.
- Lawyers and patients may wittingly and unwittingly alter health care decisions; for example, by encouraging repeat health care visits merely to document the health problem rather than to treat it.
- With worker's compensation, the patient is compensated only for lost wages and health care.
- Case closure is based on a physician statement that there has been a "healing plateau" or "end of treatment." At this time, a "permanent" restriction is made.
- Quite often the patient does not require "permanent" restrictions, even after years of "temporary" restrictions.
- "Permanent" restrictions may be modified at a later date if circumstances or health change.
- Permanent total disability is very uncommon.

REFERENCES

1. **Cocchiarella L, Andersson GBJ (editors).** Guides to the Evaluation of Permanent Impairment (5th edition). Chicago, IL: American Medical Association Press, 2001.

2. **Haig AJ, Linton P, McIntosh M, Moneta L, Mead PB.** Aggressive early medical management by a specialist in physical medicine and rehabilitation: effect on lost time due to injuries in hospital employees. J Occup Med. 1990;32:241-4.

3. **Haig AJ.** The business of dissociating pain and disabilities. Phys Med Rehabil Clin North Am. 1993;4:1-9.

4. **Haig AJ, Hadwin K, Palma-Davis L, Rich D.** Insurance case managers' perception of quality in back pain programs: results of neutral focus group studies. Am J Phys Med Rehabil. 2000;80(7):520-5. See also the commentary in Am J Phys Med Rehabil. 2001;80(7):526-7.

SECTION V

SPECIAL ISSUES

33

■ ■ ■

Stopping Physical Therapy

Lisa DiPonio, MD

Physical therapy is an indispensable tool in the management of many painful spinal disorders. The ultimate goal of physical therapy, however, is for the patient to derive benefit and eventually no longer need the services of the physical therapist. Although this goal may seem obvious, discontinuing therapy-whether because the goals of treatment (e.g., greater muscles strength) have been achieved or because the therapy is not working-may be met with resistance by the patient. For this reason, the physician needs to work with the patient to ensure that he or she understands the need to move on to the next step in the management of their back pain, as patient compliance is crucial to the success of back pain treatment.

Goals and Expectations

Patients who have unrealistic expectations about therapy are more likely to have difficulty discontinuing therapy. Before sending a patient to physical therapy, it is essential that the patient understand the goals and the limitations of the therapy. The physician must engage the patient in dialogue to determine what the patient would like to achieve with therapy. Usually patients will say, "I just want to feel better," but the physician must compel the patient to get more specific. Is the goal improved range of motion? Greater strength or flexibility? Does the patient think that therapy will make them feel 20 years younger? Unreasonable expectations need to be avoided. A time frame should be set. Therapy for very acute problems, such as an acute muscle strain, should not need more than 3 or 4 visits. Subacute problems often need 12 visits or more. Duration of treatment for chronic problems is a more complicated matter; sometimes prolonged therapy does not help these conditions, and a short course with limited goals should be agreed upon at the beginning. Finally, a follow-up visit with the physician needs to be scheduled-usually within 2 to 3 weeks after the patient has begun therapy.

Writing the Prescription

The groundwork for a successful conclusion to physical therapy begins when the physical therapy prescription is initially written. When writing a physical therapy prescription, one must keep these goals in mind and indicate them on the prescription. An open ended prescription simply stating "evaluate and treat" does a disservice to both the therapist and the patient. Such a prescription expects the therapist to perform a medical history, physical examination, and make medical decisions without the benefit of a physician's training. The physical therapy prescription must contain the diagnosis, the suspected pain generator, any precautions or expected complications, and the goals of the patient (see Chapters 20 and 24). When a relationship of trust is built between the therapist, physician, and patient, it will avoid the possibility of a patient calling you back saying "My therapist says I have a herniated disk" when you have already told the patient he has sacroiliac joint pain.

Know Your Therapists

One way to make certain that therpay is designed to achieve a set goal-and that it is discontinued once that goal has been reached-is to select an appropriate physical therapy facility in the beginning. Bad physical therapy is unfortunately a very lucrative business when unchecked. Physical therapy facilities get paid by the hour, not by the diagnosis, and payment is not linked to improvement of any kind. It is beneficial to try to get to know the reputations of the physical therapy facilities in your referral area. One can get a feel for how a facility is run by simply calling the facility and asking to speak to a therapist. Does the therapist listen to what you, the physician, have to say, or would they prefer that you simply sign a prescription that they have written? Often valuable information is ascertained by speaking with other physicians in the area, other therapists that are not in direct competition with the facility you have in mind, or by visiting the facility.

Physicians need to beware of "shake and bake" therapy facilities that encourage high volume, hands-off treatment modalities such as heat or ice packs for entire sessions followed by minimal stretches or exercise machines. Often, physicians receive multiple requests for renewal of therapies indefinitely with no set of functional goals for the patient. When receiving requests for renewals of therapy, one must always read the renewal request and make sure it corresponds to the goals set between the physician and patient. Specifically, look at what the report says the patient has been doing, and what treatments the therapist wants to continue.

Patient Follow-up

The follow-up physician visit should take place within 2-3 weeks after the patient has begun therapy. A patient ought to see some benefit within no more than 4 weeks of therapy; if they do not, then either they are receiving inappropriate treatment, the therapist is not skilled enough, or their symptoms are refractory. (See Chapter 20 for a detailed discussion of how to assess progress during the follow-up visits.)

During this visit, the physician should ask the patient if they are feeling any better, but also: "What specifically did you do in therapy?" This is another opportunity to "get to know" the therapists in your referral area. If a patient received simply hot packs and massage, followed by some group sessions, that may be an indication that the facility in question is not paying focused attention to the needs of the patient. Signs of quality therapy include working with a certified physical therapist consistently (as opposed to a PT assistant), a therapist that examines the patient at the beginning of each session, and the patient's coming out of each session with not only some pain relief but an "assignment" of exercises and/or stretches to do at home to maintain their progress. During a follow-up physician visit when a patient pulls out a small, wrinkled stack of papers with written instructions and pictures, and proceeds to explain to you their home exercise program in detail, it is a good sign. When that same patient also reports a reduction in pain and the ability to do more, it is a good indication of quality therapy.

Reasons for Stopping Physical Therapy

Although physical therapy is usually, and ideally, stopped because the patient's goals have been reached, occasionally there are other reasons:

1. When the patient has plateaued and further therapy is unlikely to change the outcome.
2. The patient is no longer deriving benefit from the therapy, either due to refractory symptoms or to noncompliance with the program.
3. The therapy is causing more pain or harm.
4. Therapy is denied or stopped by a third party payer.

The patient may not be deriving benefit from therapy for any of several reasons. Some patients are not willing to comply with a home exercise program given to them by the therapist, but instead expect to go to therapy and come out "fixed." The patient needs to understand that his or her effort is just as important if not more important than the skills and dedication of the therapist. When it is thought that the patient is not following through on home exercises, usually the best option is to discontinue therapy and explore reasons for noncompliance. Sometimes the patient doesn't understand the importance of the exercises, or misunderstands the instructions, or is fearful. Most often the reason for non-compliance is ambiguity about getting better or depression, so continued therapy without addressing these issues is fruitless.

Still other patients have symptoms that are refractory to the variety of treatments offered by the therapists. Many patients over the age of 40 have stiffness of the joints that makes them refractory to manipulation techniques. Others have muscle firing patterns that are so fixed as to be resistant to change. Upon reevaluation, the physician may decide that physical therapy is just not able to meet the needs of the patient. When that happens, physical therapy should be stopped and alternative methods of pain relief and functional improvement should be sought.

When therapy is actually causing more pain, the physician must reconsider the diagnosis and treatment plan and modify them if necessary. Is there a missed diagnosis that is putting the patient at risk of fracture, tissue injury, myocardial infarction, and so forth? Is the treatment plan too aggressive for the patient to tolerate?

How to Stop Physical Therapy

Stopping therapy when goals are reached is usually easy. Reassurance is provided to the patient and he is encouraged to continue to practice what he has learned. One should advise the patient that flare-ups will likely occur and not to throw out those exercise sheets! They will most likely be needed in the future at some point. Discontinuing therapy when goals have not been reached presents special consideration that may prove more challenging. The decision to discontinue physical therapy needs to be made with the patient "on board." If the patient does not feel that they are a part of the decision to stop physical therapy and pursue alternate means, the physician risks alienating the patient and losing their trust. At least one visit between the physician and patient will be needed to develop an alternative plan.

When advising a patient that therapy needs to be stopped, the physician should first focus on the goals that were accomplished by physical therapy. For instance, perhaps some level of pain relief or increased range of motion was accomplished. Perhaps a patient did not get complete relief, but did learn a home exercise program that they can now use both to treat future exacerbations and to continue strengthening.

After agreeing on what has been accomplished, the next step might be to try programs or methods that can help the patient achieve some of the same goals that physical therapy was meant to achieve. For instance, a swimming or walking program can achieve generalized strengthening and cardiovascular conditioning. Knowing how to apply heat or ice at home can treat muscle soreness associated with increased activities. A work hardening or functional restoration program can help the patient to change the focus from pain to function and remove the fear of pain. The physician should help the patient to develop a plan to meet the more reasonable goals. Any alternative plan to physical therapy should focus on maximizing function (examples are shown in Table 33-1).

Some patients truly enjoy the therapy and want to continue. For these patients it is useful to explore the apparent irrational wish to continue. Perhaps it is the socialization, insecurity about his or her own ability to care for the back problem, or even a wish to build up the dollar amount for a court case. These can be dealt with delicately or in a straightforward conversation, depending on the patient. At some point, it may be appropriate to point out the physician's viewpoint that therapy is a costly resource and it is frustrating for a therapist to perform meaningless work, and simply decline to refer back to therapy.

On some occasions, physical therapy is stopped when neither patient, physician, or therapist thinks it is appropriate: when insurance payments are denied or stopped. Physical therapy is too expensive for all but a few to pay out of pocket. What can a physician do to help a patient who has had the rug pulled from under them?

For one thing, the physician can encourage the patient to *move*. The vast majority of patients with back pain have no contraindication to a generalized exercise program such as a walking, swimming, or biking program. The physician can reassure the patient that exercise within reasonable limits not only will not harm them, but will help their problem in the long run. Some therapists are willing to provide simple written instructions with pictures on simple stretching and self-correction techniques. Reassure the patient that most acute and subacute back problems are self-limited, and that if they do not allow deconditioning to set in, the problem will most likely improve over time.

Finally, in some cases, although the goals of therapy have been met, patients are reluctant to give up sessions because they enjoy the the pain relief of passive therapies and become dependent on the personal attention given

---

Table 33-1   Alternatives to Physical Therapy

- Generalized strengthening program such as swimming or walking
- Focused flexibility program such as yoga
- Home modalities such as heat, ice, and home traction units
- Massage therapy
- Acupuncture
- Chiropractic
- Kinesiology, homeopathy, or other complementary treatments

them by the well meaning therapist (see Case Study 33-1). Again, for these patients it is helpful to point out that substitutes are available for the aspects of therapy that the patient enjoys. As is shown in Case Study 33-1, he or she may discover that joining a local health club, for instance, may provide the same benefit *and* pleasure, now that the goals of physical therapy have been achieved.

Case Study 33-1

A 48-year-old interior designer suffered a high lumbar radiculopathy as the result of an automobile accident. She had extensive myofascial upper and lower back pain that persisted long after her radicular symptoms had resolved. She went to physical therapy and got significant pain relief from the traction, massage, therapeutic exercise, and manipulation. Her therapist felt that the treatment had worked, and that her spine was more mobile, strong, and flexible than it had been previously. However, she enjoyed the therapy so much that even though she was independent with a home exercise program, she insisted on continuing the physical therapy because she liked the hands-on treatment. She could not understand why her therapy should be stopped because the auto insurance (ours being a no-fault state) would agree to pay for therapy indefinitely. Her therapist tried several times to discharge her but felt frustrated when her physician continued to renew the physical therapy at her request.

After much dialogue, she realized and admitted that it was not so much the manipulation that helped her as it was the fact that after her PT sessions had ended, the therapist would allow her to walk on the treadmill for 45 minutes and use the weight lifting equipment at the PT gym. She felt so good after therapy because she was exercising. She was afraid that without the encouragement of a therapist, she would lapse back into inactivity.

Her physician finally convinced her to stop the therapy on a "trial" basis and join a local health club (which her auto insurance also covered, and interestingly was much less expensive than her continuing physical therapy). She scheduled sessions with a massage therapist on her workout days. She continues to go to her health club to maintain her strength and flexibility, and massage therapy continues to help her manage the ongoing myofascial symptoms.

Recommendations

- Explain to the patient the diagnosis and the expectations of therapy.
- When writing a physical therapy prescription, indicate the diagnosis and goals of therapy.

- Schedule follow-up visits with the patient to check on progress.
- Any requests for renewal of therapy need to be checked aginst the goals that were originally set up between you and the patient.
- Finally, if therapy is no longer providing benefit, stop it. Use a positive, open dialogue with the patient, and consider other means to accomplish the patient's goals.

Key Points

- Physicians should set specific, appropriate goals and expectations for the treatment. The patient should understand these goals as well as the limitations of physical therapy.
- A follow-up visit should occur within 2 to 3 weeks after the patient has begun therapy so that the physician can check whether goals are being met.
- The patient should begin to notice improvement within 4 weeks of therapy.
- Physical therapy is usually stopped because the patient's goals have been reached. However, therapy may also be discontinued because the patient has refractory symptoms or is noncompliant with the treatment plan; the treatment may actually be causing more pain; or therapy is denied or stopped by a third-party payer.
- Patients whose goals have been met and who have therefore discontinued therapy should be advised to continue practicing the exercises that they have learned in therapy.
- When it is decided that physical therapy should be stopped because its goals are not being met, reassure patients that ongoing exercise and some alternative therapies can help them to achieve their goals.

34

■ ■ ■

Prevention of Low Back Pain and Disability

Andre Taylor, MD

Robert Werner, MD

The work of preventing back pain and back pain disability is done by primary care physicians in many roles. All primary care physicians are in a position to provide advice to patients as part of general health maintenance or after an acute event. But a very large number of internists and family medicine specialists work in industrial settings or act as consulting company physicians for smaller companies. Others are involved in community health policy. Along with the occupational medicine specialists, physiatrists, and other readers of this book whose daily work includes preventive strategies, many primary care physicians need to understand the basic principles of prevention.

Capitation and managed care, as well as an interest in alleviating human suffering, are driving primary care physicians to look more closely at disease prevention. Low back pain (LBP) will affect 60-80% of people at some point in their lives. Only upper respiratory illness exceeds LBP in time lost due to sickness; more than 19 million workers a year sustain some form of disability from low back pain, and the number of lost days associated with low back pain have been steadily increasing over the past 2 decades. A conservative estimate of the cost of low back pain to employers, including lost time for sick days as well as health care costs, is more than $30 billion (1). (The primary populations that have been used as subjects in clinical studies for the prevention of lower back pain have largely been in the occupational setting [Table 34-1]). With the ageing of the workforce in the United States, the number of injuries to the low back will only increase. The need to curtail the high health costs and costs to employers that are incurred by back pain is a forceful motivator behind current prevention strategies.

Table 34-1   Work-Related Back Injuries Resulting in Lost-Time Occurrences

Occupation	Number of Back Injuries
Registered nurses	10,702
Nurse's aides/orderlies	32,205
Construction trade workers	28,303
Machine operators	35,170
Fabricators and assemblers	13,965
Truck drivers	38,120
Equipment cleaners/laborers	68,358
Transportation and material moving workers	53,052
Freight, stock, and material-handlers	16,559
General laborers (nonconstruction)	23,070
Total lost time, work-related back injuries	319,504

Statistics established in data published by the Bureau of Labor Statistics based on the 1992 Occupational Injury and Illness Classification System and the Occupational Classification Structure developed by the Bureau of the Census. Data cited are current for the full year 1999 (2).

This chapter reviews efforts to prevent back pain and disability and the logic behind them. Although the most obvious environment in which prevention efforts take place may seem to be the health care system, workplace interventions are also important, as are public health education efforts.

Current Strategies of Prevention

Primary prevention of low back pain is defined as "prevention strategies targeted at asymptomatic individuals." Successful primary prevention strategies have included primarily ergonomic interventions such as workplace design, tool design, or administrative controls over work. Worker education, braces, exercises, and so forth, are not clearly helpful. Secondary prevention of low back pain is defined as "prevention of the exacerbation of existing back injury or the occurrence of new episodes of back pain in individuals with a history of lower back pain." Secondary prevention targets individuals with lower back pain for education, treatment or ergonomic intervention. Much of the focus of prevention efforts has been on secondary prevention since this group is associated with the highest costs. (Eighty percent of health care costs for low back pain are incurred by 20% of the population with low back pain [1].) Secondary prevention strategies consist of ergonomic assessment of the workplace, which includes a functional and a technical review of what the job tasks entails, as well as a health assessment and optimal medical management of the employee, including considering risk factors for low back pain/injury. Both primary and secondary prevention strategies can be instrumental in preventing acute low back pain episodes from developing into chronic pain with disability.

Ergonomics in the Industrial Setting

Work-Related Risk Factors

The National Institute of Occupational Safety and Health (NIOSH) established workplace guidelines for lifting because of overwhelming literature supporting the association of LBP and excessive lifting (1,3-5). They reported that overexertion was associated with approximately half of the occupational injuries reported (2). Pushing and pulling activities are associated with increased reports of LBP. NIOSH reported that 20% of all injury claims for LBP involved pushing or pulling loads (2). The risk is thought to involve higher disc loads and higher stresses on the musculature supporting the spine. Twisting is also related to higher incidence of LBP. All the above forces are associated with a higher incidence of slips and falls which in turn lead to more cases of LBP. Prolonged sitting, especially in a car or truck, has also been associated with higher incidence of LBP in several, but not all studies. Additionally full body vibration has been associated with higher reports of LBP. Excessive levels and durations of exposure to whole-body vibrations may contribute to back pain and performance problems. Several government bodies have proposed duration limits for vibration levels to reduce these problems. Although the problem of whole-body vibration and the incurrence of back pain/injury are well established, procedures for measuring and analyzing vibration are complex and therefore have are difficult to control. Table 34-2 summarizes the etiology of work injuries, demonstrating that the vast majority are related to exertion.

Table 34-2   Work-Related Back Injuries Resulting in Lost Time and Their Causational Factors

Work-Related Event Causing Injury	*Number of Lost Time Injuries*
•Contact with objects and equipment: including stepping on, being struck, rubbed, or abraded by objects and caught in or compressed by machinery.	13,437
•Falls: including jumping, slipping, and tripping.	49,311
•Bodily reaction and exertion: including bending, climbing, crawling, reaching, twisting lifting, pushing, pulling, standing, sitting, walking, etc.	343,087
•Exposure to harmful substances or environments	286
•Transportation incidents: including both public roadways and highways as well as motorized equipment on employer property.	11,110
•Fires and explosions	48
•Assaults and violent acts: including acts by humans and animals	1521

Statistics established in data published by the Bureau of Labor Statistics based on the 1992 Occupational Injury and Illness Classification System and the Occupational Classification Structure developed by the Bureau of the Census. Data cited here are for the full year 1999 (2).

The Ergonomic Process

There has been a particular focus by companies on ergonomics as a means to reduce work-related injuries. Ergonomics, the science of matching the workplace conditions and job demands to the capabilities of the working population, focuses on the assessment of work-related risk factors for musculoskeletal disorders and identifying changes to reduce those risk factors. The overall goal of ergonomic training and job modification is to enable managers and employees to identify these work-related risk factors.

One aspect of the ergonomic process involves surveillance of workers to recognize the signs and symptoms of musculoskeletal disorders so that early, if not preventative, action can be taken to reduce the severity and frequency of injury. Proactive ergonomics, on the other hand, "emphasize efforts at the design state of work processes to recognize needs for avoiding risk factors that can lead to musculoskeletal problems" (5). One such effort is an attempt on the part of employers to match and/or screen employees, based on their body types and their physical abilities, to job demands.

For an ergonomics program to be effective, it must use a tested and proven approach. NIOSH has set specific guidelines that comprise a seven-step "pathway" for evaluating and addressing musculoskeletal concerns in the workplace (6). The seven elements of this program are:

1. Looking for signs of work-related musculoskeletal disorders (WMSDs).
2. Setting the stage for action by identifying participants, expressions of management commitment to the program and encouragement of employee involvement.
3. Building in-house expertise via training, thus expanding management and employee abilities to evaluate potential musculoskeletal problems and risks.
4. Gathering and examining evidence of work-related musculoskeletal disorders using sources such as OSHA logs, medical records, and job analysis.
5. Developing engineering and administrative controls for tasks that pose a risk of musculoskeletal injury.
6. Health care management to emphasize the importance of early detection and treatment.
7. Implementing proactive ergonomic changes.

Properly and successfully implemented, an ergonomics program such as NIOSH's has the potential to yield positive results in terms a lower incidence and severity rate of work-related musculoskeletal disorders as well as produce an increase in worker productivity and product quality. While research has not definitively proven the effectiveness of interventions in a number of areas, common sense and basic science proofs suggest that these interventions will help. Nevertheless, it should be kept in mind that the OSHNA/NIOSH guidelines alone will not prevent all occurrences of low back pain.

The development of a proactive ergonomic team was a hallmark of the Ergonomic Standards that were developed and published in the Federal Register in 2000, only to be discarded by the next administration. Despite the advances in ergonomic teams in many industries and the redesign of many jobs, the attempts by industry to redesign the workstation and match the worker's physical attributes have not been very successful. This type of mixed picture of ergonomics is one of the primary reasons the Ergonomic Standards were repealed.

In the large industrial workplace, many of the highest risk jobs were redesigned to reduce the lifting requirements and reduce the pushing, pulling, and twisting, but there has not been a corresponding reduction in work related injuries. In fact, over the past 20 years, the number of work-related musculoskeletal disorders reported has dramatically increased despite the use of ergonomic teams and the development of a lifting guideline (2). This paradox seems to relate to the elimination of rate limiting jobs that had were associated with high lifting requirements and awkward movements: When redesigned with robotics or lifting assists, the rate of the production line could be increased. Therefore the reduction in lifting stress was replaced by higher repetition with the overall level of ergonomic risk being transferred from a few jobs to many jobs.

NIOSH Lifting Guidelines

The basis principles of the lifting guidelines is to reduce the force and stress on the low back, the discs and the supporting musculature (4,5,7). The load on the low back is related to the weight of the object being lifted, the relative height and tilt of the spine in addition to the distance of the object from the spine. A person would have the same load placed upon the low back when holding a 25-kg weight at their side as they would if they were holding a 5-kg weight at arms length from the body at the level of their shoulder or feet. NIOSH has developed a formula for establishing safe lifting loads for the general population based on age, gender, and height. This is used regularly in the design of industrial jobs.

More sophisticated models for rating lifting tasks in terms of reducing risks for low back disorders have been developed. The University of Michigan developed both a two-dimensional and, more recently, a three-dimensional approach to estimate the amount of compressive forces on spinal discs in the low back as well as the muscle strength needed for a person to perform the lifting task in question (8). In these studies, load weight, lift height, hand locations, and hip and joint angles for the observed lifting act were measured and serve as input for these calculations. Risk estimates are based on the percentages of the male workforce who would have the strength capacity to withstand the compressive forces that may be generated. Disk compression forces of 770 lb and greater have been identified with increasing rates of reported low back pain and thus would pose a significant hazard.

"Back School"

Many employers, most notably the health care industry where LBP is a major occupational hazard, have instituted educational programs, often called "back school" for employees (9,10,11). These programs teach the basic ergonomic principles as well as focusing on some type of fitness program to increase back flexibility and strengthening the back and abdominal muscles. In studies on the effectiveness of implementing such educational programs, the resulting change in incidence rates of low back pain, and cost effectiveness of using the programs has not been demonstrated (9,10,11).

Most studies on education programs show a change in employee behaviors immediately following the "back school," but these positive changes rapidly fall off over time and employees revert back to their former habits (9,12,13). Workers do demonstrate an increased understanding of the etiology of lower back pain and the ergonomic risks; however, this knowledge does not necessarily translate into better health outcomes. It is very difficult to have an impact on the personal health habits of a large group of workers, especially if they are not experiencing LBP. The success rate for establishing an exercise or conditioning program, as a primary prevention strategy, is quite low.

This has been studied among nurses and nurses aides, a particularly high risk group. In this population, if the ergonomic intervention involves a lifting aide or the use of two nurses for a specific transfer activity and this strategy requires more time to accomplish the task, the strategy may be ignored in favor of expediency (14). Most of the activities associated with patient transfers cannot be automated as was done in the industrial setting and therefore the options are limited.

Most recently, a completely different approach to back pain education has been shown to have remarkable results. In Norway, a country where patient education via the classic "Swedish back school" and high-quality physical therapy is the norm, Dr. Aage Indahl took an opposite approach to back pain. From the sick list in the town of Fredricstad, a random number of patients with back pain were assigned to meet for 1 hour with Dr. Indahl, with a 1/2-hour follow-up a few weeks later. Indahl's patients were instructed with great elegance, "if your back hurts, just keep on moving." "Don't pay attention to that body mechanics stuff about how to lift, your body knows what to do." Both logical and emotional arguments debunked most of the advice patients are given about their back pain. At 2 years and 7 years follow-up, Indahl's population had significantly less pain and disability (15). This approach, along with consumerism telling patients they do not usually need x-rays or surgery, has also had a great positive impact in a public health campaign in Australia. The efficacy of this approach is not only to be emulated; it teaches us something about the harm done when health care providers overmedicalize the back pain problem.

Unless there is constant reinforcement of an ergonomics program, they have been shown to have little long-term effect. Even as a secondary prevention strategy, aimed at workers with LBP, efforts intended to help change work practices and health habits have not been very successful. For many, once the acute episode of pain resolves, their compliance with the new work practice and the exercise program drops off dramatically.

Lumbar Supports

Another means of primary prevention is the use of a lumbar support to provide stability to the low back during lifting activities (11,16). The use of personal protective devices (PPDs) is one of the most controversial aspects today in the prevention of work-related LBP. By definition, a PPD provides a barrier between the worker and the hazard source on the job. Devices to prevent lower back pain and injury are among the most common PPDs used. Even NIOSH, while supporting the use of PPDs where practical, feels the use of these devices and their actual benefits is still open to question. One aspect not to be overlooked is the potential negative impact of implementing the use of PPDs. There is some evidence to show that they may actually decrease one risk factor exposure at the expense of increasing exposure to another because the worker is uncomfortable in the device or otherwise changes their physical work practices.

Studies have shown little significant evidence, if any, that back braces actually work in prevention or treatment of back pain (1,11). In contrast, a more recent epidemiological study on the use of back belts in a large, retail chain of hardware stores, found use of these PPDs reduced the rate of low back pain injuries (16). Although NIOSH believes this study does provide evidence that the use of back belts to prevent low back injury may be effective in some settings, they believe overall evidence for general applicability is inconclusive.

Case Study 34-1

A local foundry owner asks his internist/medical director whether he's heard anything about a new back belt. He's had escalating costs due to back pain, he explains. The internist performs a quick calculation: One belt per year for 500 employees, at $50 per belt, would cost $25,000. In addition, there are hassles with implementation, enforcement, and increasing the workers' perception that the workplace caused injuries. With about 25 back injuries per year, at about $10,000 per back injury, one could make a case for the back belt if it actually cut injuries by 10-20%. But that seems unlikely given the lack of evidence for any effectiveness.

Instead, the internist proposes that the foundry have an ergonomist or even the local occupational therapist tour the plant to provide recommendations. He suggests that the owner work on the punitive atmosphere regarding injuries and make light duty available for injured workers. He recommends that the foundry educate its workers on key factors about back pain: It almost always gets better regardless of treatment. It is rarely dangerous after a doctor has evaluated it. X-rays and other diagnostic tests are seldom useful. Staying active despite pain is the best way to ensure recovery.

General Health and Fitness

General health issues have been examined as a method of preventing low back pain (1,10,16). Factors such as smoking and obesity do have an association with the prevalence of low back pain. However, research studies have shown contradictory results in the association of some covariate factors and the development of back pain. For example, studies have shown that obesity is both positively and negatively correlated with the incidence of low back pain.

Implementing programs such as cessation to smoking and weight control/loss have not been shown to significantly decrease the incidence of developing low back pain or its reoccurrence in people with prior episodes of low back pain. Furthermore, the large number of covariate factors that are associated with LBP make it difficult to study the effect of a prevention strategy that changes only one factor.

The idea of preventive exercise is complex. Exercise can consist of strength, flexibility, coordination, endurance exercises to the whole body or to individual parts. Yet the nonspecific effects of exercise-fitness, mood, company morale, and so forth-may be quite important. In addition, one needs to bear in mind that an exercise program for military recruits or nurses may not necessarily apply to stock brokers or foundry grinders.

Several studies have looked at overall physical fitness and its correlation to musculoskeletal and low back pain and injury. The U.S. Navy conducted several studies on recruits after implementing its "Healthy Back Program" (13). The Navy study found that better self-reported health and physical fitness were associated with fewer low back problems.

One of the factors that conditioning is most likely to affect is muscle fatigue. Muscle fatigue is experienced when the muscles do not receive enough oxygen for the imposed workload. If job energy demands are excessive, workers may well be at greater risk of musculoskeletal injury. Fitness may condition the muscle to be more efficient in using the available oxygen and thereby reduce muscle fatigue. However, although improved fitness in general will probably decrease the incidence of developing low back pain, there is a point where increased exposure to intense training and heavy loads actually predisposes people to the development of low back pain (1).

Preplacement Physical Assessment

Several clinical investigators have reported that lack of muscular endurance causes low back injuries. Low back pain patients and those without injury not only differ in muscle strength, but also in muscle endurance. Significant flexion and extension differences and differences in trunk endurance have also been found between low back pain sufferers and health controls. Preplacement testing on which to base hiring decisions may therefore be the preferred approach to preventing work-related back injury in physically demanding jobs that cannot be redesigned. The goal is to match the worker's physiological capabilities with the physical demands of the job. Thus, this strategy seeks to control the rates of injury by selecting only those individuals with the capacity to perform a given job.

Of the preplacement tests frequently used, strength testing is considered the most effective. This test is based on the concept that there is a direct relationship between the probability of injury and percentage of strength capacity used by the worker in job performance. Thus, the greater overall physical fitness, the greater strength capacity a worker should be able to demonstrate. Studies have indeed shown strength is related to injury rate, and that a worker's likelihood of sustaining a musculoskeletal injury increased when job lifting requirements approached or exceeded the worker's strength capacity (17). For the firefighting occupation, studies have strongly indicated a relationship between the incidence of back injury and physical fitness. The reported injury rates for the least fit groups were 7.1%, middle fit 3.2%, and most fit 0.8%. Additionally, of those physically fit firefighters that did sustain low back injury, the nature and severity of injury were less costly than injuries of those who were less fit. Many studies have shown clinical evidence that fitness level and exercise training appear to be related to injury and that high levels of aerobic fitness, strength, and flexibility are inversely related to workman's compensation costs for firefighters.

With studies repeatedly showing these results, the use of preplacement screening for fitness and strength may seem logical. The caveat to that notion is that a likely outcome of implementing physical abilities testing often adversely affects female job applicants. This has opened many employers, including fire departments, to gender and Americans with Disabilities Act (ADA) discrimination lawsuits. In order to avoid costly litigation, employers must implement job analysis to illustrate the need for specific physical requirements in job applicants and why these demands cannot be corrected.

Obstacles to Prevention

OSHA and NIOSH have implemented guidelines regarding the lifting of objects in the workplace which are based on compelling evidence that lifting in an ergonomically sound manner controls factors that influence the risk of developing back pain, thereby reducing the incidence of low back pain. Obstacles to the implementation of these guidelines, however, exist. Such obstacles include their impracticality in the actual workplace environment, unwillingness on the part of the employer to comply with such guidelines, and the wage costs of expedience versus the wage costs of completing the task in an ergonomically sound manner. Furthermore, the majority of studies that have researched the implementation of these prevention programs have failed to show cost effectiveness and statistically significant, as well as clinically notable, reductions in the incidence of low back pain and injury occurrences.

Comorbid Factors

Low back pain cannot be treated or prevented in isolation. There are multiple comorbid factors, such as depression, lack of physical exercise and job satisfaction (18), that have been shown to have a correlation with the development of low back pain. Without consideration and inclusion of psychosocial factors as well as medicolegal concerns into any prevention strategy, the chance of success for that strategy is greatly diminished.

Recommendations

- Physicians who hope to prevent back pain should not rely on simply educating their patient.
- Education is helpful in preventing disability, so discussion with patients should revolve around health care consumerism and coping strategies.
- Telling workers to lift, bend, twist, and so forth in specific ways may not be effective, but ergonomic controls and administrative policies aimed toward safety and overall health are advised.

■   ■   ■

Key Points

- The direct and indirect costs incurred by back pain are significant, with more than 19 million workers each year sustaining back injury.

- One prevention strategy employs ergonomics. The goal of ergonomics is to enable managers and employees to identify work-related risk factors.
- Educational programs for workers can be used to teach basic ergonomic principles and fitness programs.
- Devices to prevent low back injury, such as lumbar supports, are another method of primary prevention.
- Preplacement testing is a useful strategy for preventing work-related injury when the job itself cannot be redesigned.

REFERENCES

1. Musculoskeletal disorders and the workplace: low back and upper extremities. Washington, DC: Panel on Musculoskeletal Disorders and the Workplace, Commission on Behavioral and Social Sciences and Education, National Research Council and Institute Medicine, 2001;303-313, 351-357.

2. Bureau of Labor Statistics Reports. Occupational Illness and Injury. Washington DC: Department of Labor, 1999.

3. Work-related Musculoskeletal Disorders, Washington, DC: National Academy of Science, National Academy Press; 1999.

4. **Levy BS, Wegman DH, eds.** Occupational Health: Recognizing and Preventing Work-Related Disease, 3rd ed. Philadelphia: Lippincott Williams & Wilkins;1994; 345-57.

5. **Halpern M.** Prevention of low back pain: basic ergonomics in the workplace and the clinic. Baillieres Clin Rheumatol. 1992;6(3):705-30.

6. NIOSH Publication 97-117. Department of Health and Human Services, Elements of Ergonomics Programs; 1997;1-5.

7. **Pope MH.** Concepts in the prevention of occupational low back pain. Contemporary Orthopedics. 1988;17(3):43-54.

8. **Raschke U.,Martin BJ, Chaffin DB.** Distributed moment histogram: a neurophysiology based method of agonist and antagonist trunk muscle activity prediction. J Biomech. 1996;29(12):1587-96.

9. **Daltroy LH, Iversen MD, Larson MG, Lew R, Wright E, Ryan J, et al.** A controlled trial of an educational program to prevent low back injuries. N Engl J of Med. 1997;337(5):322-8.

10. **Garg A, Moore JS.** Prevention strategies and the low back in industry. Occup Med. 1992;7(4):629-40.

11. **Lahad A, Malter AD, Berg AO, Deyo RA.** The effectiveness of four interventions for the prevention of low back pain. JAMA. 1994;272(16):1286-1291.

12. **Cherkin D, Deyo RA, Berg AO.** Evaluation of a physician education intervention to improve primary care for low back pain II: impact on patients. Spine. 1991;16(10):1173-78.

13. **Woodruff SI, Conway TL, Bradway L.** The US Navy healthy back program: effects on basic knowledge among recruits. Military Med 1994;159(7):475-84.

14. **Harnett S.** Work related back pain in nurses. J Adv Nurs. 1996;23(6):1235-46.

15. **Indahl A, Velund L, Reikeraas O.** Good prognosis for low back pain when left untampered. A randomized clinical trial. Spine. 1995;20:473-7.

16. **van Poppel MN, Koes BW, van der Ploeg T, Smid T, Bouter LM.** Lumbar supports and education for the prevention of low back pain in industry: a randomized controlled trial. JAMA. 1998;279(22):1789-94.

17. **Jackson AS.** Pre-employment physical evaluation. Exerc and Sport Sci Rev. 1994;22:53-90.

18. **Kendall N.** Psychosocial approaches to the prevention of chronic pain: the low back paradjgm. Best Pract and Res Clin Rheumatol. 1999;13(3):545-54.

■   ■   ■

KEY REFERENCES

Lahad A, Malter AD, Berg AO, Deyo RA. The effectiveness of four interventions for the prevention of low back pain. JAMA. 1994;272(16):1286-91.
A great review of the major preventions strategies and their effectiveness.

Musculoskeletal disorders and the workplace: low back and upper extremities. Panel on Musculoskeletal Disorders and the Workplace, Commission on Behavioral and Social Sciences and Education, National Research Council and Institute Medicine, 2001.
This bible of epidemiologic studies focuses on musculoskeletal disorders and the workplace. Addresses LBP as well as upper extremity problems in the workplace.

35

■ ■ ■

Back Pain in Children and Adolescents

Ebony Parker

Andrew J. Haig, MD

Andrew Marsh, PT

lthough this book focuses primarily on back pain in adults, primary care physicians often see children with back pain. The literature on the subject has increased explosively as we have come to find that back pain is more common in children than previously thought. Aside from the discomfort and disability that it causes, back pain is of additional importance in children because of the special health concerns it poses for this population. In children, back pain is more likely the consequence of serious disease than it is in adults. Furthermore, because of the growth process, the risk of deformity and progression is a consideration in children (1). Perhaps most important, in light of the disastrous impact of back pain on adults, is the impact of childhood back pain on future health behaviors.

Although back pain is quite common in children, there is not much research in the area. A review of the disorder and its implications may improve care and focus future research in the area. This chapter does not cover idiopathic scoliosis, an area that has been the subject of countless volumes, and it touches only briefly on malignant and systemic causes of back pain. Instead, it focuses primarily on what may be the most common complaint, "mechanical back pain."

Epidemiology

Prevalence

Though once thought to be rare, back pain in children is now understood to be a common problem. As many as one in three children will suffer from this condition at one point or another. Factors reported in association with increased prevalence of low back pain (LBP) in children are age (>13 years), female gender, parental history, participation in athletics, and time spent watching television or in physical inactivity (2,3,4).

Among school-aged children, the reported lifetime prevalence of back pain is 34.2%. In the literature the prevalence ranged from 7-63% in persons age 10-24 years. However, these numbers have a positive correlation with age, as the age of the population increases, particularly after age 13, the prevalence rate also increases (5). In a study of 1608 school children, Balague et al. reported a 12% prevalence of history of low back pain among children aged 8-12 years compared to a 32% prevalence among those aged 13-16 years (6).

With regard to gender, there is variation within the literature. While most attribute female sex as a factor for increased occurrence, (7) others report no significant difference between the two sexes (3). Balague et al. reported the low back pain prevalence of girls to be 6% higher than boys (32% vs. 38%) in their 1988 study, though in a similar study in 1994 they found only borderline differences between the two sexes. There is agreement however, that young girls tend to report back pain more frequently than their same age counterparts and have a significantly higher point prevalence with regards to pain in the previous week (6).

An abundance of literature associates a parental history of back pain as a factor for increased prevalence among children and adolescents (3,7). In one study, a child with a parental history of back pain had approximately double the risk compared to those with no history (6). Among children with no family history, 14% reported a history of LBP as compared to 21% of those with a one-parent history and 24% of those with both parents positive for treated LBP. Other literature states that up to 64% of children who admitted to LBP have had at least one parent who also suffered from the condition (9). Because a reported 80% of the adult population has experienced back pain, we can only expect to see similar occurrences within the younger generations (10).

Another factor commonly attributed to increased risk of LBP in children was participation in athletic activities, particularly those where lumbar strain, twisting, or hyperextension exists (i.e., football, gymnastics, tennis etc). In a study by Balague et al., 24% of competitive athletes reported LBP as opposed to 16% of those who participated in recreational athletic activity (5). And in a longitudinal study by the International Chiropractic Pediatric Association (ICPA), of 98 adolescents, recurrent pain was reported by 6 of 33 nonathletes as opposed to 29 of 65 athletes (11).

Not only athletic activity, but physical activity in general has been indicated as a risk factor. Taimela et al reported out of 1171 schoolchildren ages 7-16 years, 47.7% of those who were highly physically active reported LBP as compared to 25% of the moderate group and 27.6% of the low physical activity group, suggesting that both increased and decreased physical activity can lead to back pain (3).

Along with physical inactivity, time spent watching television has also been considered a factor. It has been demonstrated that the lifetime prevalence of LBP is associated with the amount of time a child spends watching television, with the prevalence increasing as the child ages (6). For those who spent greater than two hours a day enjoying this medium, the reported prevalence range from 25% to 50% (6,12). This figure is lower for those who watch less. This suggests that those who spend significant amounts of time watching television place themselves at a greater risk for back pain, which may be associated with prolonged sitting, poor posture and decreased activity that go along with the behavior (6).

Incidence

In a prospective study by Burton et al. of adolescents beginning at 11 years old and extending over a four-year period, the average annual incidence of low back pain was 16% (1a). Overall, the pain reported was mild and self-limiting (2).

Risk Factors and Prevention

Backpacks

There has been an overwhelming popular notion that backpacks are the cause or aggravator of back pain in children. Repetitive loading of the spine is a documented risk factor for low back pain among both children and adults. In schoolchildren, backpacks present a daily load with regards to repetitive motion (8). Currently, the thought exists that these backpacks represent another risk for LBP within younger populations. Whether the weight of the bag, the way in which the bag is carried, or the length of time carried are all factors that warrant further investigation.

We have just completed a study of 184 school children (13). The study measured the weight of the child and the backpack, and recorded the presence of pain. Although back pain increased with age, the % of body weight carried in a backpack had no relationship with pain.

In a study of 237 Italian schoolchildren, the average daily load carried was 9.3 kg, reaching a maximum of 12.5 kg. The percent of body-weight lifted ranged from a mean of 22 to a maximum of 36.4, with 34.8% of the students carrying more than 30% of their body-weight at least once during the week(s) of the study (8).

Because an association between backpack weight and LBP in children exists, several suggests that limits be place on how much a child can carry.

These limits are currently in place for the adult population. In Italy the labor laws dictate a maximum load of 30 kg for men and 20 kg for women. The United States National Institute for Occupational Health and Safety guidelines can be used to calculate the maximum safe weight for adults to lift under the best circumstances. Weights over 23 kg are thought to cause increased risk of back pain. The only such limit for children is the Italian labor law restricting lifting to 20 kg and 15 kg for boys and girls respectively (8). These limits, however, do not hold true in the classroom.

The French National Bureau of Education recommends a relative schoolbag weight (schoolbag weight/body weight x 100) of 10% (7). In the literature the figure ranges from 10% to 15%, though not scientifically proven (8). However, a schoolbag weight of 20% or more is positively associated with back pain requiring a visit to the physician, especially when the child walks to and from school (7). Further research is necessary in order to determine an appropriate backpack weight limit that could then be instituted in the classroom setting.

Another issue of concern with regard to preventing back pain is how the child carries his/her schoolbag. A difference in the distribution of the load on the spine is noted in whether the bag is carried on the shoulders or in the hand. The shoulder harness provides a more even distribution along the coronal plane than carrying the bag by the strap does (7).

In a study of 128 eighth graders, back pain leading to absence from school and/or sporting events was reported by 50% of those who carried their schoolbag in their hand as opposed to 11.5% of students who carried it on their shoulder (7). This suggests that students should be educated on the proper way to carry the schoolbag as a measure of prevention of back pain within the school-aged population.

A less significant factor related to back pain is the time spent carrying the bag. Students who walk to school have a higher association with pain, particularly when the backpack was equal to or greater than 20% of their body weight (7). The amount of travel between classes and number of books required for each class are also possible contributors to back pain in children and should be considered (8).

Posture

Very few kids, especially teens have good posture. This alone may cause dysfunction on the spine, especially when combined with a growth spurt. However, minor postural asymmetries are not the cause of back pain in children or adults as visible in the literature due to its lack of discussion (1). The individual posture of people is probably associated with their genetic and psychological make up (1). The child with postural problems is often corrected to "straighten up" and when the problem persists, exercises are often prescribed to strengthen the abdominal and pelvic muscles. However, the effectiveness of these exercise programs is debatable. Often there is a low compliance rate, especially among adolescents (10). The psychological effect of rewarding or punishing behavior related to back pain—thus focussing attention on illness behavior—may be the most compelling reason to avoid strong focus on active posture correction. On the other hand, passive correction—ergonomically designed seating and desks, for instance—may have merit.

It should be emphasized that the effect of body mechanic advice is unproven and challenged in adults. Respected research shows greater improvement in pain when patients are simply taught to lift and move naturally (14).

Case Study 35-1

A 5-year-old girl is brought in by her mother, who is concerned that lately the girl has been moaning and groaning and complaining of backaches. A reliable and complete review of systems indicates no fevers, night sweats, or bowel or bladder problems. She does not awaken at night with the pain. On exam she is alert, playful, and looks healthy. Neurologic and orthopedic exam are unremarkable, and you cannot reliably reproduce her tenderness. You inquire further and find that the father has recently been off of work for a back injury. The mother notes that the daughter's behavior is indeed similar to her husband's. It is a judgment call whether you proceed with a sedimentation rate or other workup, but in this case you choose to watch and have the mother call your office in a few weeks to ensure that the episode is done.

Sports

As the number of children and adolescents who participate in competitive athletic activities increase, so has the number of complaints of low back pain (15). As previously stated, increased activity increases the risk of back pain and in athletes vs. non-athletes among school-aged populations, the prevalence rates for LBP were 23.6% and 15.8% respectively. Thus demonstrating the higher risk of injury among the athletic community (5).

Athletes are particularly vulnerable to back pain brought about by acute trauma, stress fractures, spondylitic fractures and overuse syndrome. Often the pain is a nonspecific strain or of a mechanical nature (15). These conditions could be due to the tight muscles and ligaments often seen in athletes as well as weakness of certain key muscle groups, such as the abdominals. Prevention of LBP among the child and adolescent athlete should consist of instruction in technique, proper equipment and strengthening and stretching (16).

Often within the athletic population there is a tendency to over-train. They try to do too much over too short a period, which can result in overuse syndrome and injury (16). The most important role the physician can play in that situation is as advisor to the coach. A carefully designed, systematic training schedule with appropriate technique and slow progression reduce the risk of overuse and stress injuries and also promote greater physical health for the athlete (15).

A second mode of prevention is a precautionary one. Protective equipment must be appropriate when training or in competition. Properly placed mats for gymnastics is an example of such precautions that should never be overlooked as too often they can lead to serious injury (16).

The most beneficial and practical form of preventive treatment is a balanced stretching and strengthening program. Targeting both the tight and weak muscles of the athlete will increase their athletic capability as well as make them less susceptible to certain injuries (16,17). The program should consist of systematic stretches executed in a slow and consistent motion as to allow for a complete stretch, as well as weight training to increase strength and endurance, particularly in the dorsal spine, abdominals and legs (16). These measures will improve the overall health and well-being of the student athlete as well as decrease risk and promote a stronger defense against injury and other conditions which cause back pain.

Systemic Causes in Children

Systemic causes of back pain, including infection and tumor are uncommon. However, in comparison to adults, children see physicians less often for back pain, so the relative importance of ruling out systemic illnesses in greater in this population.

Diskitis

Diskitis is a bacterial infection, most commonly seen in the lower thoracic and upper lumbar disk spaces. Unlike other musculoskeletal infections, it will normally resolve spontaneously. Traditionally it is seen in children ages 1-12 years, with sixty percent of all disk space infections occurring in children six years and under, though it can occur at any age (18). The presentation of symptoms are age related and diagnosis is often delayed due to their vagueness and poor localization (1,19).

In infants the clinical features are fever, irritability and unwillingness to walk or stand. In children diskitis is a constitutional illness often with nausea and vomiting. In the adolescent, it may present as a complaint of simple back pain. There may be, a history of sore throat or upper respiratory infection preceding the diskitis (5). Usually these findings along with an elevated sedimentation rate are enough to make the diagnosis.

Early on a bone scan may show increased uptake over several vertebral levels. After two weeks or so radiographs may demonstrate disk narrowing has often occurred. Magnetic resonance imaging (MRI) scans are also useful and have been indicated as a better detector of the disease than bone scans, though they are more expensive.

If the radiographs show vertebral collapse and/or a soft tissue mass, it is wise to rule out tuberculosis of the spine as well as spinal cord compression by way of neurologic examination. Though rare, these diseases are more severe and would warrant further examination and treatment (19).

Except in the case of severe illness the literature does not advocate any treatment. However, with systematic illness an antibiotic may be used. A "panty spica" or other thoracolumbar brace to immobilize the back for 4-6 weeks may relieve discomfort (1,5).

Osteomyelitis

Osteomyelitis is a vertebral infection that most often occurs in adults, though it can also be seen in children, usually age 1 to 12 years (19). The children affected tend to be debilitated, and the older children often have a history of intravenous drug abuse (18). Patients with osteomyelitis manifest symptoms similar to diskitis, but radiographs make the erosion and collapse of the vertebral body clear. Treatment includes a biopsy and antibiotics, along with rest and possible cast immobilization. If these treatments do not prove successful, then an excisional biopsy or an anterior spinal fusion is recommended.

Tumors

Although scoliosis is beyond the scope of this chapter, a brief mention of scoliosis is called for here. Viewed from the back, a scoliosis should have a "backwards S" shape. A "forward S" curve has a high likely hood of being a tumor or other disease. While mild idiopathic scoliosis is often watched expectantly, the "forward S" deserves a serious workup.

Two forms of primary bony spinal tumors exist: Those that affect the spinal cord and those that involve the bony vertebrae or soft tissues. In children bone forming tumors are more frequent, though both are unusual. Of these, the most common are osteoid osteoma and osteoblastoma. Osteoid osteoma is a benign mass characterized by the formation of a vascular osteoid surrounded by sclerotic bone. Osteoblastomas are similar, only larger in size (5). The hallmark symptom is night pain. Others including nonspecific back pain, changes in coordination and bladder and/or bowel incontinence (though often no neurologic deficit). This pain is characteristically relieved with aspirin or nonsteroidal anti-inflammatory drugs (NSAIDs). A bone scan will best determine if a lesion is present. However, x-rays, computed tomography (CT) scans, and other imaging studies may also prove helpful. With osteoid osteoma and osteoblastoma full resection of the neoplasm is recommended.

Leukemia and lymphoma are both primary malignant neoplasms and are not commonly seen in the spine. Symptoms include pain and decreased spinal mobility. Childhood leukemia often presents with bone pain, including back pain (20). Other signs include night pain, weight loss, elevated Erethrocyte sedimentation rate (ESR) and fever (5). Bone scans prove the most successful in reaching a diagnosis.

Spinal cord tumors and malignant neoplasms are of a more serious nature, and require greater examination, yet are less frequent (1,5,17,21,22). Aneurysmal bone cysts are often present long before they are ever detected. The lesion is normally found on the posterior elements of the spine and is asymptomatic. When symptoms begin, it is usually in response to a fracture, collapse or hemorrhage of the affected area. Treatment (as with most benign tumors) is excision and, depending on the damage, bone grafting (5).

Eosinophilic granuloma is one of the few neoplasms that does not require prompt surgical intervention. Though it usually runs on a self-limiting course, in some cases it may cause collapse of the vertebral body (1). A needle biopsy is best for diagnosis and often low dose radiation therapy proves successful for treatment when needed (18).

Spondyloarthropathies

Rheumatoid arthritis rarely involves the spine. Seronegative spondyloarthropathies are a concern, however. They typically present in adulthood, but may be seen rarely in children. Chapter 19 describes their presentation and treatment. In children, especially, aggressive medication treatment and rehabilitation are important to prevent deformity (10,23).

Scheuermann disease is a familial osteochondrosis, similar in pathophysiology to the more commonly recognized Osgood Schlatter disease of the knee. It affects the thoracic spine resulting in vertebral wedging and kyphosis. The deformity is probably caused by mechanical stress of a genetically vulnerable vertebral end plate (1). Scheuermann's is reported to be the second most common cause of back pain among younger populations. Symptoms, however, are usually not severe and are reported as aggravating, but not limiting (19). In occasional cases the deformity can be disabling, leading to surgery. As with ankylosing spondylitis, rehabilitation therapies are aimed at preventing deformity, though the deformities are different in this primarily thoracic disease.

Other systemic causes which will not be discussed in any detail include fibromyalgia, myopathies causing primary muscle pain, metabolic disorders such as sickle cell anemia or porphyria. Any neuromuscular disorder may result in asymmetric movement and mechanical pain.

Case Study 35-2

A woman brings her 13-year-old son to the office for a pre-football physical examination. He says he's had a vague thoracic pain for 4 months. On exam no sacroiliac tenderness, good flexibility, and no neurologic deficit are noted. He does appear to have a mild kyphosis. X-rays show multiple schmorl's nodes (sign of disk herniation through the vertebral end plates) and some anterior wedging. The diagnosis of Scheuermann epiphisitis is made. The physician allows him to play football, but counsels him to work on trunk and neck extension strengthening and stretching exercises and encourages him to sleep on his stomach. Ibuprofen as needed is prescribed for more significant pain. He is scheduled to be seen 2 months later to encourage compliance with the exercises, monitor his use of ibuprofen, and to introduce the need for continued exercise through his growth phase. He is followed up again in about 6 months to ensure that there is no progression.

Psychosocial Causes

Psychosocial factors can be the primary cause of back pain complaints in children who have no organic spinal pathology. When careful diagnostic and physical evaluation have been done with no substantial findings or when the patients' symptoms seem to exceed the clinical findings, psychosomatic reactions should be considered (19).

Very young children rarely complain of back pain. Although systemic illness should be considered, often their complaint represents a mimicry of their parents. As children reach the later preschool age, the complaints need to be viewed as more likely related to focal pathology.

Hysteria can be associated with a typical back pain and is more often seen in adolescent girls. Often there is a family history of back pain. Treatment by cast immobilization is cited to distinguish between functional and mechanical pain, (1) though more sophisticated psychiatric approaches may be used, as well.

With a child who has had previous fractures or other severe injuries, presents with complaints of back pain child abuse should also be considered and dealt with during evaluation (5). Social clues or the specific pathology of the injury (e.g., unusual locations, associated unusual soft tissue damage, or unusual types of fractures in the limbs) should lead to inquiry.

It should be kept in mind, however, that medical conditions, though rare do exist and should not be overlooked when trying to determine a psychiatric cause (1,5,19). The interactions between psychological causes, psychological exacerbators, and psychological sequelae of back pain are important, complex, and often difficult to separate from the pathological process in the spine.

Local Spine Pathology

Spondylolysis and Spondylolisthesis

Spondylolisthesis is a condition in which one vertebra is displaced over another. Spondylolysis is a structural defect of the pars interarticularis. Together they are present in 7% of the general population, though most will never become symptomatic or require surgical intervention (24).

In children, these diseases are often discussed together because spondylolisthesis often occurs after an adolescent growth spurt where a spondylitic defect of the pars interarticularis was already present. The difference between the two is that in a spondylolysis the spatial relationship between the vertebra with the defective pars and the vertebra below remain unchanged, whereas with a spondylolisthesis there is a forward slip or movement of the affected vertebra (20).

There is a genetic predisposition to spondylolisthesis; approximately 27% of cases occur in first-order relatives, making the family history an important part of the diagnosis (5).

The onset of a spondylolisthesis is 10-15 years of age. Though some literature reports the initial defect occurring as early as 7-8 years, there is agreement that prior to 5 years of age the condition is almost nonexistent (17). The disease has a prevalence of 6% after reaching skeletal maturity. This figure is higher in boys, yet the risk for progression of the displacement is greater in girls (20).

Several etiologies for spondylolisthesis exist. Congenital and pathologic are rare and will not be discussed. Degenerative is common among the adult population, but is not relevant to our study.

In young people, isthmic spondylolisthesis is the most common. Within the isthmic type, three defects of the pars exist: Lytic fracture, where there is fibrous defect across the pars, elongation of the pars and acute fracture of the pars. The lytic fracture is the most common of the three and in an active adolescent, the more fragile pars is easy to damage, with a spondylolisthesis often caused by a stress fracture from overuse as a result of physical activity (10,17,20,24). Acute fracture is typically associated with substantial trauma and usually results in significant neurologic deficit.

The most frequent level of displacement is the L5-S1 vertebra. L4, though not as common, is also found, especially in patients with a hypomobile L5-S1 motion segment. If the displacement is severe the slippage may be palpable on examination. However, in less severe cases the defect may go undetected until adulthood when symptoms may arise (1,17).

Athletic participation is a common cause for symptoms, and there are special issues in the management of athletes with spondylolysis and spondylolisthesis (25) Briefly, spondylolisthesis or spondylolysis should be considered in young athletes with back pain. Initial diagnostics may include plane lateral x-rays. Because there is a radiation concern and most spondylolistheses are documented on that film alone, oblique films should not be obtained unless the lateral film is negative. Bone scan with single photon emission computed tomography (SPECT) imaging is more sensitive than plain bone scan. MRI is less desirable than thin slice CT scan, which can reliably indicate healing across the pars, even when the bone scan continues to light up. Traditionally athletes are kept out of the stressful part of their sport until pain resolves. Some physicians advocate bracing, as well. Although activity restriction is often advocated for persons with symptomatic spondylolisthesis, Muschik et al. followed a group of 86 young athletes with asymptomatic spondylolisthesis and found that although some improved or declined radiographically, none had onset of symptoms in almost 5 years of observation (26).

The majority of children and adolescents who have this condition will never have any significant symptoms or pain. With spondylolisthesis few will have progression of the slippage and even fewer will progress after ages 16-18. Of those that do develop symptoms, the onset is usually in the early adult years and declines thereafter. Most cases should be treated with conservative care as they will improve over time. Severe slippage may require operative intervention, which under those conditions prove successful (1,24,27).

Disk Herniation and Degeneration

Disk herniations occur rarely in the child and adolescent stages. Overall they account for 1-4% of all patients (5). A higher prevalence also exist within the male population (6). Similar to adults, the lower two lumbar disks are most commonly involved, and the pain typically radiates below the knee (1). Symptoms can also be increased by sneezing or coughing. In a study by Epstein et al. of 25 patients with disk herniation, more than 50% reported trauma as the underlying cause. However, in children this is not always the case. Accompanying herniated disk there are often other issues of the spine such as spondylolisthesis, congenital spinal stenosis, and lateral recess narrowing (19).

The natural history of disk herniations is typically benign, though this has not been well studied in children. Treatment is that of conservative care, NSAIDs, physical therapy, and psychosocial support. Physical therapy goals may include decrease in spasm and associated contractures, prevention of motor pattern alterations, reconditioning, lifestyle adaptation (perhaps with help from an occupational therapist), and education. Relative rest including a decrease in activity that would further aggravate the injury is suggested. Epidural cortizone injections are not studied in children, but are probably indicated before considering surgery. In cases where no improvement is seen, and the pain seems to worsen, surgery presents a viable option. In patients with operative disks, 90% reported good to excellent results as opposed to only 25% of those who did not receive surgery (5).

In younger patients, displacement of the posterior growth apophysis can also occur and present with symptoms similar to those produced by a herniation. Normally it is preceded by acute trauma of some type. CT and MRI scans prove most successful in visualizing the displacement to make a correct diagnosis. Though this finding is infrequent, surgical and other treatment decisions are aided by distinguishing this syndrome from disk herniation (19).

Along with disk herniation, an even smaller subgroup of adolescents suffer from disk degeneration (DD). In adults, degeneration is considered to be an inevitable and normal process of aging, not necessarily associated with pain. Although Korean War victims—young men—showed some degeneration of disks on autopsy, disk degeneration is not usually radiographically present until the 30s. In a study by Salminen et al., following eighth graders with recurrent low back pain (LBP) versus a control group without LBP, one or more degenerated disks were found in 33% of all participants at 15 years of age (2). In those with recurrent pain (subjects evaluated at 14, 18, and 23 years of age), 89% had incipient or total degeneration compared with 21% of those with episodic pain. The incidence of recurrent pain was often noted after the age of rapid physical growth into early adulthood.

The risk of recurrent and persistent low back pain was higher in individuals with early signs of disk degeneration. The young patient with degeneration is more like to experience disk disease, and in the follow-up study disk degeneration often proceeded disk herniation. In some cases, the degeneration of the disk may make it more vulnerable to everyday loading and exaggerated movement so that the patients pain may not be that of the disk at all, but rather strain in ligaments and myofascial tissues (2).

The literature suggests that nonspecific recurrent pain in adolescents may be attributed to early disk degeneration. Although this population has an increased risk for recurrent LBP, as with most back pain it is self resolving in most cases. However, as a precautionary measure it is wise to rule out other causes as the degeneration could be the manifestation of an underlying disease (2).

Mechanical Disorders

"Mechanical" back pain means localized pain made worse by movement, not associated with neurologic deficit or dangerous causes such as fracture, infection, tumor, or polyarthritis. This may be the most common cause of back pain in children, but like adults, there is no good test to objectify the lesion. The relatively unprovable differential diagnosis includes muscle strain, ligament sprain, facet joint trauma, sacroiliac joint disorders, and tears to the annulus fibrosis of the disk. Subjective diagnoses are often made by skilled therapists, osteopaths, chiropractors, and manual medicine trained MDs, based on numerous diagnostic schema. Often these diagnostic schema look far beyond the immediate cause of the pain to precipitating factors such as muscle imbalance, hip joint asymmetry, leg length inequality, and so forth. Although the truth certainly must lie among these schema, there has been only a little success in sorting out and validating components.

Often mechanical back pain presents as "overgrowth" syndrome and is seen in conjunction with a child's second growth spurt (16). The pain is generally nagging, but tolerable, intermittent and non-radiating. The diagnosis is one of exclusion after more serious causes have been dismissed. Treatment involves stretching and strengthening of the muscles in order to increase flexibility, strength and endurance. Alteration of activity may be necessary until the pain resolves (18).

Treatment

Physical Therapy

Physical therapy treatment for children with back pain is very poorly described in the literature. In general there are few special rules for treating children. However, there are several areas that require more emphasis.

The primary issue is activity level. Children seem to either be over active, or under active. For instance, the child may either be involved in competitive sports, or spend time on computers or watching television (6). Rarely is the "typical patient" one who exercises in moderation. Parental habits and pressures play a large role in the behavior of "going all out" or being a "couch potato." Typically these are the hardest to treat, either because of the lack of attention to a home program, or because of unrealistic expectation that a pill will fix a mechanical back pain issue. Regardless of this the therapist should always put the responsibility of treatment on the older child rather than the parent.

A second issue addressed in physical therapy is stabilization. Decreased coordination may be due to lack of coordination normally learned in play. In therapy, almost always, there is a need for some kind of stabilization/strengthening activities. Improved stability may avoid injury from vigorous loading. Strengthening of muscles and improving endurance through high repetition-moderate resistance training programs during the initial adaptation periods (28). However, when strengthening children, it is important to keep a good relationship between back flexors and extensors, as excessive flexor strength relates to low back pain in children (29). Balance is the key to all strengthening exercises, regardless of mechanical problems. The timing of provocative motions depends on the mechanical aspect of the particular lesion. It is recommended that mechanical correction precede a balance and strengthening program. For every flexion exercise there should be an extension exercise.

Correcting poor posture is a third area that physical therapy addresses. If one puts abnormal forces on the spine, and ask it to develop correctly, there will be a path of least resistance, which may influence alignment. In this case, early correction will be of most benefit. In combination with this, it is also important to work on proprioception within the context of posture in hopes to delay any further spinal dysfunction. If the child develops correctly, but moves incorrectly due to abnormally tight/lax structures, dysfunction will also ensue. Yoga helps children in various ways including coordination, posture through holding different poses, and developing body awareness (30). Physical therapy focusing on mechanics of the spine is very similar to adult therapy. It is theoretically possible that overstressing the developing endplates could result in inhibition of growth, however, so some moderation is indicated. As well as the pelvic angle changes in the developing body.

Medications, Injection, and Surgery

These factors are beyond the scope of this chapter. There is substantial literature on medications for pain in children (31). Injections are not studied in children, but there is an assumption that they have a similar place in children as in adults. Surgery indications and techniques are dependent on specific diagnoses that are not emphasized in this review.

Multidisciplinary Rehabilitation

Multidisciplinary rehabilitation is the hallmark of adult chronic pain management. There is little written on the format or outcomes from such a treatment for chronic back pain in children. If our knowledge of adults is any guide, there are often psychological factors which predispose to chronic pain behavior, and the chronicity of the pain and its effect on the life role of the child may lead to deconditioning, contractures, fear, anxiety, isolation, and depression. It seems intuitive that when children become chronically disabled, a multidisciplinary approach including psychology is important. Exercise is the special knowledge of physical therapists. Lifestyle adaptation is the role of occupational therapists. Psychosocial adjustment and age-appropriate communication are the job of the psychologist. Research in other areas of rehabilitation suggests that a physician leader results in better coordination of efforts. Given the crucial need to model appropriate pain behavior and disability concepts to children with back pain, psychological factors should permeate all aspects of treatment.

Management Paradigm

The diagnostic and treatment paradigm for children with back pain has not been the subject of any substantial research. The information gleaned from this chapter, along with knowledge of general pediatric principles and adult spine management principals allows us to propose a very basic approach.

Age groups are recognized as the first decision making point. Somewhat arbitrarily, children are grouped into very young (where back pain is typically serious or a social behavior), preteens (where disk herniation and athletic type trauma is less likely than in the teen years) and young teens. After age 16, aside from social contexts, back pain may follow the treatment plans for adults. Evaluation of medical causes takes importance in all groups, with infection and tumor always a consideration. But in teens, the benign natural history of most back pain allows us to hold off on definitive tests if there are no danger signs. It should be clear that for most cases of back pain in children, as in adults, an anatomically provable cause of the pain will not be found.

Conclusion

The primary care physician should be dualistic in approaching children with back pain. On one hand, he or she should be extra vigilant about potential dangerous causes. Because of the growth process, the risks of deformity and progression must also be considered. On the other hand, the first encounter with a physician is an important opportunity to teach future adults about the benign nature of back pain. The proper management of back pain, and particularly chronic pain, in children may help set the stage for preventing future illness behaviors and psychological predispositions to chronic pain in these patients when they become adults.

■   ■   ■

Recommendations

- It is of great importance to rule out serious disease in children with back pain, because such disease is the underlying cause of the pain more often in children than in adults.

- In children with a history of previous fractures or severe injuries, consider the possibility of child abuse.
- When diagnostic evaluation does not yield findings or if the child's symptoms are more severe than is expected given the findings, psychosocial causes should be considered.
- To minimize the risk of back pain, children should be educated on the proper way to carry a schoolbag.
- Children who participate in sports should be instructed to use appropriate athletic training, a balanced stretching and strengthening program, and protective sports equipment.

Key Points

- Back pain in children is more common than was previously believed. One in three children will have back pain at some point.
- The prevalence of back pain is greater in girls than in boys. Having parents with a history of back pain, participating in sports, and physical inactivity are also associated with an increased prevalence of back pain.
- Risk factors for back pain in children include use of heavy backpacks, poor posture, and participation in sports.
- Tumor, infection, and psychosocial factors are more common in young children who have back pain complaints.
- The importance of ruling out systemic illnesses is greater in children than in adults.
- Although systemic illness should be considered in very young children, complaints of back pain in preschool-aged children may represent mimicry of parents.
- Physical therapy for children with back pain is complex and poorly described.
- Although little research has been done on the optimal treatment for chronic back pain in children, it is probable that a multidisciplinary approach that incorporates psychological therapy would benefit these patients.

Acknowledgments

We thank Sabrina Starks for assistance with manuscript preparation and Edward Hurvitz, MD, and Rita Ayyangar, MD, pediatric physiatrists at the University of Michigan, for sharing their knowledge of these issues.

■   ■   ▓

REFERENCES

1. **Staheli L.** Fundamentals of Pediatric Orthopedics, 2nd ed. Philadelphia: Lippincott-Raven; 1998;9-20:73-88.

1a. **Burton A, Clarke R, McClune T, Tillotson K.** The natural history of low back pain in adolescents. Spine. 1996;21(20):2323-28.

2. **Salminen J, Erkintalo M, Pentti J, Oksanen A, Kormano M.** Recurrent low back pain and early disc degeneration in the young. spine. 1999;24(13):1316-21.

3. **Taimela S, Kujala U, Salminen J, Vilijanen T.** The prevalence of low back pain among children and adolescents: a nationwide, cohort-based questionnaire survey in Finland. Spine. 1997;22(10):1132-6.

4. **Olsen T, Anderson R, Dearwater S, Kriska A, Cauley J, Aaron D, LaPorte R.** The epidemiology of low back pain in an adolescent population. Am J Public Health. 1992;82(4):606-8.

5. **Payne W, Ogilvie J.** Back pain in children and adolescents. In: England S, ed. The Pediatric Clinic of North America, Common Orthopedic Problems, 43(4). Philadelphia: WB Saunders; 1996;899-916.

6. **Balague F, Nordin M, Skovron M L, Dutoit G, Yee A, Waldburger M.** Non specific low-back pain among schoolchildren: a field survey with analysis of some associated factors. Journal of Spinal Disorders. 1994;7(5):374-9.

7. **Viry P, Creveuil C, Marcelli C.** Nonspecific back pain in children. Revue Du Rhumatisme [Engl. Ed.]. 1999;66(7-9):382-7.

8. **Negrini S, Carabalona R, Sibilla P.** Backpack as a daily load for schoolchildren. Lancet. 1999;354(9194):1974.

9. **Gunzberg R, Balague F, Nordin M, Szpalski M, Duyck D, Bull D, Melot C.** Low back pain in a population of schoolchildren [Abstract]. Eur Spine J. 1999;8(6):439-43.

10. **Dyment P.** Low back pain in adolescents. Pediatr Ann. 1991;20(4):170-8.

11. **Research Study online.** International Chiropractic Pediatric Association. Available at www.4icpa.org/research/backpain.htm.

12. **Balague F, Dutoit G, Waldburger M.** Low back pain in schoolchildren, an epidemiological study. Scand J Rehabil Med. 1988;20(4):175-9.

13. **Young IA, Haig AJ, Yamakawa KY.** The Association Between Back Pack Weight and Low Back Pain in Children. Submitted, Pediatric Rehabilitation, August 2004.

14. **Indahl A, Velund L, Reikeraas O.** Good prognosis for low back pain when left untampered. A randomized clinical trial. Spine. 1995;20(4):473-7.

15. **Jackson D.** Low back pain in young athletes: evaluation of stress reaction and discogenic problems. Am J Sports Med. 1979;7(6):364-6.

16. **Micheli L.** Low back pain in the adolescent: differential diagnosis. Am J Sports Med. 1979;7(6):362-4.

17. **Reider B.** Sports Medicine: The School-Age Athlete, 2nd ed. Philadelphia: WB Saunders; 1996:169-83.

18. **Renshaw T.** Pediatric Orthopedics. Philadelphia: WB Saunders; 1986:56-59.

19. **King H.** Back, pain in children. In: Weinstein SL, ed. The Pediatric Spine: Principles and Practice. Vol 1. New York: Raven Press; 1994:173-83.

20. **Mason D.** Back pain in children. Pediatr Ann. 1999;28(12):727-30.

21. **Stella G, Sanctis N, Boere S, Rondinella F.** Benign tumors of the pediatric spine: statistical notes [Abstract]. Chir Organi Mov. 1983;83(1-2):15-21.

22. **Frassica F, Waltrip R, Sponseller P, McCarthy E Jr.** Clinicopathologic features and treatment of osteoid osteoma in children and adolescents [Abstract]. Orthoped Clin North Am. 1996;27(3):559-74.

23. **Brewer E, Giannini E, Person D.** Juvenile Rheumatoid Arthritis, 2nd ed. Philadelphia: WB Saunders; 1982:111-4:241.

24. **Kahanovitz N.** Diagnosis and Treatment of Low Back Pain. New York: Raven Press: 1991;80-81, 105-107.

25. **Stinson JT.** Spondylolysis and spondylolisthesis in the athlete. Clin Sports Med. 1993;12(3):517-28.

26. **Muschik M, Hahnel H, Robinson PN, Perka C, Muschik C.** Competitive sports and the progression of spondylolisthesis. J Pediatr Orthoped, 1996;16(3):364-9.

27. **Fysh P.** Pediatric Low Back Pain: Case Report. DC Archives; 2000. Available at www.chiroweb.com/archives/10/15/26.html.

28. **Faigenbaum AD, Westcott WL, Loud RL, Long C.** The effects of different resistance training protocols on muscular strength and endurance development in children. Pediatrics. 1999;104(1):e5.

29. **Newcomer K, Sinaki M.** Low back pain and its relationship to back strength and physical activity in children. Acta Paediatrica. 1996;85(12):1433-9.

30. **Raghuri P, Telles S.** Indian J Physiol Pharmacol. 1997;41(4):409-15.

31. **Golianu B, Krane E J, Galloway KS, Yaster M.** Pediatric acute pain management. Pediatr Clin North Am. 2000;47(3):559-87.

■   ■   ■

KEY REFERENCES

Mason D. Back Pain in Children. Pediatr Ann. 1999;28(12):727-30.
 A good general review of the topic.

Staheli L. Fundamentals of Pediatric Orthopedics, 2nd ed. Philadelphia: Lippincott-Raven; 1998;9-20, 73-88.
 An extensive text of pediatric orthopedics with substantial discussion about back pain.

36

■ ■ ■

Athletes with Back Pain

Richard W. Kendall, DO
Michele Bird, PT

A s has been shown in previous chapters, low back pain is quite prevalent in the adult population. Athletes are no different and certainly not immune to episodes of low back pain. In fact, low back pain ranges from 30% of college football (1) and professional tennis players (2) to 90% of professional level golfers (3). However, it is important to remember that athletes are people, too. They can have tumors, arthritis, and infections as reasons for lower back pain. In this chapter, we plan to discuss common injury mechanisms, general diagnostic and treatment considerations in specific injuries, and rehabilitation strategies for recreational and elite athletes with low back pain.

Pain Generators

Numerous studies have reported on the possible sources of pain in the lumbar spine. Many of these have involved asymptomatic subjects who have undergone injection of irritants into various anatomic structures of the lumbar spine with documentation of pain response. It is generally agreed upon that the lumbar vertebrae, intervetebral disk, the various ligamentous structures, facet joint capsule, sacroiliac joint, segmental nerve root, and paraspinal muscles all can be sources of pain in the lumbar spine.

Injury Mechanisms

Injury to the lumbar spine, as well as all musculoskeletal injuries, can be broken into two major groups: macrotrauma and microtrauma. Macrotrauma is usually related to a single destructive event leading to tissue failure.

Table 36-1   Lumbar Spine Injury Types

Macrotrauma	Microtrauma
• Vertebral fracture	• Spondylolysis
• Intervertebral disk herniation	• Facet joint pain
• Spinal cord injury	• Myofascial pain syndromes; muscle strain

Microtrauma or overuse injuries are associated with repetitive loading of a tissue and failure of reparative processes to heal that tissue. Examples of each type are included in Table 36-1.

Macrotrauma Injuries

Vertebral Fracture

Though uncommon, spine fractures are potentially serious injuries. Although on-field evaluation and management of spinal injuries is beyond the scope of this text, a number of athletes may present to your office without prior evaluation after significant trauma. Full history and examination, including neurologic evaluation should be completed on all individuals. If a history of trauma is elicited, plain radiographs should be used to evaluate for alignment and fracture. Common mechanisms for compression, burst, and posterior element fractures include falls from height, high-velocity deceleration, forced hyperextension and hyperflexion. Commonly, these are associated with skiers, snowboarders, skateboarding and cycling, but can occur in all sports, especially those that involve apparatus. The presence of fracture on plain radiographs, warrants further evaluation with CT scanning to evaluate the full extent of the fracture. If there is associated neurologic changes, immobilization and magnetic resonance imaging (MRI) evaluation of the soft tissues should be done promptly.

Compression fractures with less than 25% height loss may be managed with analgesics, activity restrictions, and bracing in a Jewitt brace or thoracolumbo-sacral orthosis (TLSO) for 6 weeks. Compression fractures with greater than 40% or greater height loss should be further evaluated for middle or posterior column involvement. In addition, these should be referred for consideration of development of kyphotic deformity. Initial treatment should involve analgesics, activity restrictions and bracing. If pain persists after 6 weeks, further evaluation for disk injury, facet pathology or neural injury should be done.

Disk Herniation

Disk injury is associated with trauma in up to 60% of cases in the general population. Injury to the disk may include internal disk disruption, annular tears, protrusions, and herniations. In younger athletes another cause of pain can be end plate fracture and formation of Schmorl's nodes. Common mechanisms include axial loading and rotation, high compression force, and hyperflexion. Pain from the intervertebral disk has been described as dull, achy, deep, and pressure. This may be referred to the hip or buttock, thigh, knee, leg, calf and ankle in a nonspecific distribution. Conversely, pain from neural structures is usually described as shooting, burning, and stinging, and tends to be in a precise, localized distribution in the extremity. Evaluation should consist of history and physical examination, with detailed neurologic examination in the lower extremities. Strength deficits may be subtle, especially in strong athletes, so side to side comparison is crucial. Additionally, many athletes may be hyperflexible, which can cause confusion with range-of-motion (ROM) testing and specific provocative testing. Segmental examination and abnormal patterns of hip, pelvic and knee ROM should be noted. With a specific history of trauma, plain radiographs for evaluation of fractures and alignment, is the initial step. If suspicion of disk injury or radiculopathy, MRI evaluation is recommended (see Chapter 12). MRI is also recommended in evaluation of an athlete with chronic LBP with or without radicular symptoms, which has not responded to appropriate analgesics and therapy over 4-6 weeks.

Initial treatment should include activity restriction, ice, and analgesics. Nonsteroidal anti-inflammatory medications should be the mainstay of treatment, though may need to be supplemented with short-term use of narcotics for breakthrough pain. Caution should be taken in prescribing medications, especially in athletes subject to drug testing evaluations. Different drug tests are used in different sports and at different levels of competition. Especially with high-level athletes, the treating physician is encouraged to inquire of the governing body of the sport or look on their Web page for rules. Associated muscle spasm or hypertonicity is effectively treated with physical modalities such as heat and cold packs, or ultrasound, as well as short-term use of diazepam, cyclobenzaprine, or methocarbomol (more on these medications can be found in Chapters 13 and 29).

Microtrauma Injuries

Spondylolysis/Spondylolisthesis

Most commonly, spondylolysis is associated with repeated extension and/or extension and rotation movements. Many athletes will complain of a specific episode of pain with this type of movement during training or competition. This can occur with repetitive loading of the pars interarticularis and facet joints, such as a fatigue fracture, as well as a final single event resulting in the fracture. Wiltse, Newman, and Macnabb classify spondylolysis in five categories (Table 36-2) (5). In the athletic population type II is the most commonly seen, though in older athletes the type III may be more frequent. There is some association with hereditary factors

---

**Table 36-2   Classification of Spondylolisthesis by Wiltse, Newman, and
          Macnab**

- **Type I *Dysplastic*:** associated with congenital abnormalities.
- **Type II *Isthmic*:** a lesion in the pars occurs.
- **Type III *Degenerative*:** associated with long-standing segmental instability.
- **Type IV *Traumatic*:** acute fractures in the neural arch other than at the pars inter-articularis.
- **Type V *Pathologic*:** associated with generalized or local bone disease.

(type I), congenital anomalies, such as spina bifida occulta, and age. The
incidence of spondylolysis ranges from 3% to 6% in the general population
and 15% or greater, depending on the specific sport, in the athlete. Sports
with high rates of spondylolyis include Javelin throwers, high jumpers,
gymnasts, divers and football lineman (4). The most common site involved
is the L5 vertebra, followed by L4, however uncommonly the L2 and L3
vertebra can be involved.

Clinical presentation usually involves a history of a forced or repetitive
extension movements and onset of pain. This may be unilateral or bilateral.
Pain can be reproduced with extension and extension/rotation movements.
Pain is usually limited to the back with infrequent radicular pain symptoms.
A step-off may be palpated along the spinous processes. Neurologic examination is usually normal, however there may be a myotomal or dermatomal
pattern, particularly in cases that neuroforaminal narrowing occurs.

Diagnosis of spondylolysis is certainly not standardized. Clinical history
is an important part in deciding which diagnostic tests to order. Important
factors to consider are clinical suspicion of a fracture, the sensitivity of the
diagnostic test, amount of radiation exposure, cost and the extent information desired. Plain radiographs, computed tomography (CT) scanning, nuclear medicine imaging, and magnetic imaging have all been evaluated in
the diagnosis of spondylolysis/spondylolisthesis.

Although anteroposterior (AP), lateral, coned down lateral, and oblique
radiographs have been considered the mainstay in evaluation of spondylolysis, they may not detect a significant number of fractures. In addition, the
presence of a spondylolysis seen on plain films may simply be an old finding, as up to 5% of children aged 5-7 have asymptomatic fractures.
However, in an athlete with a recent history of trauma and back pain these
films may rule out other fractures, as well as detect any spondylolisthesis.
Cost is relatively low and radiation expose can be limited by obtaining AP,
lateral and coned down lateral views. Oblique views may be added for further evaluation of questionable lesions.

Planar bone scan with single photon emission computed tomography
(SPECT) has had an increasing role in the evaluation of spondylolysis.
Advantages with bone scan with SPECT include localization of the lesion
to the area of the pars, as well as giving some estimation of age of the
lesion. Though new lesions will have increased uptake, these lesions can

be "positive" for up to 1 year after injury. This can, however, help differentiate old asymptomatic lesions from recent trauma. A spondylolytic lesion seen on plain radiographs, but not on nuclear medicine scanning, will necessitate further diagnostic workup for other causes. Disadvantages of nuclear medicine scans include high cost, radiation exposure and in some cases accessibility.

Benefits of computed tomography include evaluation of the vertebrae in axial and sagittal planes, allowing further assessment of the facet joints, intervertebral disks, central canal, and neuroforamen. Disadvantages include high dose of radiation, relatively high cost, and low sensitivity, unless thin slices are used. Perhaps the best use of CT scanning is in assessing age and healing stage of a lesion.

Case Study 36-1

A college-aged female gymnast was referred for left-sided lower back pain, worse with extension. Presumed diagnosis was spondylolysis of L5. She did not complain of radicular pain, paresthesias, or weakness. Plain radiographs and bone scan did not detect an area of fracture. CT scan of the lumbar spine showed multiple levels with disk dengeneration and facet hypertrophy. At L5 there was a left paracentral disk bulge, facet hypertrophy, causing severe neuroforaminal narrowing. She did not have significant improvement with 3 months of rest and physical therapy. She was sent for L5 transforaminal epidural steroid injection at L5 on the left. She became pain-free, progressed in physical therapy workouts, and was able to return to sport.

Benefits of magnetic resonance imaging include full evaluation of soft tissue and neural structures. This is important in reinjury as well as in when plain radiography and bone scans do not detect a fracture. Additionally, there is no radiation dose, which may be important over the life of young athletes. Disadvantages include cost, timely accessibility, and physical size limitations.

Spondylolisthesis is an additional concern if present. For those with less than 25% slip on initial presentation, the risk of further slip is low. Hensinger et al. (5) have identified those at greater risk for increased slip (Table 36-3). Depending on the severity of slip, symptoms, and the child's activity, some recommend that children and adolescent patients should be evaluated every 6-8 months with spot lateral radiographs, through growth spurts for development of and/ or progression of slippage. For those with less than a 25% slip, activity restriction, hamstring stretching, and abdominal strengthening will usually be successful in reducing pain and improving function. Healing occurs in 30% or less of the lesions, even with rigid bracing. For those cases where activity limitation is not successful after 4 weeks, a rigid brace, such as Boston overlap or TLSO, may be used. For those patients with slip greater than 50%

Table 36-3   Risk Factors in Spondylolisthesis for Pain, Progression, and Deformity

Clinical risk factors
- Younger age
- Female patient
- Recurrent symptoms
- Hamstring tightness if associated with gait or postural deformity.

Radiographic risk factors
- Type I greater risk than type II
- Greater than 50% slip
- Increased risk with increased slip angle
- L5-S1 instability with rounded sacral dome and vertical sacrum.

or failure of conservative measures, surgery should be considered. Though never reported in the literature, cauda equnia syndrome from acute progression of a stable spondylolisthesis is of theoretical concern. This may be better evaluated by a sports medicine professional on a sport by sport basis.

Facet-Mediated Pain

The lumbar facet or zygapophyseal joint bears up to 20% of load in the lumbar spine of a normal young individual. The facets limit motion in the lumbar spine, especially in the axial (rotation) and coronal (side-bending) planes. Facet injury is most common in sports with repeated extension and rotation movements (swimmers, gymnasts, golfers). Early hypertrophy of facet joints of hypermobile segments or in athletes with sports requiring extremes of ROM (gymnasts, butterfly and breast stroke swimmers) can cause pain with or without referral. Commonly, referred pain does not extend below the knee, though in athletes with facet hypertrophy and disk bulging this may cause intermittent nerve root irritation in positions in which the neuroforamen is narrowed. Evaluation with plain radiographs may show sclerosis or hypertrophy of the facets, however MRI is likely the better choice as this may show active inflammation within the joint capsule, neuroforamenal narrowing, presence of synovial cysts, as well as evaluation if the intervertebral disk.

Case Study 36-2

An elite college-aged male swimmer presents with complaints of thoracolumbar pain more on the right side and worse with extension. There is no radicular pain and no report of numbness or tingling. The pain has increased over the season, and now 1 week before the national championships this pain limits his performance. Neurologic examination was normal. There was an increased lumbar lordosis and thoracic kyphosis. Lumbar extension and rotation to the left was limited due to tenderness. Plain radiographs showed sclerosis and hypertrophy of the right L3 facet. Due to the upcoming national championship event, an intra-articular steroid injection was performed. This relieved his pain and allowed him to compete pain-free.

Treatment includes nonsteroidal anti-inflamatory medications, activity restriction, and relief of biomechanical loading of the joint. Flouroscopically guided, intra-articular steroid injections may be beneficial for short-term use of pain control in conjuction with a therapy program. Bracing and lumbar traction may also give short-term relief and can be tried within a therapy program.

Myofascial Syndromes

Perhaps the most common etiology of back pain in athletes is the various myofascial or muscle strain syndromes. These can result not only directly from trauma, such as contusions, strains or tears, but also from overuse and training errors. Athletes often have unique biomechanical issues specific to their sport, which must be addressed prior to return to play. Many of these are due to training errors or poor technique, and can be corrected with close contact between a manual therapist or athletic trainer and coach.

Restrictions to Play

Generally speaking, athletes should able to perform full ROM and sport specific activities pain-free before returning to competition. Although this may seem a fairly simple guideline, athletes may have difficulty following these restriction. Potentially more serious injuries such as spondylolysis and spondylolisthesis, disk herniations, vertebral fractures, and radiculopathies should have restriction from competition and sport-specific training until pain-free ROM and stability of the involved segment is assured. Myofascial pain syndromes of a chronic nature may also need specific restrictions and decrease in training load until symptoms are relieved.

Rehabilitation Strategies

Treatment and rehabilitation strategies are similar to those of the injured worker. Generally these can be broken down into four stages:

- Stage 1 is activity restriction and relative rest, for tissue healing and attention to reduction of pain.

- Stage 2 involves passive and active range of motion in pain-free range and correction of biomechanical restrictions and kinetic chain inequities.
- Stage 3 begins progressive general strength and endurance exercises and reconditioning.
- Stage 4 continues reconditioning with sport-specific exercises and slow return to activity.

There are many similarities for applying physical therapy to athletes with back conditions and for applying to those of the general population with the same types of back conditions. The main differences are athletes need to restore range of motion, strength, flexibility, and endurance beyond that of the general population and in sport-specific activities to meet the demands of their practice and competition. For example, a gymnast would need to achieve flexibility beyond what would be considered within normal limits, and a football player would need to achieve strength beyond normal limits as well.

Physical modalities such as ice, heat, massage, and stretching can be started in the training room or by the athlete at home to help reduce pain and inflammation after the injury. However, professional physical therapy should be sought for conditions that cause minor or major limitations in training, practices, or performances that are not resolved with home treatments.

Stage 1

Stage 1 includes goals for decreasing pain and inflammation, with tissue healing. Although discussion of tissue repair mechanisms and time frames are beyond the scope of this chapter, general guidelines of pain-free motion prior to progressing to the next stage can be followed. The athlete may need to take time off of his or her sport if unable to perform the activities of the sport, the condition worsens, or he or she fails to respond to initial treatment. Bed rest, if used, should not last longer than 2 days. The effects of bed rest and immobilization results in generalized deconditioning and muscle atrophy. Consideration of cross training for sustained cardiovascular conditioning should be given.

Modalities used in the initial stage of rehabilitation by a physical therapist include cryotherapy, ultrasound, and electrical stimulation. Manually trained physical therapists may also include manual therapy/joint mobilization techniques for pain relief and soft tissue mobilization and manual muscle stretching. These techniques are described in Chapters 20 and 24

In the acute phase of physical therapy for disk herniation, the goal is a little more specific. If the athlete is experiencing radiation of symptoms, then the goal is to centralize the symptoms to the low back and eliminate the leg symptoms first. Some positioning options may be, prone lying, supine lying, lumbar extension, lumbar flexion. Manual, mechanical, or self-traction may also be useful in centralizing the symptoms.

Stage 2

Stage 2 of rehabilitation is to restore muscle flexibility and joint range of motion. This can begin 2 days to 6 weeks after the onset of symptoms, with fractures, herniations, and spondylolysis being toward the longer duration. A full pain-free range of muscle stretching should begin with the affected tissues. Skilled physical therapy of manual therapy, joint mobilization, and soft tissue techniques may also be continued during this period. The athlete will need to be performing self-mobilization exercises to improve and maintain proper joint ranges of motion performed 2-3 times a day, not including before and after practice and even during their training sessions.

Stage 3

The third stage of rehabilitation is to begin increasing muscle strength and endurance. The response of the athlete throughout this phase will determine their return to competition. The athlete should continue their flexibility and self-mobilization exercises, as well as likely needing joint mobilization with manual therapy techniques throughout this phase. Trunk stabilization exercises should be started at this point. With the goal being to increase strength of the abdominal muscles, specifically the transversus abdominus, as well as the quadratus lumborum, multifidi, and rotatores muscles in the back. The exercises should be advanced to continually challenge the athlete in multiple planes of motion, increased resistance and duration to improve endurance.

Stage 4

The final stage of rehabiliation should transfer these exercises to sports-specific activities and training. These training methods may include, pulleys, sport cords, medicine ball training, and plyometrics.

Return to activity should involve a progressive resumption of activities and involve specific motions performed in the individuals sport. Return to sports competition should only be when the athlete has pain-free range of motion in all activities, restored strength, preinjury endurance levels, and demonstration of sport-specific tasks without pain, swelling, inflammation, or substitution patterns.

Recommendations

- Rehabilitation of the athlete may require a more extensive approach toward strength and endurance prior to safe return to sport.
- There are four stages in rehabilitating the athlete, starting with tissue healing and progressing to sport-specific strength and conditioning.

- Athletes should be able to perform full ROM and sport-specific activities pain-free before they may return to sports competition.
- Similar to nonathletes, failure to progress with therapy or a return of symptoms should trigger reconsideration of the athletes diagnosis and enjoin further work-up.

■   ■   ■

Key Points

- Athletes commonly have low back pain, but not all back complaints are caused by the sport.
- Spondylolisthesis, fracture, herniated disk, facet arthrits, and myofascial causes are common in athletes.
- Rehabilitation progresses gradually to a level closely approximating that of the actual sport before competition is recommended.

■   ■   ■

REFERENCES

1. **McCarroll JR, Miller JM, Ritter MA.** Lumbar spondylolysis and spondylolisthesis in college football players: a prospective study. Am J Sports Med. 1986;14:404-6.
2. **Feeler LC.** Racquet sports. In: Hochschuler SH; ed. The Spine in Sports. Philadelphia: Hanley & Belfus; 1990:143.
3. **Duda M.** Golfers use exercise to get back in the swing. PhysSportsmed. 1989;17:109-13.
4. **Rossi F.** Spondylolysis, spondylolisthesis and sports. J Sports Med Phys. Fitness. 1978;18:317-40.
5. **Wiltse LL, Newman PH, Mcnabb I.** Classification of spondylolysis and spondylolisthesis. Clin Orthop Rel Res. 1976;117:23-9.
6. **Heinsinger RN.** Spondylolysis and spondylolisthesis. J Bone Joint Surg. 1990;71A:1098-1102.

■   ■   ■

KEY REFERENCES

Hochschuler SH, ed. The Spine in Sports. Philadelphia: Hanley & Belfus; 1990.

Kibler WB, ed. ACSM's Handbook for the Team Physician. Baltimore: Williams & Wilkins; 1996.

Kibler WB, Herring SA, Press JM. Functional Rehabilitation of Sports and Musculoskeletal Injuries. Aspen, CO: Pro Ed;1998.

37

■ ■ ■

Back Pain in Pregnancy

Diane Rufe, MHS, PT

Back pain during pregnancy is a common complaint too often left untreated due to the belief it is an accepted part of pregnancy. Most studies determine the incidence of back pain in pregnancy to be approximately 50% (1-3). It typically occurs in the second trimester, most frequently between the fifth and seventh months of pregnancy (2). Not only is back pain a frequent complaint, but it is also one of the leading causes of sick leave during pregnancy.

Another common misbelief is that the back symptoms of pregnancy always disappear upon delivery of the baby/fetus. According to Svensson, 10% of chronic low back pain patients report their initial back symptoms occurring during pregnancy (4). One also must consider that this patient population has limited pharmacological avenues to address their symptoms as well as limited ability to have diagnostic tests performed to confirm the etiology and diagnosis of their symptoms. For these reasons, it is even more important primary care physicians recognize that back pain symptoms in pregnancy are typically easily treatable. Giving pregnant patients an avenue other than medication to manage their symptoms (exercise, supportive techniques, pacing strategies) and working with them to avoid or modify activities that are precipitating factors in the development of symptoms significantly enhances the woman's sense of control and understanding of the symptoms. By addressing back pain in pregnant women, we can hopefully avoid sick leave during pregnancy and prevent the patients from having recurrent back symptoms postpartum (5).

Risk Factors

The most frequently documented risk factors for back pain in pregnancy are 1) history of back pain prior to pregnancy, 2) smoking, 3) prior pregnancies, and 4) vocational factors requiring heavy physical labor, frequent bending or lifting, or prolonged sitting or standing work posture (1,2). Interestingly, Ostgaard did not find weight gain to be a risk factor for developing back pain in pregnancy (6).

Etiology

There are several widely accepted contributing factors to back pain in pregnancy. The most common are joint dysfunction, muscle imbalance, and ligamentous laxity. In most cases, it is a combination of at least two of these factors that result in lumbar back or posterior pelvic symptoms with the pregnant patient. For the purposes of this chapter, posterior pelvic pain and lumbar symptoms will be collectively referred to as back pain.

Joint Dysfunction

Either hypomobility or hypermobility of the thoracic spine, lumbar spine, pubic symphysis, and sacroiliac joints can contribute to complaints of back pain. The sacrum or the hemi pelvis can rotate out of normal alignment. The laxity of the sacroiliac joints has been discussed as a cause of posterior pelvic pain (described as pain inferior to the lumbar spine) in pregnancy by Berg and Kristansson (1,7). Fortin has studied the referral pattern of the sacroiliac joints in both asymptomic and symptomic volunteers (8). His studies reveal the sacroiliac joint referral pattern is inferior and lateral to the ipsilateral sacroiliac joint along the upper buttock, lateral hip, and lateral proximal thigh (8). Berg reported sacroiliac dysfunction was discovered in two-thirds of patients with severe back/pelvis symptoms in pregnancy (1).

Muscle Imbalance

Janda's work in non-pregnant patients has demonstrated that some muscles have a tendency to develop tightness, whereas other muscles develop weakness (9). With back pain specifically, it is crucial to appreciate that the gluteus medius, gluteus maximus, and abdominals weaken and that the tensor fascia lata, quadratus lumborum, gastroc-soleus, hip flexors (iliopsoas, rectus femoris, tensor fascia lata), piriformis, and paraspinals develop tightness (9).

The piriformis muscle can be affected by not only the hormonal ligament and joint laxity of the pelvis but also the potential of inefficient use of the gluteal-musculature (which are major stabilizers of the sacroiliac joints). The combination of these factors can contribute to overload of the piriformis resulting in increased tone and muscle tightness. Often joint dysfunction, whether hypo or hypermobility and muscle imbalance occur together and thus both areas should be addressed simultaneously in a treatment program.

Hormonal (Relaxin) Ligament Laxity

There is inconsistency in the literature regarding when relaxin levels peak in pregnancy. According to MacLennan relaxin levels are highest during the first and second trimester then drop in the third trimester (10). There is agreement that there are increased relaxin levels during second pregnancies compared to the first pregnancy (11). Also, there are increased levels of relaxin with twin pregnancies as opposed to single pregnancies (10).

Hormonal ligament laxity occurs throughout the body during pregnancy and for a period of time after delivery. Some degree of ligament laxity lingers until after nursing has stopped. The laxity puts joints in a vulnerable position for strain injury and malrotation from imbalanced loads or end range of motion. In addition to the ligament laxity, the stabilizing force of abdominal musculature is comprised by the growing fetus.

It is important that pregnant women are educated as to what the hormonal ligament laxity is, when it occurs, that it affects the entire body and its presence after delivery. This information can facilitate making an educated decision regarding sports, impact aerobics, lifting heavy loads, and performing activities which place their joints at a new possibly excessive end-range.

Musculoskeletal Evaluation

During the physical exam, it is important to reproduce the patient's symptoms (to help focus treatment to the appropriate structure) and to determine what functional limitations the symptoms are causing.

Some key areas of evaluation are the following.

1. Posture
   - Is lumbar lordosis excessive or decreased?
   - Is thoracic kyphosis increased or decreased?
2. Range of motion: lumbar spine
   - Are there significantly limited segments resisting flexion, extension or side bending?
   - Do any of the test movements increase or decrease symptoms?
3. Tone of piriformis muscle

To assess for muscle spasm or increased muscle tone of the piriformis muscle, the patient can be positioned side lying with pillow between knees and ankles. The piriformis muscle attaches onto the anterior surface of the sacrum and then crosses the buttock horizontally to insert on the greater trochanter. Palpation of piriformis should include deep palpation near the lateral border of sacrum, palpating along the muscle belly and to its attachment onto the greater trochanter. Increased tone of one or both piriformis muscles can be a result of sacroiliac dysfunction (hypo or hypermobility), faulty muscle recruitment of gluteus medius or maximus, or a result of faulty body mechanics.

Evaluation of the Sacroiliac Joint

There are many avenues to evaluate for hypomobility or hypermobility of the sacroiliac joints. Many manual therapists use a combination of tests to identify the side of dysfunction (stork test, standing flexion test, and seated flexion test). In addition, they determine the direction of restriction of movement by following changes in position of bony landmarks during flexion, extension and rotation of the spine. Therapists and physicians with extra training can determine abnormalities of joint play, alignment and muscle balance. If one is not familiar or trained in the appropriate way to perform these tests, symptom provocation test is also helpful in evaluating for sacroiliac dysfunction and symptoms. This test has been referred to by several different terms- painful femoral compression test; thigh thrust test; or the PPPT (posterior pelvic pain provocation test). The test is performed with the patient supine and on the affected side the hip flexed to 90 degrees. The clinician stabilizes the opposite iliac crest while exerting pressure vertically throughout the flexed thigh. A positive test is reproduction of the patients pain (buttocks/sacral area) (7). Kristiansson et al found this test to have "good diagnosis discriminatory power" and was shown to have "high sensitivity and specificity". Kristianson did demonstrate the combination of tests yielded the most useful results included the painful femoral compression test, tender PSIS, tender sacrospinous ligament, painful lumbar movements and lumbar tenderness.

Muscle Lengths and Neural Tension Tests

It is important to assess muscle length of the hamstring, piriformis, quadratus lumborum, psoas, gastrocnemius, iliotibial band, and to check for neural tension signs such as straight leg raising (SLR) and femoral nerve test.

Palpation

Key areas to palpate include the thoracic and lumbar paraspinal muscles, piriformis muscle, iliotibial band (especially as it interfaces with the quadriceps and hamstring). Evaluate for symmetric alignment by palpating key bony landmarks such as the anterior superior iliac spines, superior borders of the pubic symphysis, sacral base, and medial malleoli. If asymmetric, there is likely a musculoskeletal malalingment problem.

Functional Limitations

Gathering information regarding functional limitation can be helpful in determining the structure(s) resulting in the patient's symptoms. For example, if the symptoms occur typically during transitional movement (transferring supine to sit, rolling left and right in bed, transferring sit to stand) it would be crucial to assess for lumbar spine and sacroiliac joint dysfunction. Symptoms occurring primarily in the morning and subsiding one to two hours after waking, inquiring about sleeping positions may be of benefit. If the symptoms occur after prolonged standing, prolonged walking or consistently occur at the end of the day, muscle fatigue is likely a factor and pacing strategies should be discussed with the patient.

Treatment

Treatment of back pain that occurs with pregnancy should consist of patient education regarding supported positions, pacing strategies, and body mechanics. Physical therapy may include a treatment plan consisting of exercise, joint mobilization, and soft tissue mobilization.

Body Mechanics

Simple reminders such as avoiding lifting bent at the waist with straight legs and to avoid bending forward combined with twisting (a very vulnerable position for the lumbar spine and sacroiliac joints). Instead instruct them to bend their knees when lifting or bending forward and to avoid twisting. Remind patients to think of using proper body mechanics not only with heavy loads but also with the repetitive activities such as loading the dishwasher, dryer, sweeping, and vacuuming. Keeping elbows at ones side when vacuuming or sweeping helps to minimize flexing and rotating at the trunk. In addition, walking forward and back similar to a mini lunge creates weight shifting and full body movement as opposed to repetitive flexion and extension across the low back and pelvis during these activities.

Maternity Braces

To determine if a patient would benefit from a maternity brace try unweighting the abdomen and stabilizing the pelvis. First, with the patient standing, the clinician places both hands under the abdomen and gently lifts up to partially unweight the patient's abdomen. For the second test, the patient is standing while the clinician simultaneously places a hand around each iliac crest at the level of the anterior inferior iliac spines and compresses both hands towards each other. If either of these tests decreases the patient's symptoms a trial of a maternity brace would be worthwhile.

There are many maternity braces on the market today. They vary signif-icantly in price, size, and ease of use. Some simply support under the ab-domen and along the lateral pelvis, while others also provide a strap traveling above the belly. The more extensive and supportive braces are helpful with patients carrying more than one child. Though helpful, some people do not tolerate the elastic, and the more encompassing the brace, the hotter it will be. The less extensive type of brace may pose fewer chal-lenges for warm weather climates.

To ensure a proper fit of the three-strap type brace, one should loosely fasten the strap under the abdomen and then firmly fasten and snug both side straps. Do not overtighten the abdominal strap, as it is the snugging of the side straps that actually provides the back and pelvic support. Experience has shown that the maternity brace provides the most benefit when worn during standing or walking activities. The brace should be taken off if the patient will be sitting for more than 15 to 20 minutes.

Maternity braces worn correctly typically decrease the intensity of symptom and often delay the onset of symptoms throughout the course of the day (1,5). Beatty's study determined use of the "Mother-To-Be" mater-nity brace did not acutely affect the hemodynamics of the fetus and mother (12). The fetal heart rate, maternal blood pressure, and maternal cardiac output were monitored in this study before, during, and after wearing the brace while standing and sitting (12). In addition, the subjects did report a decrease in symptoms while wearing the brace (12).

Supported Sleeping Positions

Instruct the patient in supported sleeping positions including a pillow be-tween her knees and ankles, thus bringing the top knee nearly in the same plane as the hip (Figure 37-1a, 37-1b). She should be instructed to support top arm and upper trunk with a pillow placed either horizontally or verti-cally along her chest and under her top arm. A small towel roll should be placed under her neck (inside the pillow case) to support head and neck.

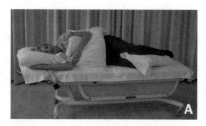
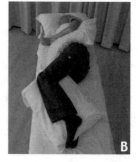

Figure 37-1   Supported sleeping positions.

Supported Sitting Posture

If the patient has a sitting job, the use of a lumbar roll is helpful in decreasing the intensity and frequency of symptoms. In addition, it often helps prevent the posterior pelvic symptoms which occur with sit to stand transfers. The inflatable type of lumbar rolls is preferred best with the pregnant population to help accommodate for their changing body posture. Lumbar rolls should be placed in the small of the back.

Taking frequent posture breaks should be strongly encouraged. The posture break should be used as a prevention tool as well for symptom management. The patient should take a posture break after each hour of sitting whether or not symptoms have occurred that day. A posture break simply consists of a change in position such as a short walk around the desk or to a water fountain or a brief stretch into lumbar extension in standing.

Support for Standing and Walking

The patient who experiences pain with standing should be instructed in pacing activities (e.g., interrupt standing with short periods of sitting). The patient should also be instructed to perform a stretching exercise for her low back paraspinals, preferably in a hands and knees position. Lastly, the use of a maternity brace should be considered.

The patient who experiences buttocks pain with prolonged walking should be advised to purchase a maternity brace to offer additional pelvic support. The brace should be worn while walking. The patient should be told to be certain to wear new supportive walking shoes that provide appropriate shock absorbing qualities. Instruct the patient in piriformis stretches (20-second hold time, repeat 3 times) and a gluteal strengthening exercise (hands and knees position—extend hip).

Case Study 37-1

A 32-year-old woman had some back pain in her first pregnancy that spontaneously resolved. When pain developed 4 months into her second pregnancy, she patiently waited it out. By month 7, the pain had become excruciating. It radiated down into her right toes, and her Achilles' reflex disappeared. She had some bladder incontinence that may have been pregnancy related. No x-rays were taken. An MRI showed an equivocal bulge at L5-S1. An EMG revealed paraspinal denervation, confirming that this was a radiculopathy, not uterine pressure on the lumbar plexus.

Diskectomy while pregnant or early caesarian delivery were contemplated, but serial exams showed that the nerve damage did not progress. She was kept comfortable with physical therapy, massage, ice, and activity avoidance. A week prior to delivery, she practiced positioning and pain relief on a delivery table. To avoid pressure on the disk during delivery, she was coached to not bear down, and epidural anesthesia was used. A bolus of corticosteroids was injected with the anesthetic for long-term therapeutic benefit. She required opiate analgesia the week after delivery, but with the help of a lactation consultant was later able to nurse.

Physical Therapy

If basic instruction in posture, stretching, and pacing activities does not improve the patient's functional status or as above if the case has complicating factors, a referral to physical therapy is recommended. The evaluation should include assessment of range of motion, muscle strength, muscle firing recruitment patterns, muscle tone, posture, alignment, joint accessory motion, gait, and functional limitations. Reproduction of the patient's symptoms can help to guide appropriate treatment. The treatment plan for a patient with low back or posterior pelvic pain (PPP) in pregnancy would include: Exercises to address muscle tightness, muscle weakness, and faulty muscle firing patterns, joint mobilization, and techniques to decrease muscle tone, spasm or guarding. This could include soft tissue mobilization, positional release, and strain counter strain. Exercises in side lying or in the hands and knees position (Fig. 37-2) are emphasized, as supine exercises are not recommended after the third month of pregnancy. The goal of the treatment is to improve the patient's function and to independently manage symptoms. In addition, physical therapy will provide further instruction in proper posture including use of lumbar roll, use of a maternity brace, instruction in proper body mechanics for job, household, and childcare tasks. Functional goals might be to sleep through the night, walk 30 minutes, and be able to care for a toddler. (A sample physical therapy program and the specific exercises used is given in Table 37-1.)

Physical therapy treatment for the patient with back pain in pregnancy typically can be completed in four to eight sessions. Most patients seem to be highly motivated to participate fully in therapy for several reasons: 1) they know there are not many pharmacological options, 2) the options in diagnostic testing are very limited when pregnant, 3) they fear significant

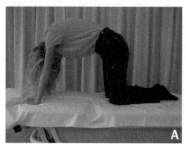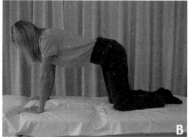

Figure 37-2 The "cat-camel." A, Spine flexion (the "camel"). B, Spine extension (the "cat" stretch).

Table 37-1   Physical Therapy Program for the Pregnant Patient with Low Back Pain

Should include the following: education (proper body mechanics, use of maternity brace, supported sleeping, proper posture), a home exercise program (to address muscle length, muscle strength, increased muscle tone/spasm, and joint dysfunction), and manual techniques to address joint dysfunction and muscle tightness.

Proper Body Mechanics

- Supine to sit transfer—1) Roll onto your side; 2) drop your feet off the edge of the bed; 3) push up with your hands
- Lifting
- Job tasks
- Child care tasks
- Avoid bending conbined with twisting
- *Reminder.* Poor body mechanics with highly repetitive light loads can be a contributing factor to development or reoccurence of low back pain.

Maternity Brace (information of 2003)

- The Ultimate Maternity Brace® ($13 at Motherhood Maternity Stores)
- Prenatal Cradle® ($50; 1-800-383-3068)
- Mother-To-Be® ($39.95 from Saunders Group; 1-800-456-1289)

Posture Education

- Use of lumbar roll
- Instruction in neutral spine posture breaks every 30 minutes

Muscle Tightness

- Hamstring stretch (Figure 37-3)
- Piriformis stretch—1) In a seated position, using your left hand, slowly bring your right knee toward your left shoulder; 2) do not twist/rotate your trunk; 3) a stretch should be felt across the right buttocks; 4) hold 20 seconds and repeat 3 times each side
- Paraspinal stretch (cat-camel) (Figure 37-2)
- Paraspinal stretch (seated)
- Psoas stretch (front of the thigh stretch)—1) In a standing position with the left leg in front of the right, stand up straight; 2) tuck your buttocks underneath you; 3) tuck your stomach in; 4) start with your weight on the right [back leg]; 5) slowly transfer your weight to left leg; 6) a stretch should be felt in the front of the right thigh; 7) hold 20 seconds and repeat 3 times each leg

Supported Sleeping

- See Figures 37-1A and 37-1B for supported sleeping positions
- Place pillow between knees and ankles

Muscle Weakness/Faulty Muscle Recruitment

- Gluteus medius strengthening (Figure 37-4)
- Gluteus maximus strengthening (Figure 37-5)

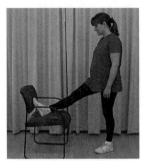

Figure 37-3   Hamstring stretching for pregnant women.

symptoms during labor, and 4) they do not want to be limited because of back pain when they have a newborn.

Case Study 37-2

A 27-year-old woman complained of right sacroiliac joint area pain, right buttocks pain, and occasional right posterior thigh symptoms. Her pain began at 18 weeks of pregnancy and she entered physical therapy at 20 weeks. She reported difficulty with sleeping due to pain, care of her 3-year-old child, vacuuming, prolonged walking, transferring sit to stand and supine to sit, and increased symptoms at the end of the day. Tylenol does not reduce her symptoms. Exam revealed restricted lumbar mobility, hypermobility of right sacroiliac joint, slight restricted left sacroiliac joint mobility, increase muscle tone and tenderness of the right piriformis muscle (which produced her buttocks symptoms), tightness of bilateral psoas muscle, and impaired firing of the gluteus medius and maximus muscles.

Physical therapy treatment consisted of instruction in supported sleeping position, proper body mechanics for household, lifting, and childcare tasks, pacing strategies, instruction for piriformis muscle stretches, lumbar spine and sacroiliac mobility exercises, gluteus medius and maximus muscle retraining, and use of a maternity brace.

At the end of six physical therapy sessions, there was significant reduction of the piriformis muscle tenderness, improved gluteal muscle firing and strength. She reported sleeping through the night and was without functional limitations except for an increase of symptoms on days she did not pace herself and over did it. When sacroiliac or buttock symptoms did occur, she was able to eliminate the home exercises.

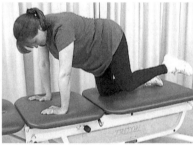

Figure 37-4   Knee adduction "squeezes" for the pelvis.

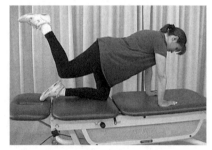

Figure 37-5   Exercises to stabilize the spine. One leg or one arm is lifted at a time.

Caution

If a patient presents either during pregnancy or postpartum with pain primarily at the pubic symphysis and/or along the medial thigh, it is important the patient be evaluated for osteitis pubis. Place this high on the differential list if the patient has not responded to conservative treatments. During examination, differentiate between pain arising from the adductor tendon (tendonitis) versus symptoms arising from bone itself (osteitis pubis). If symptoms are unilateral, palpate the asymptomatic or less symptomatic side first then assess the symptomatic side. Follow the adductor muscle then tendon to the bony origin. Sharp pain elicited at the bone is a positive indicator of osteitis pubis. The mainstay of treatment is 180 degrees opposite most treatment; it is resting the area and controlling inflammation. (This is in essence virtually the "opposite" of treatment ofmost back pain pregnancy, which focuses primarily on exercises tailored to restoring function.) If the patient is pregnant, the treatment would include frequent icing of both the bone and tendons, rest including not stretching of the legs, no walking or exercise, no stair climbing, no lifting, and anti-inflammatories depending on what trimester they are in. Postpartum patients should receive a bone scan to confirm the diagnosis. Overactivity will severely delay healing. Treatment can take 3 to 6 months. Return to activities should be gradual.

Outcomes

Given a course of physical therapy, patient compliance with home self-treatment exercises, supported sleeping, attention to proper body mechanics, and the use of a maternity brace, a large majority of pregnant women are able to independently manage their symptoms and have improved function. Noren et al. found a reduction of sick leave by 50% in the intervention group for lumbar pain and posterior pelvic pain during pregnancy (5). The intervention group was offered five visits with a physical therapist, which consisted of teaching an individualized program of exercise (no passive treatment) as well as instruction in posture, body mechanics, and relaxation (5). Education regarding back care and body mechanics was found also to be beneficial in the Orvieto study (13). Ostgaard found that physical therapy and an education program during pregnancy for those with back pain improved long-term function and lowered the rate of recurrent symptoms (14).

Recommendations

- A little education about body mechanics and posture (e.g., proper sleep supported, a few simple stretches) can often yield significant symptom reduction and functional improvement.
- The key elements to treatment of back pain during pregnancy are identifying precipitating factors and correcting them (e.g., patient is lifting her 2-year-old child incorrectly) and identifying avenues to self-manage symptoms (e.g., pacing strategies, maternity braces, stretches, self-treatment techniques).
- Several key structures to evaluate are piriformis tone, sacroiliac joint mobility, and lumbar spine mobility.
- If physical therapy is needed, the treatment typically consists of only four to six sessions. The patient is educated in strategies for symptom self-management for comfort, increased function, and prevention of sick leave during pregnancy. These strategies are also used for decreasing back symptoms postpartum.

■　■　■

Key Points

- The most common causes of back pain in pregnancy are joint hypomobility and/or hypermobility, muscle imbalances, and ligament laxity.
- Treatment consists of postural education for sleeping, sitting, and walking, possible use of a supportive maternity brace, and instruction in proper body mechanics.
- More involved cases will need physical therapy to deal with muscle imbalance, and joint dysfunction and to teach more advanced exercises and pacing strategies for independent management.
- Addressing back pain during pregnancy will improve quality of life, minimize sick leave during pregnancy, and minimize symptoms postpartum.

■　■　■

REFERENCES

1. **Berg G, Hammar M, Moller-Nielsen J, Linden U, Thorblad J.** Low back pain during pregnancy. Obstet Gynecol. 1988;71:71-5.
2. **Fast A, Shapiro D, Ducommun E, et al.** Low back pain in pregnancy. Spine. 1987;12:368-71.

3. **Mante J.** Back pain in the childbearing year. In: Grieves Modern Manual Therapy: The Vertebral Column. New York: Churchill Livingstone.

4. **Svensson HO, Andersson GB, Hagstad A, Jansson PO.** The relationship of low back pain to pregnancy and gynecologic factors. Spine. 1990;15:371-75.

5. **Noren L, Ostgaard S, Nielsen TF, Ostgaard HC.** Reduction of sick leave for lumbar back and posterior pelvic pain in pregnancy. Spine. 1997;22:2157-60.

6. **Ostgaard H, Anderson G, Karlson, K.** Prevalence of back pain in pregnancy. Spine. 1991;16:549-52.

7. **Kristiansson P, Svardsudd K.** Discriminatory power of tests applied in back pain during pregnancy. Spine. 1996;21:2337-44.

8. **Fortin JD, Dwyer AP, West S, Pier J.** Sacroiliac joint: pain referral maps upon applying a new injection/arthrography technique. Spine. 1994;19:1475-82.

9. **Janda V.** Evaluation of muscular imbalance. In Liebenson C, ed. Rehabilitation of the Spine: A Practitioner's Manual. Baltimore: Williams and Wilkins; 1996:97.

10. **MacLennan A, Nicolson R, Green R.** Serum relaxin in pregnancy. Lancet. 1986;ii:241-3.

11. **Calguneri M, Bird H, Wright V.** Changes in joint laxity occurring during pregnancy. Ann Rheum Dis. 1982;41:126-8.

12. **Beaty CM, Bhaktaram VJ, Rayburn WF, Parker MJ, Christensen HD, Chandrasekaran K.** Low backache during pregnancy. J Reprod Med. 1999;44:1007-1011.

13. **Orvieto R, Achiron A, Ben-Rafael Z, Gelernter I, Achiron R.** Low back pain of pregnancy. Acta Obstet Gynecol Scand. 1994;73:209-214.

14. **Ostgaard H, Zetherstrom G, Roos-Hansson.** Back pain in relation to pregnancy: a 6-year follow-up. Spine. 1997;22: 2945-50.

▓   ▓   ▓

KEY REFERENCES

Beaty CM, Bhaktaram VJ, Rayburn WF, Parker MJ, Christensen HD, Chandrasekaran K. Low backache during pregnancy. J Reprod Med. 1999;44;1007-11.

This article provides information regarding the fetal and maternal effects of the maternity brace and its pain-reducing aspect.

Kristasson P, Svardsudd K. Discrimatory power of tests applied in back pain during pregnancy. Spine. 1996;21:2337-44.

This article addresses the most useful combination of exam techniques when evaluating back pain in pregnancy. It also discusses several treatment options.

Ostgaard H, Zetherstrom G, Roos-Hansson. Back pain in relation to pregnancy: a 6-year follow-up. Spine. 1197;22:2945-50.

This article discusses the effect physical therapy had on back symptoms during pregnancy and the extent to which those skills carried over postpartum.

38

■ ■ ■

Back Pain in People with Disabilities

William M. Scelza, MD

Christopher M. Brammer, MD

Patients presenting with back pain as their chief complaint will often have a unique combination of various co morbidities that may or may not be contributing factors to the back pain. One subset of such patients are those with disabilities, either congenital or acquired. With pre-existing limitations on function, the patient with disabilities may have greater impairments and decline in their functional status in comparison to a patient without any prior limitations, perhaps a reflection of a deceased ability to adapt and compensate. For this reason as well as for others, the clinician should review any history of back pain with the disabled patient, whether the pain is the chief complaint or not. The clinician should not disregard typical causes of back pain when making a diagnosis in patients with disabilities. However, although the clinician should approach these patients in the same manner as nondisable patients, there are special considerations that need to be addressed.

In this chapter, we discuss several categories of disabilities and identify key aspects that need to be thought of first. It is of utmost importance to know the patients past medical history, baseline physical examination, and capabilities. These items may certainly play a large role of the etiology of their pain and guide the clinician to the diagnosis. At the same time, it is important to remember that people with disabilities are just as susceptible to the common cause of back pain as the general population and these diagnoses must also always be considered.

Case Study 38-1

A 45-year-old female with a past history of spastic diplegic cerebral palsy presents with neck pain. She has a difficult time eating because her head and neck cannot flex. This has been present for the past few years. There has been no trauma. The pain is localized to only the paraspinal area without radiation into her upper extremities. There are no reports of weakness or other neurological deterioration.

Examination reveals increased spasticity in all four extremities, though this could be considered mild. Her cervical spine is in an extended position and slightly rotated to the right. It is difficult to passively flex or rotate her cervical spine. She seemed to have exacerbating pain on further cervical spine extension. Cervical extension and rotation did not cause any radicular symptoms. Muscle stretch reflexes of the biceps and triceps tendons were brisk at 3+. Muscle strength is 5/5 in her upper and lower extremities.

There is no evidence of acute radiculopathy or myelopathy.

Diagnostic imaging is indicated at this time. Magnetic resonance imaging (MRI) of the brain was performed to exclude any focal lesions that may be contributing to the dystonia. It was found to be normal. X-rays films of her cervical spine, including extension and flexion and oblique views, showed multilevel facet arthritis without any fracture or tumor invasion. Treatment of the dystonia and spasticity of the cervical spine included local botulinum toxin to the cervical extensors and right sternocleidomastoid muscle, which is generally repeated every 3-6 months. After the first injection, a course of sustained passive stretching was begun. Wheelchair seating was changed to include a hard cervical collar to facilitate neutral positioning. Positioning in regard to her wheelchair seating is important, and adding a neck support may be beneficial. Her spasticity improved to the point where she was able to feed herself and look forward without placing abnormal stress on the posterior elements of her cervical spine. Her pain decreased substantially in the ensuing weeks.

Neuromuscular Disease

Many studies have shown decreased strength of abdominal and spinal muscles in patients with low back pain (1-3). Often, it is difficult to describe the initial mechanism leading to functional deterioration of the spine. One mechanism begins with intrinsic back pathology (i.e., degenerative disk disease, facet arthopathy, spinal stenosis). This can lead to a physiologic guarding, both intentional and reflexive. Disuse and muscle deconditioning follow this.

In describing a second potential mechanism of spinal degeneration, patients with neuromuscular diseases, such as muscular dystrophy, spinal muscular atrophy, anterior horn cell disease, or even postpolio syndrome can present initially with progressive weakness of the paraspinals, thoracic and abdominal musculature. This weakness begins a progressive cascade in which further stresses are placed upon the structural elements of the spine, including the facet joints, vertebral disks and the spinal ligaments. This can accelerate the degeneration of these spinal structures similarly to changes seen in weightbearing joints of weakened lower extremities in neuromuscular disease patients. These degenerative changes of the spine, as described above, can indeed be the pain generators of the patient's chief complaint.

In either of the two presented scenarios, a decompensating cycle begins where weakness and deconditioning leads to further spine degeneration; and further degeneration with disabling pain leads to guarding, disuse and further weakness; thus perpetuating the cycle. It is however difficult to arrest this cycle, especially in a patient with a neuromuscular disease. Strengthening and conditioning in this population is especially challenging with ongoing muscle degeneration. A narrow window of exercise intensity, which maintains fitness, is believed to exist, although it is not specifically defined in general neuromuscular diseases, let alone specific diagnoses. Exercising at too low an intensity can contribute to disuse atrophy and too high an intensity causing overuse weakness. Moderate exercise training at approximately 40% of maximal resistance is felt to be an adequate level for training; no additional exercise benefits are achieved with a high resistance program (4-8). This proposed strengthening program, which studied extremity strengthening in slowly progressive neuromuscular diseases, perhaps can be extrapolated to designing conditioning programs of the spine in a similar population. Adequate studies in this population are grossly lacking.

Scoliosis

Patients with neuromuscular disease, as well as other diseases, may present with scoliosis of the spine, however in much higher percentages compared to normal populations (9). Much experience has been gained from the treatment of idiopathic scoliosis, which accounts for 85% of patients with scoliosis. Bracing and conservative care of the scoliosis may slow the progression of the curve, but is not effective in arresting. Recommendations for bracing are beyond the scope of this chapter, but braces are generally considered when the angle of the deformity is greater than 20 degrees but less than 40 degrees. Though the precise time to intervene with surgical intervention varies from clinician to clinician, spinal fusion will typically be considered with obliquities greater than 40 degrees as measured by the Cobb method, as long as pulmonary function tests are at least 40% or greater of predicted values.

In comparison to the idiopathic scoliosis varieties of infantile, juvenile, and adolescent, the clinician viewing an adult patient with neuromuscular disease will see progression of the scoliosis into adulthood, osteopenia, and increased pelvic obliquity with progression of the systemic disease (10). Regardless of whether the scoliosis is of idiopathic or neuromuscular type, pain is not usually related to the scoliosis except in cases of moderate-severe scoliosis of 45 degrees or more. The pain presents as facet joint pain on the concave side and paraspinal muscle pain and spasm on the convex side (11,12). However, one must consider degenerative spine disease to be the primary cause of the scoliosis. In scoliosis caused by degenerative disease, the pain generator may indeed be related to commonly associated pain generators (as facet arthropathy, compression fractures with osteopenia, and degenerative disk disease) found in nonscoliotic patients.

Uncommon in the scoliotic patient, pain in the spine should prompt the clinician to consider the possibility of tumor invasion, high-grade spondylolisthesis, neurofibromas and other diseases of the spine, such as multiple myeloma, as seen in the nonscoliotic patients. Patients with a history of spinal instrumentation and fusion may present with pain from hardware failure (see below).

Seventy-one percent of people with a history of polio often have myofascial or muscle overuse pain according to Agre et al. (13). This pain may be secondary to postpolio syndrome or progression of degenerative spine disease. Often patients with a history of polio can have difficulties with sleep contributing to and even being the primary cause of myofascial pain (see Chapter 29 for more information on the use of antidepressants in patients with pain).

Treatment options for the pain can vary depending on the pain generator. Deep heating modalities can help with pain relief as well as improve tissue flexibility. Initiation and progression of segmental stretching and exercises are helpful in maintaining flexibility and biomechanical efficiencies. Though exercise has not been shown to correct spinal deformities, it may improve conditioning and strength which may aid in off loading degenerative spine structures that are pain generators. One must be assured that optimal seating has been established if their patient is a wheelchair user (see below). For myofascial pain in the midst of poor sleep, a trial of tricyclic antidepressants such as amitriptylline or nortriptylline may improve deep stages of sleep, thus lessening myofascial pain.

Spinal Cord Injury

Spinal cord injury (SCI) carries a number of potentially serious causes of back pain. These patients are insensate below the level of injury, so they may have difficulty localizing or describing pain or may not have any complaints at all. A small change injury to the spinal cord can have a dramatic effect on the patient's level of impairment will have a major impact on their ability to maintain independence and move about the environment. Thus periodic examinations of the key muscles and sensory dermatomes as outlined by the American Spinal Injury Association (see Figure 38-1) guidelines are necessary to provide a baseline and thus clue one in to a worsening spinal cord lesion (14).

Case Study 38-2

A 35-year-old male with 18-year history of a traumatic T-4 SCI is now having numbness in his right little finger. He has not had any recent injury, and the symptoms have come on insidiously. The patient had a spinal stabilization with fusion and Harrington rods at the time of his accident but does not report back pain. There has been no report of new weakness, and he remains independent with the use of a manual wheelchair. He works full-time.

When reviewing the differential diagnosis of this patient, one must think of the unique etiologies that may be present. A syrinx, for example, may be progressing rostrally and this will be the first presentation. Little weakness may be noticed as the thoracic myotomes provide no upper extremity innervations (except T-1). Advanced degenerative arthropathy above the level of spinal stabilization can contribute to radiculopathy. The physical exam could help aid in detecting progressive loss of sensation if comparisons can be made to previous careful exams. Advancing sensory level, new muscle weakness, or other upper motor neuron signs and must be compared to patient's baseline. Thus clinicians are encouraged to record sensory level using landmarks (e.g. "3 cm below the nipple") rather than neurologic constructs (e.g. "T4 sensory level") Electromyography could be quite helpful to rule out a radiculopathy or ulnar mononeuropathy, which would be quite common in a long-term wheelchair user. An MRI would be the best choice to rule out syrinx. In this case a syrinx was not found on MRI, but on electrodiagnostic studies an ulnar neuropathy at Guyon's canal in the wrist was noted. The patient was given special padding in his wheeling gloves and symptoms resolved over the next month.

Types of Pain

For people with spinal cord injury, the nature of pain can give a clue to its cause and the location of the pain generator (15). For nocioreceptive or mechanical pain, the lesion is usually above level of injury. Trauma and overuse are typical causes. Neuropathic pain above the level of the spinal cord injury suggests focal neuropathy/radiculopathy. Neuropathic pain at or below level can be due to segmental radicular pain, incomplete injury, or phantom pain. Visceral pain is vague and poorly localized. It can be a clue to a serious process (i.e., fracture or acute abdomen) and must have high

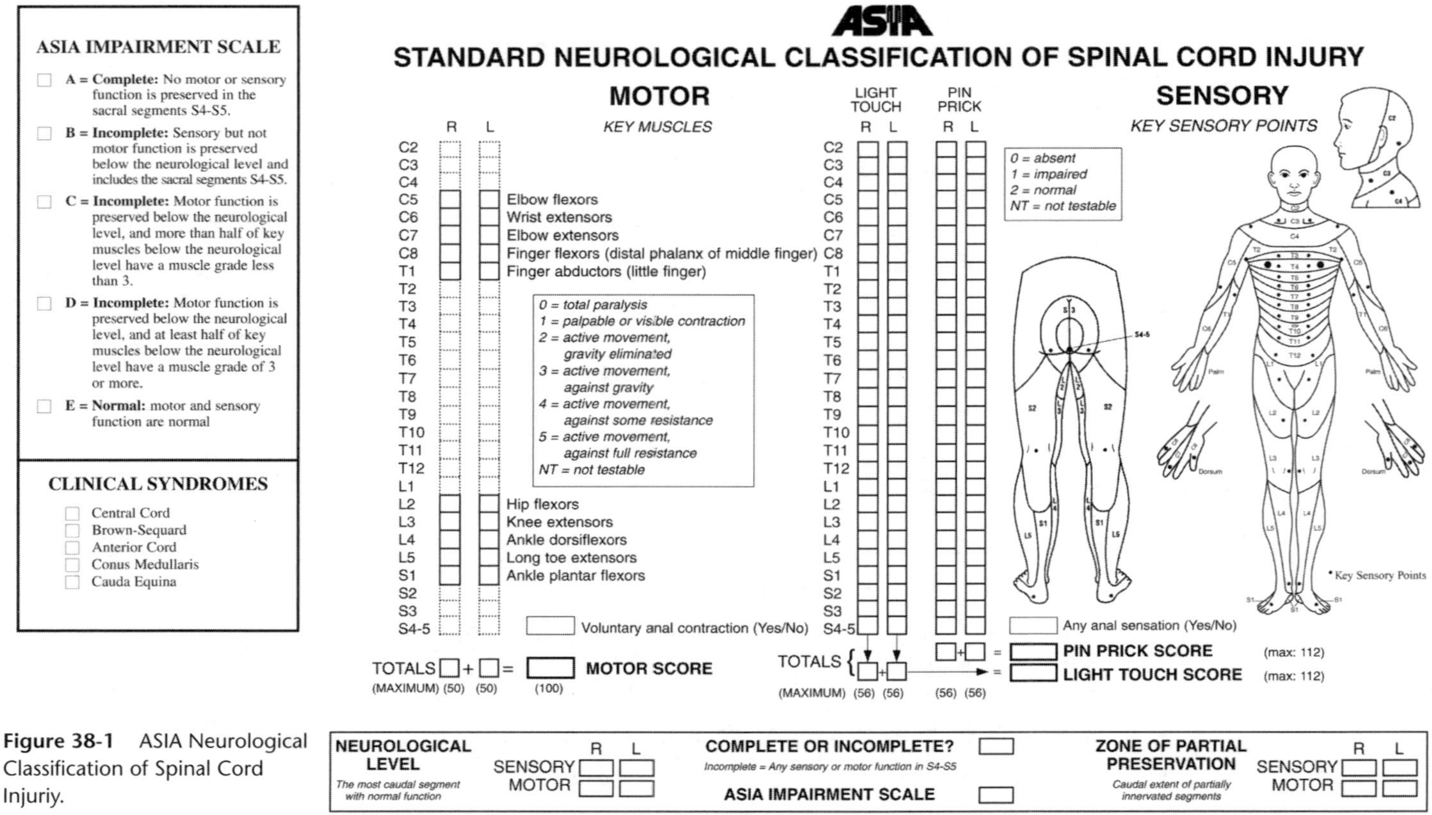

Figure 38-1 ASIA Neurological Classification of Spinal Cord Injury.

level of suspicion in insensate patients who may not have significant complaints.

Syringomyelia (Syrinx)

This is a condition in which a cystic fluid filled cavity exists within the spinal cord and may migrate rostrally. It must always be suspected in SCI. This is often secondary to the traumatic injury to the spinal cord or exists as a congenital anomaly as in patients with myelodysplasia. Approximately 3-4% of persons with traumatic SCI develop a syrinx which is clinically significant (16). Syrinx may present at any time in the life of a person with a spinal cord injury. It often will start as an ascending pattern or radicular type pain or parasthesias, gross motor deficit, or increased spasticity. The syrinx may also descend causing pain, weakness, and neurogenic bladder/bowel as well. This may be progressive and lead to further cord compression and neurological damage. An enlarging syrinx may also contribute to progressive scoliosis. Magnetic resonance imaging is the diagnostic test of choice and neurosurgical consultation is indicated.

Charcot Spine/Hardware Failure/Infection

Many patients have had previous spine surgery with fusion and instrumentation. Excessive stress above and below the fusion can cause weakening, hardware failure, and instability of the spine, especially in areas which are insensate (17). This occurs most frequently 1-2 levels below the fusion. Insensate patients may not always complain of pain but rather will notice a grinding sound, deformity, or neurological deterioration. Instrumentation may be a seed for infection and this may also lead to pain, spinal instability, or indolent/florid sepsis. Plain/dynamic radiographs, computed tomography (CT) scan, MRI, and laboratory studies are helpful in diagnosis and acute surgical consultation and further spine stabilization or irrigation/debridement may be indicated to prevent further disability. Osteoporotic fractures and scoliosis may be a cause of pain in the SCI population. Appropriate wheelchair seating support, bracing, and appropriate postural exercises can be used as primary treatment and prevention, as well as medical management of metabolic disorders such as osteoporosis.

Autonomic Dysreflexia

A serious and potentially life-threatening condition in SCI patients with injury levels of T-6 or above. It is characterized as an unopposed sympathetic outflow and hypertensive crisis (remember SCI patients usually can normally run systolic blood pressure in the 90s) and end organ failure. Patients will often be flushed above level of injury with signs of vasoconstriction below. Irritation from any noxious stimulus below the spinal cord lesion can bring it on. Signs/symptoms include hypertension, tachy/brady-cardia, pounding headache, vague or general feeling of fatigue and unwell, or have no complaints at all. Most common cause is distended bladder/kinked catheter. The primary treatment is typically not antihypertensives, although they are used in an emergency. Most often the clinician identifies and removes the noxious stimulus. This can be a challenge as the stimulus is often below the lesion and thus not localized by the patient.

Multiple Sclerosis

Multiple sclerosis (MS) is an inflammatory disorder of the central nervous system characterized by demyelinating lesions in the brain and spinal cord. Over the course of the disease a variety of neurological signs and symp-toms may be present. Weakness, fatigue, gait abnormalities, and spasticity are all very disabling to the patients. Pain may present as anything from a dull aching sensation in the low back to lancinating neuropathic pain to the trunk or extremities. Lhermitte's sign, an electric shock sensation radiating down the spine with forced flexion/extension of the head, is frequently present in MS patients but does not signify structural lesion (18). Heat in-tolerance from exercise or a hot shower for example may also increase the fatigue and weakness. This fatigue and prolonged weakness can further contribute to deconditioning, predisposing one to overuse injuries. Other sources of pain in the MS population may be overuse injuries from pro-longed weakness. Treatment is usually conservative with physical therapy, orthotics, and analgesics. Gross spinal pain or instability is not directly as-sociated with MS, so other diagnoses should be explored.

Myelodyplasia

Defined as a congenital defect of the developing neural fold during embry-onic development, myelodyplasia may range in severity of an asympto-matic incidental finding to paralysis (usually in lumbosacral region). The symptomatic defects are usually surgical fixed shortly after birth and neuro-logic deficits usually do not improve. Patients often have cognitive deficits, relating to hydrocephalus or type II Arnold-Chiari brainstem malformations. These may lead to difficult history taking. Children and adults with irritabil-ity, lethargy or fever may have shunt dysfunction which requires prompt evaluation. Patients have often had multiple surgeries with instrumentation, so subsequent surgical complications such as fracture, infection, or hard-ware failure must be considered in the differential diagnosis.

A tethered spinal cord, typically asymptomatic, can also be a cause of pain. Lumbosacral tumors and scarring are other complications in people with myelodysplasia (19). With these, traction of the spinal cord in a growing child may produce worsening radicular pain/paresthesias, new weakness, bladder/bowel dysfunction, and progressive scoliosis. MRI is an appropriate diagnostic test. Symptomatic tethered cord may need surgical release.

Central Nervous System Injury and Spasticity

As a result of upper motor neuron injury to the brain or spinal cord, patients can exhibit spasticity, defined as a velocity-dependent increase in tone. This can be seen in patients with conditions such as cerebrovacular accidents, traumatic brain injuries, cerebral palsy, and spinal cord injuries. Because one has spasticity does not automatically require treatment and intervention. Treatment is usually reserved for patients with spasticity-impairing activities of daily living, uncontrollable pain, or difficulty in ambulation, transfers or positioning.

Spasms can be painful. Also, because spasms can be difficult to control, it is not uncommon to have spasticity lead to improper positioning, especially in wheelchair dependent patients. Poor positioning, spasms, and limited range of motion can contribute to the development of contractures, particularly in muscles crossing two joints, such as the rectus femoris. Abnormal positioning and compensatory postures can lead to abnormal stresses placed on structures of the spine. These become pain generators.

Attempts to control the spasticity should be manage by clinicians with sufficient experience. Management strategies always begin with less invasive actions such as stretching regimens, tone-reducing orthotics, and modalities such as cold and heat. If these measures are not helpful, antispasticity medications and neuromuscular junction blocking agents can be tried. These include baclofen, dantrolene, lorazepam, tizantidine, botulinum toxin, or phenol/alcohol denervation.

Proper assessment of wheelchair seating must occur. If spasticity cannot be relieved with the above measures, accommodations for the abnormal postures must be made (see below).

Orthotics, Prosthetics, and Assistive Devices

Patients with disabilities often use a variety of assistive devices (i.e., wheelchairs, orthoses, braces, prosthetic limbs) in their everyday lives and will often require them indefinitely. A study by Ehde et al. shows nearly 25% of lower extremity amputees experience severe back pain that interferes with daily activities (20). Thus, proper use and fit is essential to their use and prevention of injury. Prosthetic limbs that may be too long or too short can put unequal stresses on the spine and pelvis, causing premature arthritis, scoliosis, or mechanical back pain. Long-term use of a wheelchair or crutches may lead to overuse injuries such as rotator cuff tendonopathy or carpal tunnel syndrome. Ankle foot orthoses (AFOs) have been known to put excess pressure over the fibular head and cause a peroneal mononeuropathy and foot drop. Wheelchair seating that encourages poor posture and little back or head support may lead to muscle strain, arthritis, progressive scoliosis, and potentially restrictive lung disease. The wheelchair seat should be reviewed. Sling-type seating in patients with poor trunk strength or scoliosis is not optimal and can contribute to the scoliotic curves. Often, to compensate for scoliosis, patients will require a custom-molded seat that accounts for scoliotic curves, contractures, and spasticity seen in patient populations such as cerebral palsy and spinal cord injury. A wheelchair with a tilt feature, though expensive, may help offload degenerative structures causing pain.

▦   ▦   ▦

Recommendations

- To promote strengthening and conditioning, moderate exercise training at approximately 40% of maximal resistance is best. Exercise regimens at too low or too high an intensity should be avoided in patients with disabilities.
- Make certain that orthotics, prosthetics, and assistive device are used properly. For patients who use a wheelchair, make certain that the patient has adequate seat support.
- For patients with spinal cord injury, examination of key muscles and sensory dermatomes to provide a baseline and periodic examinations thereafter are needed to monitor spinal cord lesions.
- In patients with multiple sclerosis, overuse injuries require conservative treatment with physical therapy, orthotics, and analgesics.

▦   ▦   ▦

Key Points

- In persons with neuromuscular disease, weakness and deconditioning lead to further spine degeneration.
- Baseline and periodic neurological examinations will aid in diagnosis of progressive neurological deficits that may cause more disability.
- Knowledge of history of disability, past procedures, assistive devices, and functionality will be crucial in determining etiology of pain.
- It is important to remember that people with disabilities can and do have common causes of back pain.

- Factors associated with disability may require unique intervention strategies (i.e., spasticity management) before standard therapy programs can be implemented for back pain.

▪   ▪   ▪

REFERENCES

1. **Addison R, Schultz A.** Trunk strengths in patients seeking hospitalization for chronic low back disorders. Spine. 1980;5:539.

2. **Alston W, Carlson KE, Feldman DJ, et al.** A quantitative study of muscle factors in the chronic low back syndrome. J Am Geriatr Soc. 1966;14:1041.

3. **McNeill T, Warwick D, Andersson G, Schultz A.** Trunk strengths in attempted flexion, extension, and lateral bending in healthy subjects and patients with low back dysfunction patients. Spine. 1984;9:588.

4. **Aitkens SG, McCrory MA, Kilmer DD, Bernauer EM.** Moderate resistance exercise program: its effect in slowly progressive neuromuscular disease. Arch Phys Med Rehab. 1993;74:711-5.

5. **Kilmer DD.** The role of exercise in neuromuscular disease. Phys Med Rehab Clin North Am. 1998; 9:115-25.

6. **Kilmer DD, Aitkens SG, Wright NC, McCrory MA.** Response to high-intensity eccentric muscle contractions in persons with myopathic disease. Muscle Nerve. 2001;24:1181-7.

7. **Kilmer DD, McCrory MA, Wright NC, Aitkens SG, Bernauer EM.** The effect of a high resistance exercise program in slowly progressive neuromuscular disease. Arch Phys Med Rehab. 1994;75:560-3.

9. **Wright NC, Kilmer DD, McCrory MA, Aitkens SG, Holcomb BJ, Bernauer EM.** Aerobic walking in slowly progressive neuromuscular disease: effect of a 12-week program. Arch Phys Med Rehab. 1996;77:64-9.

10. **Boachie-Adjei O, Lonner B.** Spinal deformity. Pediatr Clin North Am. 1996;43:883-97.

11. **Murphy KP.** Scoliosis: current management and trends. Physical Medicine and Rehabilitation: State of the Art Reviews. 2000;14:207-19.

12. **Gerbino PG, Micheli IJ.** Back injuries in the young athlete. Clin Spots Med. 1995;14:571-90.

13. **Hoeffel C, Gaucher H, Hoeffel JC, Galloy MA, Arnould V.** Painful scoliosis. Klin Padiatr. 1977;209:78-83.

14. **Agre JC, Rodriquez AA, Sperling KB.** Symptoms and clinic impressions of patients seen in a postpolio clinic. Arch Phys Med Rehabil. 1990:70:367-70.

15. **American Spinal Injury Association.** International Standards for Neurological Classification of Spinal Cord Injury, Revised. Chicago: American Spinal Injury Association; 2000.

16. **Bryce MB, Ragnarsson KT.** Pain after spinal cord injury. Phys Med Rehabil Clin North Am. 2000;11:157-68.

17. **Goetz L, Priebe M.** Posttraumatic syringomyelia. eMedicine Journal. 2001;2:1-14.

18. **Standaert CJ, Cardenas DD, Anderson PA.** Charcot spine as a complication of traumatic spinal cord injury. Arch Phys Med Rehabil. 1997;78:221-24.

19. **Adams RD, Victor M, Ropper AH.** Multiple sclerosis and allied demyelinative disease. In: Adams RD, Victor M, Ropper AH; eds. Principles of Neurology, 6th ed. New York: McGraw-Hill; 1997:902-27.

20. **Molnar GE, Murphy KP.** Spina bifida. In: Molnar GE, Alexander MA; eds. Pediatric Rehabilitation, 3rd ed. Philadelphia; Hanley & Belfus; 1999:219-44.

21. **Ehde DM, et al.** Back pain as a secondary disability in persons with lower extremity amputations. Arch Phys Med Rehabil. 2001;82:731-4.

39

Low Back Pain in the Older Patient

Henry C. Tong, MD

Back pain is common in older persons, and this population is increasing. Older patients present with diseases, disability, and goals that are often different from those of younger patients. Primary care clinicians need to understand the unique aspects of the diagnosis and care of back pain in older persons. This chapter begins with a discussion of epidemiology then reviews diagnoses common in the older population. Notable aspects of the history and physical examination in older persons with back pain are covered, followed by diagnoses and treatment of specific diseases. The chapter ends with a discussion of special considerations in management of geriatric pain and disability.

Epidemiology

Many studies have shown that back pain disables 60% to 80% of American adults during their lifetime. Within a given year, up to 50% will complain of back pain, although the majority of persons with back pain do not seek care (1). However there have been fewer studies evaluating the prevalence of back pain in people greater than 65 years old. One study evaluated the 1037 surviving members of the original Framingham Heart study, ages 68-100 (2). This study noted a 48.6% annual prevalence of back pain symptoms. Back pain "on most days" was experienced by 22.3% of this group. This prevalence was slightly higher among women, but did not vary with respect to age (68-80 vs. 81-100 years old). These rates are similar to those reported in previous studies of back pain in working age adults (3).

Even though the prevalence and incidence of back pain in older adults does not seem to significantly increase with age, the occurrence of arthritic lesions in the low back does. In asymptomatic subjects, it has been shown that for those younger than 60 years, the prevalence of herniated disks is 20%, and prevalence of any significant abnormality was 27-33%, whereas for those older than 60 years, the prevalence of herniated disk was 36-40%, the prevalence of a significant abnormality was 57-67%, and the prevalence of spinal stenosis was 21% (4,5). This high prevalence of spine lesions in the asymptomatic population makes it clinically difficult to determine if a specific lesion is causing a patient's symptoms.

Thus, in the younger patients, the precise cause of pain is rarely identified (6,7), whereas in older patients, while back pain is also usually nonspecific, there is a slightly greater incidence of systemic conditions or malignancies causing the pain.

General Approach to Diagnostic Studies

Clinicians should be aware that older adults have an increased risk for malignancy in the spine and osteoporotic compression fractures of the spine. Because of this, there is a lower threshold to obtain an x-ray study to screen for these lesions. An anteroposterior and lateral lumbar spine film is also 70% sensitive at detecting the aortic calcifications (8). If the patient has a history suspicious for cancer (history of cancer, fever, pain worse at night, or unexplained weight loss), myelopathy, or cauda equina syndrome (bower incontinence, bladder incontinence, perianal numbness and tingling, foot drop or weak ankle push off), then a more comprehensive imaging study (MRI or CAT scan) should be considered. A Westergren sedimentation rate may be ordered if there are concerns of cancer or polymyalgia rheumatica.

Axial Back Pain

Lumbar Strain or Sprain

As with working-age adults, musculoskeletal back pain in the older adult is fairly common and usually self-limited. *Lumbar strain or sprain* usually resolves in a few weeks with relative rest and appropriate analgesic medication. A clinician should not recommend bed rest but may authorize it for a maximum of two days if the pain indicates it (9,10). There have been very little data that physical therapy may help the initial recovery, but one study has shown that a lumbar stabilization program for an acute first time back pain can reduce the number of patients with a second episode by 50% (11).

Compression Fracture

Although osteoporosis is common in older patients, especially women, it by itself rarely causes any symptoms until a pathologic fracture occurs. The most common pathologic fracture in the spine related to osteoporosis is a vertebral compression fracture. This may be associated with a fall or may occur with minimal trauma (e.g., getting out of bed). The pain is usually acute and is increased with trunk flexion. The pain usually subsides over 6-8 weeks. If clinically indicated, a bone scan or MRI may help determine if the fracture is recent or old.

Treatment options for acute lumbar compression fractures include a trial of bracing, analgesic medications, calcitonin nasal spray, physical therapy. The rehabilitation program should avoid severe flexion exercises to avoid causing another compression fracture. For acute compression fractures, treatment with vertebroplasty or kyphoplasty may be considered but these treatments are fairly new and need to be evaluated with a randomized controlled trial (12).

In addition to direct treatment of the compression fracture, the osteoporosis that causes such fractures may be addressed. There are many treatment options for osteoporosis such as hormone replacement therapy, raloxifene, oral bisphonate, calcitonin, calcium supplementation/ vitamin D. The optimal medication regimen for osteoporosis is beyond the scope of this chapter.

Polymyalgia Rheumatica

This occurs usually in patients over 50 years of age with acute onset of pain and stiffness in the neck, upper back, shoulders, and low back. There is a high association with temporal arteritis, characterized by fevers, headaches, vision changes and jaw claudication. Patients usually have a Westergreen sedimentation rate >40 mm/h and dramatically improve with low-dose prednisone (13).

Degenerative Disk and Joint Disease

Degenerative disk and facet joint changes are common in all people over age 50, even those without back pain. Thus, even when there is radiologic evidence of arthritis in the spine, if the older patient has signs or symptoms suggestive of potentially dangerous causes for the back pain, these should be ruled out before attributing the pain to degenerative changes.

If degenerative disk and joint disease are determined to be the cause of the back pain, treatment should begin with physical therapy (McKenzie approach, manual therapy, lumbar stabilization) and an analgesic medication. If these do not help, then a trial of facet injections or referral to a spine surgeon should be considered.

Spinal Stenosis

Spinal stenosis may be associated with degenerative disk disease and facet arthritis, which may cause axial back pain and neurogenic claudication (leg cramping and weakness with ambulation, as discussed in detail below). Spinal stenosis does not necessarily cause back pain, however, as radiologic evidene of this condition has been noted in 21% of asymptomatic persons older than 60 years. As for degenerative disk and joint disease, teatment of spinal stenosis should begin with physical therapy (McKenzie approach, manual therapy, lumbar stabilization) and the use of analgesics. If the pain is not relieved, a trail of facet injections or referral to a spine surgeon may be necessary.

At press time we have just completed a prospective trial of diagnostic tests and functional assessments in persons with spinal stenosis, low back pain, and control subjects (Tong HC, Haig AJ, Geisser ME, Yamakawa KSJ, Miner JA. Comparing pain severity and functional status of older adults without spinal symptoms, with lumbar spinal stenosis, and with axial low back pain. In preparation.). We found that seniors with spinal stenosis and axial low back pain are more disabled than than seniors without spinal problems. However, they compensate so their total weekly walking distance is not as significantly decreased.

Spondylolisthesis

This is defined as an anterior (anterolisthesis) or posterior (retrolisthesis) translation of a vertebral body compared to the level above or below it. The prevalence in the adult population has been estimated to be about 6% and was noted to be unchanged with increasing age (14). A small amount of slippage has not been associated with back pain, but a slippage >25% has been associated with back pain. Back pain in spondylolisthesis is believed to be related to stress on the intervertebral disk, fibrocartilage mass or the spinal ligaments (15). In older age, degenerative spondylolisthesis becomes more common. It is the result of facet joint arthritis causing hypermobility of spinal segments. The isthmic spondylolisthesis that may have occurred in a younger age may now interact with degenerative arthritis changes to compromise the spinal canal, causing spinal stenosis. Spinal surgery at a younger age may have damaged the ligaments or paraspinal muscles, causing spinal slippage, too.

If there is motion with the flexion-extension films or the patient has symptoms of gradual neurologic compromise, refer to a spine surgeon. If these are not noted, then nonsurgical management can be tried. First consider physical therapy (range of motion of hip flexors and lumbar stabilization [16]) and an analgesic medication. The therapist should avoid back extension exercises that hyperextend the lumbar spine. If these do not help then a trial of an epidural injection at that level or referral to a spine surgeon is appropriate (17).

Abdominal Aortic Aneurysm

Abdominal aortic aneurysm occurs in 4% of people over 50, more common in persons with evidence of intermittent claudication (8). Most patients are asymptomatic, but 10-15% of these patients have back pain, often associated with abdominal pain. The physical examination may reveal a pulsatile abdominal mass in half of the patients.

Malignancy

The most common neoplastic cause of back pain is metastatic disase to the vertebral column. The most common causes are breast, prostate, lung, or renal cancer.

The most common spinal cancer is multiple myeloma. Magnetic resonance imaging (MRI), computed tomography (CT), and bone scans are all very sensitive for spinal malignancies (except for multiple myelomas, which may not be detected by a bone scan). These patients should be referred to a specialist (medical oncologist or radiation oncologist). If spinal stability is questioned, also refer to spine surgeon.

Pain Radiating to the Leg (Sciatica)

Lumbosacral Radiculopathy

Lumbosarcral radiculopathy is characterized by leg pain that is greater than the back pain, caused by nerve root entrapment and compression and nerve tissue inflammation. It usually is associated with neurologic symptoms such as burning, numbness, or dyesthesias (pins and needles sensation). There may be associated neurologic signs such as sensory change in a dermatomal distribution, muscle weakness in a myotomal distribution, or decreased reflex.

Compared with younger persons, older patients more commonly present with higher level disk herniations, as in many older persons the lower lumbar disks have already undergone degeneration. These higher level disk herniations may be harder to detect due to a number of factors. Anterior thigh pain may be present, rather than more classic posterior pain radiating below the knee in lower disks. The "standard" straight leg raise test may be negative, with the "reverse" straight leg raise test being positive in about 50% of cases. (The reverse straight leg raise test involves lifting the bent knee of a prone patient to cause anterior radiating pain.) Motor loss (hip flexors) and reflex change (patellar reflex or none) may have an unusual, unreliable presentation and may be difficult to detect. High lumbar disk herniations are more likely than other disk herniations to be in far lateral positions, making it difficult to detect with routine MRI (up to 50% of surgically proven lesions may be missed). Nevertheless, electromyography can sample the high lumbar paraspinal muscles, so it has a fairly high sensitivity if appropriate techniques are used.

Initial treatment of this condition consists of physical therapy, analgesic medication and adjunctive pain medications (e.g., low-dose amitriptyline or gabapentin). If the pain is severe, consider an epidural injection or referral to a spine surgeon (17). If there is weakness noted (excluding mild great toe weakness), referral to a spine surgeon should be considered.

Lumbosacral Plexopathy

This rarely occurs spontaneously and is usually related to a history of pelvic trauma (e.g., fracture or hip surgery).

Neurogenic Claudication/Pseudoclaudication

This is related to central canal spinal stenosis (may be due to disk herniation, spondylosis, facet arthritis, ligamentum flavum hypertrophy, spondylolisthesis, or space occupying lesion). The exact pathophysiological mechanism is not known, but there are theories based on ischemic, nutritional, and mechanical models. This is classically described as symptoms of leg pain, numbness, and/or weakness when standing or walking and are relieved by sitting for a few minutes (18).

The research study that we have completed at press time includes the largest cohort of asymptomatic older persons ever tested with lumbar MRI. Surprisingly, masked radiologists saw some central or lateral recess changes that could relate to stenosis in about 80% of older persons without spinal stenosis or radiating symptoms. It is important to note that, although not perfectly sensitive, electrodiagnostic testing had 90-100% specificity depending on the group studied, and there was no statistically significant difference in MRI canal diameter between the asymptomatic and symptomatic group (10). A number of subjects in whom the clinician suspected stenosis were actually found to have polyneuropathy or myopathy in this study. This new information makes it critical that clinicians not treat the MRI scan findings, but rather use tests like electrodiagnostics to compliment history and physical examination in making decisions about radiating pain or claudication in older people.

The initial treatment may consist of physical therapy (walking, stretching hip flexor muscles, and manual therapy), analgesic medication, and an adjunctive pain medication such as low-dose amitriptyline or gabapentin. An epidural injections may be considered if the symptoms are disabling or the patient is not responding to noninvasive treatments. If the patient does not respond to these, and the pain is disabling, than a referral to a spine surgeon to consider surgical decompression is recommended (17).

Osteoarthritis of the Hip

This usually causes pain in the groin or lateral hip region, but may also present as buttock or deep thigh pain. The earliest physical finding in hip osteoarthritis is loss of internal rotation; with progressive disease, range of motion is limited further in all directions, and significant functional limitation occurs (20).

Trochanteric Bursitis

This is an inflammation or irritation of the subgluteus maximius bursa overlying the greater trochanter. It can be seen in all age groups, but has a peak incidence of 30-60 years (21). This is characterized by pain in the lateral thigh with focal tenderness to palpation over the greater trochanter. This is associated with tightness of the iliotibial band (Ober's test), and weakness of the hip adductors and gluteus medius muscle (21).

Cauda Equina Syndrome

This is characterized by decreased functioning of the S2-4 nerve roots usually due to a compressive lesion such as a herniated disk. The presenting symptoms are bladder incontinence, perineal numbness ("saddle anesthesia"), and leg weakness. It occurs in less than 0.04% of subjects with low back pain (22) and is not known to occur in higher frequency in the older patient with back pain. However, this differential should always be screened during the history and physical, as it is one of the few surgical emergencies. Is has been shown that outcome with surgical release within 48 hours has better outcomes compared to surgical release after 48 hours of symptom onset (23). Older patients with cauda equina syndrome or myelopathy should be referred to a specialist emergently for management (23).

History and Physical Examination

The basic history and physical examination should be focused on three things: determining the likely causes of the back pain as best as possible, determining what dangerous lesions should be ruled out, and determining the barriers to recovery.

In the older patient, it is also important to determine the patient's current functioning level and identify comorbid problems that may impair function and recovery. Patients who are living alone or are caring for a sick spouse will need to be independent and safe with their basic activities of daily living (dressing, eating, ambulation, toileting, bathing) as well as their "instrumental" activities of daily living (shopping, finances/paying bills, cooking and cleaning, yard work, transportation, and caring for spouse). Comorbid problems are important to evaluate, as the back pain alone may not be disabling, but the combination of severe asthma or knee arthritis in addition to back pain may be debilitating. These problems may also affect how likely the patients are able to participate or benefit from therapies (e.g., severe congestive heart failure with neurogenic claudication will increase the risk of surgical decompression). Comorbid problems may also dictate the optimal treatment plan. For example, a patient with ischemic heart disease should be optimally managed medically before starting a functional restoration program; conversely, improving a patient's trochanteric bursitis with physical therapy and injections will maximize a patient's outcomes with a cardiac rehabilitation program.

In the older person, comorbid conditions also need to be taken into consideration when one is determining the functional outcome of spine surgery. For example, surgical relief of neurogenic claudicationmay not improve the quality of life of a person who is limited from ambulating more than 40 feet by chronic obstructive pulmonary disease.

Addressing Functional Abilities

There is no literature on the disability caused by back pain in older persons, but there is every reason to believe that back pain is associated with severe disability in some older people. In general, older people have decreased functional abilities compared to younger people. In addition to the magnitude of the disability, the nature of the disability is likely different. Seniors are physically different from younger persons. The social roles of seniors often do not include work or child rearing responsibilities, but this is not an absolute.

Our group studied a group of 37 elderly persons with significant chronic back pain and disability referred to a tertiary care spine program (24). Experience with this group is useful in understanding the nature of disability. We found that older persons with back pain may have substantial physical impairment and disability. Their health related quality of life is greatly decreased in relation to the U.S. population as a whole. They are different from younger adults with chronic pain; e.g., they have less fear of pain, less depression, and different life goals.

The complexity of factors that relate to their quality of life suggests that a multidisciplinary approach, such as the one presented here, is necessary to optimize care. Figures 39-1 to 39-4, from a study performed at The University of Michigan, provide graphic demonstration of disability and quality of life issues for older persons with complex back pain disability. In

Figure 39-1, it is remarkable that less than half of these patients were completely independent in bathing and lower extremity dressing. Not shown in these figures is the amount of assistance needed to accomplish these tasks. In fact, the data showed that very few patients relied on human help, but instead they sought assistive devices or compromised their activities. Most patients are not completely independent in any aspect of functional mobility, as shown in Figure 39-2. About a third of patients needed the assistance of another for community ambulation, and 20% required another person to help with stairs.

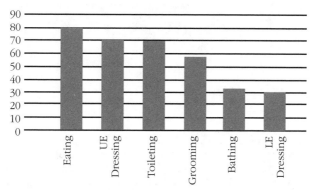

Figure 39-1   Self-care independence in older persons with complex back pain. (Data from Haig AJ, Geisser ME, Bade S, et al. Back Pain and Disability in Older Persons. Multidisciplinary Comparision to Working Age Persons. American Academy of Physical Medicine and Rehabilitation Annual Assembly. San Francisco; 2000.)

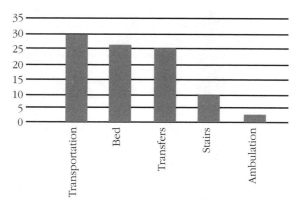

Figure 39-2   Functional mobility in a population of older persons with significant back pain disability. (Data from Haig AJ, Geisser ME, Bade S, et al. Back Pain and Disability in Older Persons. Multidisciplinary Comparision to Working Age Persons. American Academy of Physical Medicine and Rehabilitation Annual Assembly. San Francisco; 2000.)

Back pain disability is associated with failure in activities that allow older persons to live independently in their own home, as shown by Figure 39-3. More patients were completely unable to perform many of these tasks, even with human assistance. For instance, 5% of people could make

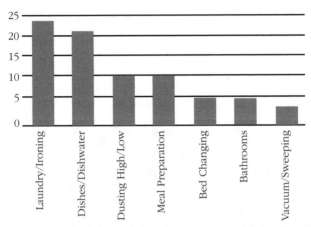

Figure 39-3   Home activities in a population of older persons with significant back pain disability. (Data from Haig AJ, Geisser ME, Bade S, Miller Q, Yamakawa K. Back Pain and Disability in Older Persons. A Multidisciplinary Comparison to Working Age Persons. American Academy of Physical Medicine and Rehabilitation Annual Assembly, San Francisco; 2000.)

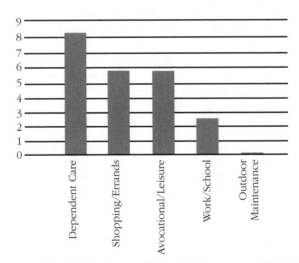

Figure 39-4   Outside life activities in a population of older persons with significant back pain disability. (Data from Haig AJ, Geisser ME, Bade S, Miller Q, Yamakawa K. Back Pain and Disability in Older Persons. A Multidisciplinary Comparison to Working Age Persons. American Academy of Physical Medicine and Rehabilitation Annual Assembly, San Francsisco; 2000.)

their bed independantly, and (not shown here) about a third (32%) were completely unable to make their bed, even with assistance. Figure 39-4 shows more advanced life activities. Not all of these activities pertain to all seniors. Nevertheless, the inability to perform shopping or to maintain the yard limit the quality of life of older persons.

Still, the nature of disability is different in older people. One older scientist, on reviewing this data, said "we're like Teflon. We just slide by the disabilities." In contrast to people who must work or care for children, older people may just "slide by," slowly loosing independence without anyone noticing the losses, attributing the isolation and inability to accomplish life tasks to their age.

Symptomatic Treatment and Treatment of Function

Deconditioning

Most patients with *chronic* disabling back pain are inactive. Older persons often start in suboptimal physical condition, they deteriorate quickly with rest, and recover more slowly than younger persons. Deconditioning in this population can lead to falls, functional decline, and social isolation. Older women especially may not have had previous experience with exercise.

In some patients, the deconditioning may be as disabling as the pain itself. All patients with subacute and chronic back pain should be encouraged to stay active and participate in an aerobic type activity at least 3 days per week. Low-impact activities such as walking, chair aerobics, and pool activities may be done daily. If needed, working with a comprehensive rehabilitation program (e.g., functional restoration program) can improve the patient's functioning and quality of life.

Depression

Although our population of older patients with chronic back pain seemed to have less depression than our group of work disabled younger persons, depression is still present in a large number of patients. Sometimes the depression is difficult to detect, masquerading as dementia, somnolence, or social isolation. Suicide is a risk, especially in older men with pain. Antidepressant medications and counseling are effective treatments.

Decreased Activities of Daily Living

Occupational therapy can evaluate the tasks they cannot do, and then work with patients on compensatory strategies (e.g., alter mechanics of activity, pacing, ergonomic changes, or use assistive devices) to help them live independently.

Decreased Balance

For patients with decreased balance, a simple home exercise program taught by physical therapy can improve balance and safety. Other possible interventions include using an assistive device (cane or walker) or home safety evaluation (can be done by an occupational therapist or visiting nurse).

Decreased Sleep

Work with the patient on good sleep hygeine. With caution, some nonaddicting medications can be used for sleep. Low-dose amitryptaline is commonly used. Imipramine may be as effective with pain and slightly less sedating. Either pill may cause increased CNS, balance, and bladder changes in older persons (see Chapter 29 for more information on antidepressants in patients with pain).

"Whole Patient" Rehabilitation

We have experimented quite successfully with a multidisciplinary approach to rehabilitating older people with complex back pain disability. In a process called the "Senior Functional Restoration Program," older people first undergo a multidisciplinary assessment somewhat analogous to the Spine Team Assessment noted in Chapter 27. If their needs go beyond the abilities of individual treatment efforts noted above, they enroll in an 8-week, 2 hours per day, 3 days per week program involving occupational therapy, manual physical therapy, exercise, psychological counseling, and educational lectures. Qualitative information and some uncontrolled data show substantial improvement in both function and quality of life with this approach.

Conclusion

Because back pain is disabling in this increasing population, primary care providers should become familiar with unique aspects of management. Medical complexity relates to both the chances of more significant spinal disease and the interaction of other medical problems with treatment and rehabilitation. On one hand, because work and family burdens are often less, back pain may be less of a crisis, but on the other hand, back pain is associated with a number of slow losses in function that can lead to dependence and institutionalization. Minor back aches are common, but when associated with disability, back pain should be treated aggressively.

Recommendations

- It is important to determine the older patient's current level of functioning and identify comorbidities that may impair function and recovery.
- Comorbid conditions also need to be considered to help determine the functional outcome after spine surgery.
- Radiography is more likely to be necessary in older patients, because older adults are at greater risk for spinal malignancies and osteoporotic fractures.
- Minor backaches are common, but when associated with disability, back pain should be treated aggressively.
- Deconditioning is more difficult to overcome in older adults, making it that much more important that these patients be encouraged to stay active.
- Electrodiagnostic testing, not imaging, should be used to confirm the presence of neurologic disorder.

Key Points

- Because older persons are at greater risk for dangerous or disabling back disorders, diagnostic testing strategies may be different and more aggressive than in younger persons.
- Spinal stenosis, higher level lumbar disk herniation, compression fracture, and arthritis in hip or facet joints may cause back complaints more commonly in older people.
- The physician may need to ask older people specifically about functional deficits.
- Multidisciplinary rehabilitation is a valuable tool for older people with more complex or severe disability.

REFERENCES

1. **Lahad A, Malter AD, Berg AO, Deyo RA.** The effectiveness of four interventions for the prevention of low back pain. JAMA. 1994;272(16):1286-91.
2. **Edmond SL, Felson DT.** Prevalence of back symptoms in elders. J Rheumatol. 2000;27(1):220-5.
3. **Loney PL, Stratford PW.** The prevalence of low back pain in adults: a methodological review of the literature. Phys Ther. 1999;79(4):384-96.

4. **Boden SD, Davis DO, Dina TS, Patronas NJ, Wiesel SW.** Abnormal magnetic-resonance scans of the lumbar spine in asymptomatic subjects. A prospective investigation. J Bone Joint Surg Am. 1990;72(3):403-8.

5. **Jensen MC, Brant-Zawadzki MN, Obuchowski N, Modic MT, Malkasian D, Ross JS.** Magnetic resonance imaging of the lumbar spine in people without back pain. N Engl J Med. 1994;331(2):69-73.

6. **White AA 3rd, Gordon SL.** Synopsis: workshop on idiopathic low-back pain. Spine. 1982;7(2):141-9.

7. **Nachemson A.** The lumbar spine: an orthopedic challenge. Spine. 1976;1:59-71.

8. **Mazanec DJ.** Evaluating back pain in older patients. Cleve Clin J Med. 1999;66(2):89-91, 95-99.

9. **Abenhaim L, Rossignol M, Valat JP, Nordin M, Avouac B, Blotman F, et al.** The role of activity in the therapeutic management of back pain. Report of the International Paris Task Force on Back Pain. Spine. 2000;25(4 Suppl):1S-33S.

10. **Deyo RA, Diehl AK, Rosenthal M.** How many days of bed rest for acute low back pain? A randomized clinical trial. N Engl J Med. 1986;315(17):1064-70.

11. **Hides JA, Richardson CA, Jull GA.** Multifidus muscle rehabilitation decreases recurrence of symptoms following first episode low back pain. In: Proceedings of the National Congress of the Australian Physiotherapy Association. Brisbane; 1996.

12. **Watts NB, Harris ST, Genant HK.** Treatment of painful osteoporotic vertebral fractures with percutaneous vertebroplasty or kyphoplasty. Osteoporos Int. 2001;12(6):429-37.

13. **Klippel JH, ed.** Primer on the Rheumatic Diseases, 11th ed. Atlanta: Arthritis Foundation; 1997.

14. **Virta L, Ronnemaa T, Osterman K, Aalto T, Laakso M.** Prevalence of isthmic lumbar spondylolisthesis in middle-aged subjects from eastern and western Finland. J Clin Epidemiol. 1992;45(8):917-22.

15. **Wiltse LL, Rothman LG.** Spondylolisthesis: classification, diagnosis, and natural history. Semin Spine Surg. 1989;1(2):78-94.

16. **O'Sullivan PB, Phyty GD, Twomey LT, Allison GT.** Evaluation of specific stabilizing exercise in the treatment of chronic low back pain with radiologic diagnosis of spondylolysis or spondylolisthesis. Spine. 1997;22(24):2959-67.

17. **Wong DA, Errico T, Saal J, Sims W, Watters W.** Clinical guideline on low back pain. Rosemont and LaGrange, IL: American Academy of Orthopedic Surgeons; 1996.

18. **Verbiest H.** A radicular syndrome from development narrowing of the lumbar vertebral canal. J Bone Joint Surg Br. 1954;36B:230-7.

19 **Haig AJ, Yamakawa KSJ, Tong HC, Quint DJ, Hoff JT, Chiodo A, et al.** A Comparison of Electromyography and Magnetic Resonance Imaging in Older Persons with Lumbar Spinal Stenosis, Low Back Pain, and no Back Complaints. Accepted for presentation, International Society for Physical and Rehabilitation Medicine, Sao Paolo Brazil, April 12-14, 2005.

20. **Schnitzer TJ.** Osteoarthritis (degenerative joint disease). In: Goldman L, Bennett JC, eds. Cecil Textbook of Medicine, 21st ed. Philadelphia: WB Saunders; 2000:1550-4.

21. **Shbeeb MI, Matteson EL.** Trochanteric bursitis (greater trochanter pain syndrome). Mayo Clin Proc. 1996;71(6):565-9.

22. **Deyo RA, Rainville J, Kent DL.** What can the history and physical examination tell us about low back pain? JAMA. 1992;268(6):760-5.

23. **Ahn UM, Ahn NU, Buchowski JM, Garrett ES, Sieber AN, Kostuik JP.** Cauda equina syndrome secondary to lumbar disc herniation: a meta-analysis of surgical outcomes. Spine. 2000;25(12):1515-22.

24. **Haig AJ, Geisser ME, Bade S, Miller Q, Yamakawa K.** Back Pain and Disability in Older Persons. A Multidisciplinary Comparison to Working Age Persons. American Academy of Physical Medicine and Rehabilitation Annual Assembly, San Fransisco, November 2-5, 2000.

▪   ▪   ▪

KEY REFERENCES

Grobler LJ. Back and leg pain in older adults. Presentation, diagnosis, and treatment. Clin Geriatr Med. 1998;14(3):543-76.
   A surgeon's perspective on evaluation and management of geriatric back pain.

Lazaro L, Quinet RJ. Low back pain: how to make the diagnosis in the older patient. Geriatrics. 1994;49(9):48-53.
   A good general article on the issues of back pain in this population.

40

■ ■ ■

Administrative and Policy Issues

Joseph Niester, MHA

Andrew J. Haig, MD

Back pain is in the unenviable position of being one of the largest expenses in the health environment, costing society billions of dollars each year in medical and lost wage expenses. Employers, insurers, and health care system administrators struggle with this subjective complaint that is associated with highly variable cost and disability. Physicians often have responsibilities as administrators. This chapter provides a brief outline of some of the administrative issues and solutions in back pain management.

Back Pain in a Health Care System

Back pain management occupies a disproportionate amount of health care system administrators' time. One reason is that the American health care system values back pain in highly capricious ways. For instance, if disability is caused by work, the worker's compensation insurer is typically liable for lost wages as well as health care costs, but if the problem did not happen at work, the patient and indirectly the employer, but not the worker's compensation insurer, absorbs the cost of disability. Because 4/5 of the cost of back pain is associated with disability from work, rather than actual health care expenditures, the value that employers and insurers place on back pain is different from that they place on other diseases.

A second important reason is that the care of back pain is the purview of many different providers within and outside of a health care system. Table 40-1 lists different health care providers who have a stake in the management of back pain. There is not a rational relationship between the importance of back pain to each type of provider, the power of each type

Table 40-1   Health Care Provider Groups with a Stake in Back Pain Management

• Internal medicine	• Anesthesiology
• Family medicine	• Occupational medicine
• Emergency medicine	• Pediatrics
• Orthopedic surgery	• Physical therapy
• Neurosurgery	• Occupational therapy
• Physical medicine and rehabilitation	• Psychology
• Rheumatology	• Chiropractic
• Neurology	• Alternative providers

of provider within the health care system, and the optimal structure of back pain management within the system. For example, primary care physicians see the vast majority of patients with back pain within most systems, but they typically are less concerned with the details of clinical management or disability outcome than others. Orthopedic and neurosurgeons have a great stake in the triage of back pain, and because of the income they bring into the system, are individually powerful players. But at most 5% of back pain gets an operation, and the rate of operation for low back pain in the United States is twice that of other industrialized nations. Physical medicine and rehabilitation has substantial expertise and a high stake in back pain management, but since there are only a small number of providers and these do not individually generate operating room income, their influence on the health care system is disproportionately small.

A third reason is the uneven flow of cases through the system. Primary care physicians may hang on to patients beyond their level of expertise, then refer the patient to surgeons, whom they consider the back experts. Most modern surgeons have little training or interest in nonsurgical treatment. They feel that they get too many nonsurgical referrals and are burdened by postoperative management that they cannot bill for. At the same time, they are worried about loosing potential surgical cases if they decline referrals. Similarly, anesthesiologists, neurologists, and rheumatologists may hang on to a disproportionate number of less appropriate cases in order to keep a supply of referrals for injections, electrodiagnostic procedures, and general clinic volumes. Because physicians are paid "piecemeal" for their work, throughput is very important. It takes less time in clinic to order a thousand-dollar MRI or renew a $200/hour physical therapy referral than it does to explain why they are not needed.

Depending on the realities of a health care system and the administrator's role, he or she may want spine care to be triaged differently. At the University of Michigan, the original design for our spine program used physical medicine and rehabilitation as the main triage point. Figure 40-1 shows the general flow of patients. This model places responsibility for total system quality and cost effectiveness on the physiatrists within the Physical Medicine and Rehabilitation (PM+R) Spine Program.

System-Wide Back Pain Interventions

A number of actions can be taken within a health care system to decrease the cost and disability associated with back pain (Figure 40-2).

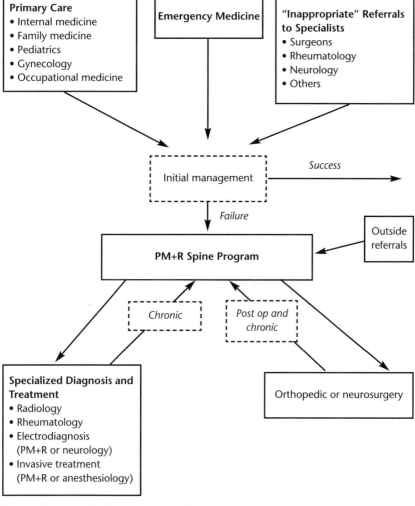

Figure 40-1   Idealized flow of patients through a health care system.

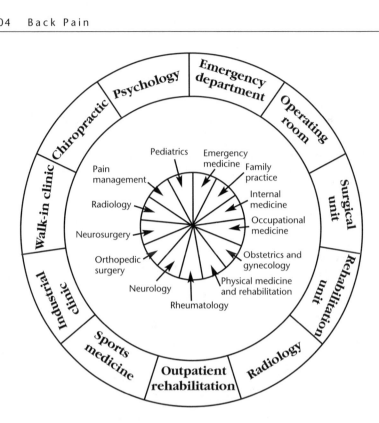

Figure 40-2   Physician specialties that see back pain on a daily basis, surrounded by the health care facilities that are involved in back pain management.

Education is a powerful tool. Patient and community education has been proven to decrease inappropriate utilization of services. The emphasis is not so much on prevention as it is on intelligent health care consumerism-when to see a doctor, when to get x-rays, when to get surgery. For primary care physicians, education about appropriate use of diagnostic tests, therapy, medication, and invasive treatment (perhaps using this book!) can make a difference, especially when tied to daily practice habits. Group exercise/education programs can treat specific populations without using expensive individual therapist referrals. We have had success with a geriatric spine exercise group, a general spine exercise group, a seating clinic, a pregnancy and back pain clinic, and others.

Another important action is elimination of roadblocks to appropriate care. This can take a number of forms. One protocol provides two daily open slots to the emergency department for after-hours use. Another marketed a two visit PT program for acute back pain to increase appropriate referrals to therapy while decreasing the total number of therapy visits. Other ideas include subspecialty clinics-a sciatica clinic, a postoperative clinic, and so forth. The Spine Team Assessment, described in Chapters 25 and 27, has been a key solution to chronic back pain. All physicians in the system are encouraged to refer all patients with more than 3 months of disability to the Spine Team Assessment. Rehabilitation Team Assessments, LLC, has developed software protocols to help health care systems adopt the Spine Team Assessment protocol (see www.rehab-team.com).

Administration of a Spine Program

A coordinated spine program is in increasingly popular solution to the back pain problem. In addition to being a facility that can be used to provide access to appropriate care as described above, a spine program provides high visibility and credibility to an expert team that has been charged with changing the system. The intellectual and financial benefits of participation attracts hard to find high quality specialist physicians and allied health professionals. Because of the importance of this kind of facility within a health care system, we will describe the workings of a spine program in greater detail below.

Place Within the System

Revenue sharing may be a large obstacle. Depending on how budgets are managed in the system, some departments may be unwilling to share financial gains or expenses. The surgery department does not want to lose any of its revenue generated from spine surgeries, the radiology department does not want to lose control over the use of necessary scanning equipment (and the revenue they generate), and anesthesiology may not want to give up revenue from spinal injections. Additionally, other departments do not want to be held accountable for some of the overhead expenses that are necessary to properly run a spine program (i.e., case management services).

Another challenge is the possibility of disagreement among the health disciplines as to what protocols (if any) should be used to diagnose and treat back pain. When do you use a specialist instead of a primary care physician? When is surgery indicated? Who needs to make the decision on surgery? There may be disagreement as to the process that should be followed for patients with back pain who want to enter into the system. Is there coordinated scheduling from a centralized location or service that must be used as a "front door" to the system? Is there an internal case management function to track patients who enter the system and to aid in communication? Do patients or providers that contact any part of the health system get a different message as to how back pain will be handled?

As part of a larger health system, the goal of a spine program should be to rationally manage the patients in the system who have back pain. In this situation, it is likely that there already is plenty of business inside the system to keep your program busy. The goal is not necessarily to attract new patients, but to provide care to existing patients in the most effective manner. As an example, it might be valuable to a health system to off-load non-operable back pain patients from a surgeon's schedule to allow them to spend more time in the OR. If attracting new patients is not the focus, the priority for the spine program is to develop support for and participation in a consolidated and unified approach to back pain treatment that will be "controlled" from a centralized place (your spine program).

A first step in this process is to get the key players to agree to an organized approach to back pain, including developing and adhering to a unified message to patients and referring providers on how to access the system. The ideal situation would be to have a centralized location that can provide all back pain services in one place. If the "one-stop shopping" physical location can not be achieved, then operational coordination should be the next goal. This would include a centralized triage and scheduling service that would be the "first stop" for all patients entering the system. The drawback to a spine program providing only operational coordination, however, is that it then becomes easily viewed as an overhead center in the eyes of the health system. If the spine program that provides mainly coordinating services is financially evaluated purely as a separate entity, without accounting for the value provided to all parts of the system, the program will have a more difficult time proving it is successful.

It thus becomes very important to determine the value of a spine program, and how all the different players in the health system will define its value. In general, qualities of any program that provides value to the healthcare system include the following:

- Improve the quality of care (patients are getting better).
- Increase patient and referring provider satisfaction (patients are more satisfied with the care they receive, less running around the system, improved communication about services that are provided).
- Enhance customer service (friendliness, ease of navigating the system, questions are answered).
- Improve access (timely appointments, convenient hours and locations, parking).
- Help get sick patients back to work a quickly as possible (good for selling to employers, insurance companies, workers' compensation).
- Provide financial gains (services cost less and are more profitable).
- Decrease the use of more expensive treatments (therapy instead of surgery).
- Reduce "return" referrals for the same services (repeated referrals for PT).
- Direct patients to the most appropriate location for service (download the surgeons).

- Increase the amount of business coming into the system (get surgeons more surgeries).
- Create potential for market differentiation from competitors ("we have a spine program and they do not," creates a potential draw for new customers to come into the system).
- Provide research opportunities (for the spine program and for other services).

Proving Value

In the administration of a spine program, it is a necessary goal to determine how your particular program can measure and prove any or all of these aspects of value. In the case of financial value, this may seem relatively easy to measure. However, it is important to take a system-wide approach to reporting financial benefits, so that the program is not judged only on what happens within the four walls. The other aspects of value are often more difficult to measure and quantify. A concentrated effort needs to be made to position the program as a source of value to the system on the "softer" issues (satisfaction, utilization rates, administrative improvements, etc.). To do this, it becomes important to understand how value is defined for each of the key stakeholders that affect the operation of your program. Each party may want to see something different to prove value, so you need to know who you are going to interact with and how *they* determine the value of your program. Above we have listed the valuable qualities in general. Below is a brief summary of issues that are more important to some of the specific key parties involved in the operation of a spine program.

Hospital and/or Health System Administration

- Budget issues (are you making money, losing money).
- Are there access issues (can people get timely appointments, are you helping wait times in other areas. e.g., surgery).
- Coordination of services (provide a unifying force for all back pain issues).
- Satisfaction of referring providers (they know where to go for their back pain questions or to whom to send their patients).
- Patient satisfaction (are they happy, will they tell others they are happy or upset).

Department Administration (Physical Medicine and Rehabilitation, Surgery, Primary Care, Radiology, Anesthesiology)

- Issues are similar to those that are meaningful hospital administrators.
- Will have more "turf" related issues.
- Some departments have more clout than others, based usually on their worth to the system (research power, financial power, provide a unique service to the community).

Insurance Companies

- Proof of high-quality care.
- Lower cost for the condition (the combination of services and/or controls you have that will reduce the overall cost of back pain-less surgery, less repeat referrals for the same service, getting patients back to work).
- Access (avoid long wait times).
- Documentation of services (tell us what you did and why you did it).

Case Managers/Employers

- Returning the patient to work as quickly as possible.
- Help someone transition to a new line of work (improve mental outlook, adapt to new work).
- Timely appointments.
- Thorough communication and documentation.
- Questions answered quickly.

Internal Staff (Physicians, Faculty, Therapists, Support Staff)

- Positive work environment.
- Opportunity for research.
- Opportunity to make money.
- Professional challenge.
- Team environment.
- Security.

Patients

- Quality of care ("getting better," reduced pain, increased function).
- Ease of access.
- Questions are answered.
- Fears reduced.
- Coordination of services, navigation of the system.
- One-stop shopping.
- Friendly, caring atmosphere.
- Knowledge of specific case across all disciplines (questions aren't repeatedly asked).

If value as each player perceives it can be defined and demonstrated, a spine program can be comfortably positioned as a successful part of a health system.

Customer Service

It is important to understand the role customer service plays in the delivery of back pain services. Patients who have back pain often feel that they are lost in the system, that the world is against them, and no one is helping them. Customer service should be viewed as the opportunity to make a positive impression in the minds of your patients and other customers.

Support personnel must have a clear understanding of the role that they play and the tremendous impact they can make on a patient's overall perception of the program. It is also important that the support staff feel that the clinical professionals in the program support them. Physicians who keep on schedule, listen compassionately, and respond to patient requests promptly are important.

Internal Administration

Administrative infrastructure will vary, but most spine program administrators are paired with a medical director. This pair answers to both a hospital administrator and one or more physician clinic administrators. The spine program administrator is responsible for maintaining the program's internal budget, often under the guidance and expectations of a department administrator and/or hospital administrator. The program administrator will also have responsibility for personnel hiring, coaching, and evaluation. They will help to set the tone for the overall work environment for the staff, and will help to create a positive environment that will maintain a high level of employee moral. This is not just an afterthought task, but something that can play a big role in the performance of the program. High employee morale is likely to translate into low employee turnover, which can result in better continuity. The program administrator will also deal with many customer service issues such as phone wait times, appointment errors, canceled or changed provider schedules, and overall patient and/or provider complaints.

Besides these typical administrative tasks, the program administrator can help provide an understanding of the overall business environment of the health system. Because other areas have administrators who are involved in decisions that might impact the operation of your spine program, it is helpful to have someone on your side who can "speak the language." The program administrator can help navigate the health system and can work to position the spine program for success by developing key relationships with hospital and department administrators.

The medical director must have credibility with the community physicians, and must be compensated sufficiently that program goals are valued above clinical income. Internally he or she leads development of protocols and insures quality of care, both in the physician clinics and in the therapy areas. The medical director's most challenging internal task may be ensuring that the program is cost-effective. Individual staff typically do not take ownership in the cost of the services they provide, but feel very strongly about the quality of their work and the work habits they have developed. Externally the medical director interacts with community physicians, insurers and insurance case managers. He or she is often a figurehead in public relations programs. Even in a private sector program, it is ideal if the medical director brings some academics to the program-research papers, visiting

students, and continuing medical education (CME) conferences greatly enhance the view of the program in the eyes of the community.

Corporate Medicine

Physician medical administrators for corporations (or, corporate physicians)
have great influence over the quality of care and cost provided to their
workers. There are three areas of intervention that deserve comment:
Prevention, return to work, and acting as a catalyst for improved community care. Prevention and return to work are discussed in earlier chapters
(Chapters 14 and 34). The substantial role of the corporate physician in the
local health care system cannot be overestimated.

Corporate physicians typically have better access to health care system
leaders than the physicians within the system themselves do. Yet they are
not typically mired in the politics of the local health care referral pattern.
They can, therefore, act as a voice of reason. Corporate physicians should
consider encouraging formation of local spine programs, with structure
based on quality and cost, rather than political influence. The corporate
physician can request that health care systems develop multidisciplinary
triage protocols and limited, well-defined therapy protocols for acute back
pain, for instance. In addition to simply encouraging change, the corporation might consider funding small grants or awards for research into local
issues in spine care. By letting the community know that effective health
care is valued by the corporation, the political meaning of such funds far
outweighs the actual money spent.

Payer Considerations

Any physician who is involved in the paying side of health care is quite familiar with the problem of back pain. Policies regarding back pain can be
rethought in relationship to the issues discussed in this text. Perception of
quality of care for back pain is highly variable among consumers, and
therefore can be changed. Payers should therefore consider consumer education, even more than prevention, as a major goal in cost cutting.

As with employers, insurers can have great influence on the quality of
care within local health care systems. By setting metrics for quality, pro-
moting quality, cost-effective care, and supporting small local quality projects, insurers may have substantial impact. Goals might be referral of all
chronic and all nonemergent potential surgical patients through a nonsur-
geon, perhaps a physiatrist. Subsequently, better control can be made over
use of x-ray, therapies, and so forth.

Rehabilitation services are often the victim of insurance coverage
"dumbsizing" rather than "downsizing." Clearly, rehabilitation therapies do

have an effect on pain, and probably they help prevent surgery. Policies and enforcement should emphasize the nature of therapy and the control exerted over the quality of therapy. Brief interventions for acute back pain, rather than the standard "1 month" or "annual 20 visits" quotas may be appropriate. Restriction of therapy for chronic back pain, except in the context of a well developed multidisciplinary plan, with specific goals and time frames, may be one appropriate cost cutting measure. Perhaps one of the biggest mistakes in regard to back pain is the frequent restriction of psychological intervention to a specific group of contracted providers. Substantial literature suggests that team intervention is more effective than parallel play here. Brief psychological counseling is substantially more effective when it is done by a counselor who is part of the physical therapy team.

Spine Care and Health Care Policy

The political and legal context of back pain cannot be ignored. Politically active clinicians should be aware of a number of issues: Back pain is ubiquitous, but back pain disability is largely a cultural phenomenon, driven by those who make money from it-physicians, alternative providers, and attorneys. The need to "prove" causation and disability, and the perceived rewards for doing so, in contrast to the disastrous consequences of true disability without compensation, make back pain a high stakes game for Americans. On one hand, nationalized or ubiquitous health care coverage acts as a safety net, and decreased these tensions. On the other hand, as our European colleagues are finding, unfettered access to care with little barrier to disability payments proves very costly, especially with an aging population.

Perhaps the best tool society and government has to prevent back pain disability is consumer education regarding health care. This education must go beyond anatomy and physiology. It should include prognosis and appropriate use of diagnostic and treatment modalities. People need to know the micro economic aspects of back pain-who makes money off of your disease, and how do they do it. Finally, the legal veil over the rewards for back pain can be removed. People can be made aware of the odds of winning the legal "lottery" for various types of back pain in various situations, in different communities, the average amount paid, and the percent going to the attorney, for instance. Consumers who know how to not be afraid, not be cowed into inappropriate treatment, and not be "ripped off" by the legal system will seek out the best care. To be most effective, this education should start early—before the first backache. That means junior high! Government, political, medical, and social agencies can make a difference.

PATIENT HANDOUT

What You Need to Know
About Back Pain

■   ■   ■

Andrew J. Haig, MD

In the "old days," people with back pain usually went to their doctors and did whatever they were told. Research in the last 10 years has shown that this approach is not ideal. Patients who take charge of their care are most likely to succeed in alleviating their back pain. To take charge, however, you must understand your medical problem and the choices you have. As doctors, nurses, and therapists, we can guide you in learning more about your problem, but obviously we cannot know your pain, your lifestyle, or your priorities as well as you do. And almost all of the decisions in back pain depend on weighing these factors. So you need to get educated! There are many useful books and Web sites available. But perhaps begin with this Patient Handout.

What Is Back Pain?

Back pain is very common—so common that almost everyone you will meet will have had some personal experience with back pain at some point in their lives. Sure, back pain runs in families—everyone's family! More than half of all people get their first episode as a teen. Almost all adults go through a period where they may miss work for a few weeks because of a backache. Many older persons do not have to do physical work every day, but the pain of a "bad back" can interfere with the lives of older persons, too. No matter what your age, when back pain strikes, it can often make your normal day-to-day life unpleasant or even impossible. Even if we "cure" you, you can expect occasional backaches to continue to be a part of your life, just as they are a part of everyone else's.

People who experience back pain have many different stories. You may have heard your neighbor complain about a pain in the lower back, stiffness in the neck, or even shooting pain down an arm or a leg that feels like it starts somewhere in the back. Most back pain results from problems associated with the muscles, nerves, or bones around the spine.

People with back pain often worry that they have something horribly wrong with their backs—something that might cause death or paralysis, or something that is caused by some other hidden illness, like cancer. In fact, dangerous causes of back pain are rare. They are reliably found with a physical examination along with various tests that can be performed. If you are worried about something dangerous, it is important to discuss these concerns with your doctor.

What Happens to All These People with Backaches?

It really depends on how long the pain has been around.

A new backache: *Acute* back pain is pain that has just happened, usually within a few days. Most people who see a health care provider with a new backache will just get better—with or without treatment. We hope our medicines and therapies speed up the process, but just like the common cold, acute back pain will pass. A careful examination can help eliminate worries about more serious problems. X-rays and other tests seldom provide information that would change treatment. Since they cost money and expose people to radiation, most people with acute back pain should avoid getting an x-ray. Our main job as doctors and therapists is to support people with acute back pain and to teach them ways to avoid pain in the future.

Pain that hasn't gone away yet: Some patients have back pain that lasts more than 6 weeks. This is called *subacute* pain. Most will also get better with time, but at 6 weeks, we typically begin to think about more advanced diagnostic tests, such as an MRI Scan, CT scan, electromyography (EMG), bone scan, or blood tests. Depending on what we find and how the person is dealing with the pain, we may begin to think about more intensive treatments, such as injections, surgery, or intensive physical therapy. If the person is missing work or school, this is the time that gradual rehabilitation to return to activities—even despite the pain—may begin. By being more aggressive at this stage, we hope to avoid a patient having pain that won't go away.

Pain that won't go away: The few people whose pain disables them from their work or usual life activity for 3 months or more have *chronic* pain. In the very long term, they may get better, but they've run out of miracle cures, and they're often running out of patience. Their medical history is often more complex. They may have tried and failed at surgery, or their doctors have told them that they are not "surgical candidates." By this time, they are often so out of shape due to inactivity that they couldn't go about their usual life even if their back pain was cured. Their muscles and joints are often very tight. They may have suffered through many frustrations—disappointing promises of a cure or problems with their jobs, their finances, and the disability system. Their relationships with family and friends may be stressed, and they may have begun to lose hope. Anxiety and depression are very common.

For persons with chronic pain, a team of experts is the best way to care for the patient. The team is usually lead by a physiatrist—an MD or DO who is a specialist in Physical Medicine and Rehabilitation. The physiatrist tries to be sure that no reasonable cure has been missed, sometimes consulting with specialists in orthopedics, neurosurgery, rheumatology (arthritis), anesthesiology pain specialists, radiologists, and others. The physiatrist then assembles a rehabilitation team, which might include a physical therapist, occupational therapist, exercise physiologist, psychologist, and a job and lifestyle expert "rehabilitation counselor." The team approach focuses on rehabilitation—getting the person back to his or her life despite the disability that the back or neck problem has caused. It's amazing (and hard for some people to believe), but a good rehabilitation team can get most people with the worst pain back to work and play, help them feel less down in the dumps, and keep them going. The teamwork is the key. Just a doctor or a therapist alone is a real compromise.

How Do We Find Out What's Wrong with Your Back?

The patient usually tells us! It turns out that the best single test to find out what's wrong is the patient's story about what happened. That's why we ask our patients lots of questions about their pain and their medical history. A detailed examination confirms what the health care provider suspected. In most cases, we're pretty sure of what's going on without any other tests.

Why not get a test anyway, just to be sure? Many experts agree that a solid "anatomical proof" of the cause of back pain can be found in less than 1 out of 5 back pain patients. No test shows torn muscles, sprained ligaments, or a host of other "soft tissue" causes of pain. Diagnostic tests, such as x-ray, MRI, CT scan, bone scan, EMG, and blood tests, sometimes show that the cause of pain has a name, like herniated disk, spinal stenosis, or spondylolysthesis. But it is very important to understand that almost every cause of pain we can see on diagnostic tests is also found in people who have no pain at all. Spinal arthritis happens in all of us. Disk herniations that cause no pain still show up on scans. So your health care provider needs to be sure the test findings make sense with your pain and examination. It's bad medicine to treat an x-ray instead of the patient.

Common Diagnostic Tests

X-ray: Everybody thinks we get a lot of information fromx-rays for back pain, but in fact we usually don't. X-ray takes pictures of the bones but does not see the disks between the bones, the nerves, the muscles, or other causes of pain. It rarely provides information the doctor couldn't have found out by examining the patient. X-ray sometimes provides confusing information. For example, "arthritis" on an x-ray is usually just the normal aging process of the spine and may not be related to pain at all. X-ray exposes gonads to a little bit of radiation. On the other hand, x-ray is not too expensive and can find broken bones and other major problems.

CT (computed tomography) scan: This is a special x-ray in which a computer fine-tunes the images and slices them up so that disks, nerves, ligaments, tendons, and muscles can actually be seen. More things can be seen with a CT scan than with a normal x-ray, so it can be more confusing. In fact, one third of people with no pain at all have "significant" findings like disk herniations on their CTs. These findings may have no impact on the pain a patient is having or may be no bother at all to the patient. So a doctor has to look at the patient—not just the CT scan—to make sense of its findings. This test is a little more expensive than regular x-ray and exposes the patient to a little more radiation, but it is a painless procedure.

MRI (magnetic resonance imaging): This test is very like a CT scan, except that a magnet (with no radiation) is used. It gives more detail, so it is sometimes even more confusing. Depending on the age of a patient, up to two thirds or more of people without pain have changes in the spine that show up on an MRI. This test is fairly expensive, not painful, and is safe for most people (though some don't like the closed-in feeling as they're lying on the machine, and others with metal implants can't go under the magnet). MRIs do become useful if there is concern about infection or fracture or if the pain has lasted long enough that an "invasive" treatment (injection or surgery) is being considered.

EMG (electromyography): EMG is a test in which a physician uses small electric shocks and needle insertions into muscles to "map out" where nerves are pinched. It doesn't provide pictures like CT, MRI, or x-ray, but is actually better at finding where nerves might be pinched due to changes in the spine. Unlike the other tests, a well-done EMG is normal in people who have no disease, So it is often used to decide what's happening when the MRI or CT isn't giving a straight answer. EMG is a little painful, but it is as safe or safer than all the other tests mentioned here (due to lack of radiation exposure). The cost of this procedure is moderate.

Bone scan: This test finds out if bones have been damaged by fracture, infection, tumor, or arthritis. It involves injecting a small amount of radioactive dye (not a high dose of radiation) and taking pictures of where it goes in the body. A bone scan takes part of a day to perform, but it is not painful and is moderate in price.

Diagnostic injections: If a body part hurts and a doctor numbs it up, the pain will temporarily go away. Doctors may use x-rays to help insert a needle in a place where pain might come from. If the injection of anesthetic numbs the pain, that place may be where the problem is. Cortisone, an anti-inflammation medicine, is often injected with the anesthetic to get rid of the inflammation (painful swelling) that often is the cause of pain. Common injections include "epidural" injections, which inject medicine to stop inflammation and pain in the spinal canal; "facet" injections, which get rid of swelling in the small facet joints in the back; and "sacroiliac" injections, which get rid of inflammation and pain in the joints around the "sacrum" bone, a triangle shaped bone at the bottom of the spine. Serious problems related to the needle insertion into the spine or the medicine used are very uncommon. Most of the different injections help in the short term, but research is not conclusive on whether they help in the long term. We don't know whether two or three injections are better than one injection. This procedure is moderate in price, and it can be a little painful.

Blood tests: There are hundreds of blood tests that test different chemicals in your body. Some of these chemicals are around when there is arthritis, an infection, or another problem. Doctors may choose different blood tests to find out about different diseases that may be causing your back pain.

Possible Treatments for Back Pain

At some point, the patient will need to choose how to treat his or her back pain. People usually think that their doctor finds their diagnosis, then looks up the "best" treatment in some book. With back pain, it doesn't work that way. If the patient doesn't have an emergency (i.e., fracture, infection, cancer, or rapidly progressing weakness) nothing "has" to be done. The patient is the expert on how much a back problem hurts and how much treatment time, pain, cost, or health risk is "worth it." The patient's opinion on how to proceed is very important. To make an informed decision, the patient needs to understand the treatment possibilities that are available.

It is hard for patients and even good clinicians to tell which treatments really work. Most people with back pain get better with or without medical intervention, so they and their doctor may think some treatment had an effect when it really did not. Even a sugar pill has a strong temporary effect on pain. Remember that besides being a patient you are a consumer. And, as a consumer, you need to remember that back pain is a $40 billion dollar a year business and that some people may want to make money off of your pain.

Fortunately, there are only a certain number of treatment categories available to choose from.

Surgery: It seems tempting to just take out the busted parts when the back is hurting badly. But people aren't like cars. You can't just replace a broken part of the body with a new part and have everything run smoothly. When you have surgery, you actually have to damage perfectly good parts (i.e., muscle) to get down to the damaged part. And unlike a car, in many cases the damaged body part will heal itself over time and doesn't need to be removed. That is why 95% of back problems are not treatable with surgery. Disk herniation is the most common reason for surgery, but most spine surgeons don't operate on a disk herniation unless the patient has failed to be helped by everything else (injections, physical therapy, medicine, and time), isn't willing to wait out a cure, and has their emotional act together to tolerate the surgery and the recovery period that must follow.

People who were "cured" by surgery, but now have worsening pain, often surprisingly wish for even more surgery. Many of our patients have had multiple back operations, yet research shows that these complex fusions and similar procedures usually are no better than a little education and therapy. The fact is that with few exceptions, re-operating on a "failed back surgery syndrome" causes even more problems. Still, for selected patients with the right problems, surgery can make a big difference.

Injections: Injections of anti-inflammation steroids (not the kind that some athletes abuse) into certain areas of the spine can help certain back problems. The most common injection is an epidural steroid injection. Injections probably help with pain that radiates below the knee from a pinched nerve in the back or pain that radiates into the arm from a neck problem. Other injections that can be made into the little "facet joints" in the spine, the the disk, or the pelvis-back joint (sacroiliac joint) are commonly performed, but are less proven to be effective. Spinal injections are outpatient procedures. Some people worry about needles in the back, but in fact the safety record of steroid injection is quite high. These injections are many times less dangerous than back surgery, for instance.

Medications: A number of drugs have been shown to be effective for acute (new) pain. They never cure chronic (long-standing) pain, but sometimes the right drug can cut the amount of chronic pain by a third or so. Medications for pain work best when they are taken at scheduled times, rather than "as needed." The medications often build up strength in the blood stream over a few days or weeks, so the doctor may ask a patient to keep taking a prescription until they are sure the drug has an effect. If there are troublesome side effects with a new pain medicine, it is usually best to stop the medicine and call the doctor's office for advice on what to do next. With chronic pain, doctors can't easily predict which medication will work best for an individual, so patience is needed. The good news is that there's nothing mysterious about whether a medication is working. The patient can tell. If the patient isn't sure, sometimes the doctor will stop and then restart the medication to see if things get worse and then better again.

A few types of medicine used for back pain are described below.

Acetaminophen (i.e., Tylenol): This is a very safe drug and it is fairly effective. People with liver problems who drink moderate-to-large amounts of alcohol and older people should be cautious about daily use without their doctor's permission.

NSAIDs (non-steroidal anti-inflammatory drugs): Over-the-counter aspirin, ibuprofen (Motrin, Nuprin, and other brand names), naproxen (Aleve and other brand names), and about 20 other prescription medications are NSAIDs. They all help with back pain. Doctors choose them based on cost to the patient, ease of use, and side effects. Bleeding or ulcers from the stomach area are some possible side effects. If one drug doesn't work, it may help to try another. Some should be avoided by people with liver or kidney problems. A few newer ones can be used safely by people who haven't tolerated this type of medicine in the past.

Steroids: These are very strong anti-inflammation medications based on natural chemicals the body secretes. They are not used commonly by mouth, but in some cases are used for a short time for severe back problems. Short-term use—an injection or a week or so of pills—is usually quite safe, but long-term use can cause all kinds of problems.

Opiates: These are medicines related to morphine and codeine. Because of problems with addiction, drowsiness, and other side effects, these pills are usually avoided. However, some persons with severe acute pain and a few persons with chronic pain may be helped by these medicines.

Muscle spasm medicines: The medications include Flexeril, Soma, and others. Some patients swear *by* them, and a few swear *at* them for the drowsiness they may cause. There's little research to say they actually slow muscle spasm—usually the only effective treatment for spasm is to stretch out the spasm—but research shows that a few of them may help with pain.

Chronic pain pills: There are a number of medications which may be quite helpful for chronic pain. They come from all kinds of drug families—antiseizure drugs and antidepressants, among others. They share with each other the ability to stop the brain and the spinal cord from abnormally amplifying the pain signals coming through your nerves. They usually take a few weeks to begin to work, so they're just used for long-standing pain. Amitriptyline (Elavil), an antidepressant, and gabapentin (Neurontin), an antiseizure drug, are most commonly used, but there are many others.

Pills for other problems: Treating depression, anxiety, sleep disorders, and other medical problems can make a big difference for persons with chronic pain. A clinician who is looking at "the whole patient" may prescribe medications for these problems in addition to medicine to help control pain.

Passive therapies: This type of treatment can be defined as things that are put on you or done to you without someone actively participating in your care. Examples include hot packs, cold packs, ultrasound, iontophoresis, phonophoresis, and electrical stimulation. Passive therapies usually make you feel good, but the good feelings usually don't last, and these types of treatments can be quite costly when used by a physical therapist. Most reputable physical therapists either don't use passive therapies or use them just briefly at the beginning of an aggressive therapy session to loosen up tight muscles. However, these therapies can help you get through the day, so people with back pain are encouraged to learn how to safely use, for example, hot and cold on their own at home.

Manual medicine: Manual medicine includes things like manipulation or more gentle stretching of specific tight areas with the help of a trained expert. There is substantial research that says this can help certain back problems. Chiropractors, some osteopaths, some physical therapists, and a few MDs know how to do it. Not all physical therapists have sufficient training in manual medicine. How do you tell if your local therapist is an expert in manual medicine? Ask questions. Ask how many advanced courses they have attended. Ask what percentage of their patients are manual medicine patients. Most experts agree that when you are in therapy—whether with a physical therapist, chiropractor, osteopath, or MD—you should notice a substantial improvement within a month of starting. They should be spending substantial time teaching you how to treat yourself. And they should only spend minimal time using the "passive therapies" described above. Research shows that manual medicine without a specific home exercise program is less effective than manipulation alone. Experts feel that most manual treatments can be taught to the patient. So a good practitioner should show you how to put him or her out of business!

Active exercise: This is our secret weapon against disability. Most people with pain, especially back pain, are afraid to move. Early on, especially before they get permission to get going, that may make sense. But if they don't get past the fear, they become weak, their muscles tighten up, and they lose endurance. Their pain worsens as the day goes on, and they have difficulty doing things they used to be able to do. So active exercise—weight training, aerobics, stretching, and so on—can make a big difference. Exercise certainly increases strength and endurance to do active things. It also helps with the mental part—fear and depression that can result from inactivity. Sometimes the exercise fixes the area with "myofascial pain." On their own, people sometimes do too much or too little— for example, exercising one group of muscles but forgetting other important parts. Motivation is tough, especially early on when everything seems to ache and hurt. It's rare for exercise to be the wrong thing, but many patients need coaching from an exercise physiologist or physical therapist to help them get started with an exercise program.

Lifestyle adjustment: There are smart ways to do things and dumb ways. There are things you love to do, things you need to do, and things you really can give up. When pain interferes with activity, an occupational therapist is an expert on how to get around the problem. Sometimes they suggest adapting your home or workplace to make it easier for you to be active. Sometimes they provide devices which make the work easier. Sometimes they just teach you how to pace yourself so you don't burn out. Changing the world around you to fit your problem is smart. But forget about all of those instructions on how to lift or bend. It turns out your body knows more than your brain does about how to move best when your injured. We often ask patients to make a list of 50 ways their back interferes with their lifestyle. Then we find solutions. When we get stuck, we ask an occupational therapist to help out.

Psychological support: No question about it, back pain stinks. For many patients, it is overwhelming enough that they become depressed and anxious. Others aren't depressed, but feel trapped by their circumstances. Still others are seeking new ways to look at their lives and their relations now that they have to live with chronic pain. Expert pain psychologists help many of the patients in our clinic deal with the complex and common problems.

Team rehabilitation: Two heads are better than one. A lot better. In fact, research has shown that patients who have no cure in sight but who undergo an intensive team "Functional Restoration Program" are twice as likely to return to work as those who don't. Other chronic pain programs are less physically intense and are the right choice for many other patients. Research shows that team rehabilitation results in less disability, better physical conditioning, less depression and anxiety, fewer doctor visits, and overall life improvement compared to usual treatment. If you are disabled by pain for more than 3 months, team rehabilitation is a must.

Alternative medicine: There's so much we can't prove about back pain that it makes sense some good treatments are "unproven" or come from places outside of the traditional medical system. Yet some ideas are pretty far-fetched, and some can harm you or your pocketbook. Don't be shy to discuss alternative treatments with your health care provider. You may be surprised to find that he or she has a good handle on the dozens of types of alternative treatments available in your community.

Living with the pain: Despite the fact that we can't cure some cancers, AIDS, and other diseases, some people insist that there must be a cure for their pain. It's not always true. These people go from doctor to doctor, enduring painful tests and treatments, and collecting side effects, debt, and frustration. Sometimes they are so focused on their *disability* that they can't see their *abilities*. The fact is that pain often takes its own course—it gets better on its own early on, or, when it's chronic, it sticks around no matter what we do medically. Although patients are free to choose not to be treated, we can help them to live a good life despite the pain.

Index